Overview Map Key

Part One NORTHEAST OF MADISON

Part Two SOUTHEAST OF MADISON

Part Three SOUTHWEST OF MADISON

Part Four NORTHWEST OF MADISON

Other Menasha Ridge Press Paddling Guides

The Alaska River Guide

Canoeing & Kayaking Florida

Canoeing & Kayaking Georgia

A Canoeing & Kayaking Guide to Kentucky

A Canoeing & Kayaking Guide to the Ozarks

Canoeing & Kayaking New York

Canoeing & Kayaking West Virginia

Carolina Whitewater

Paddling the Everglades Wilderness Waterway

Paddling Long Island and New York City

CANOEING & KAYAKING SOUTH CENTRAL WISCONSIN

60 Paddling Adventures Within 60 Miles of Madison

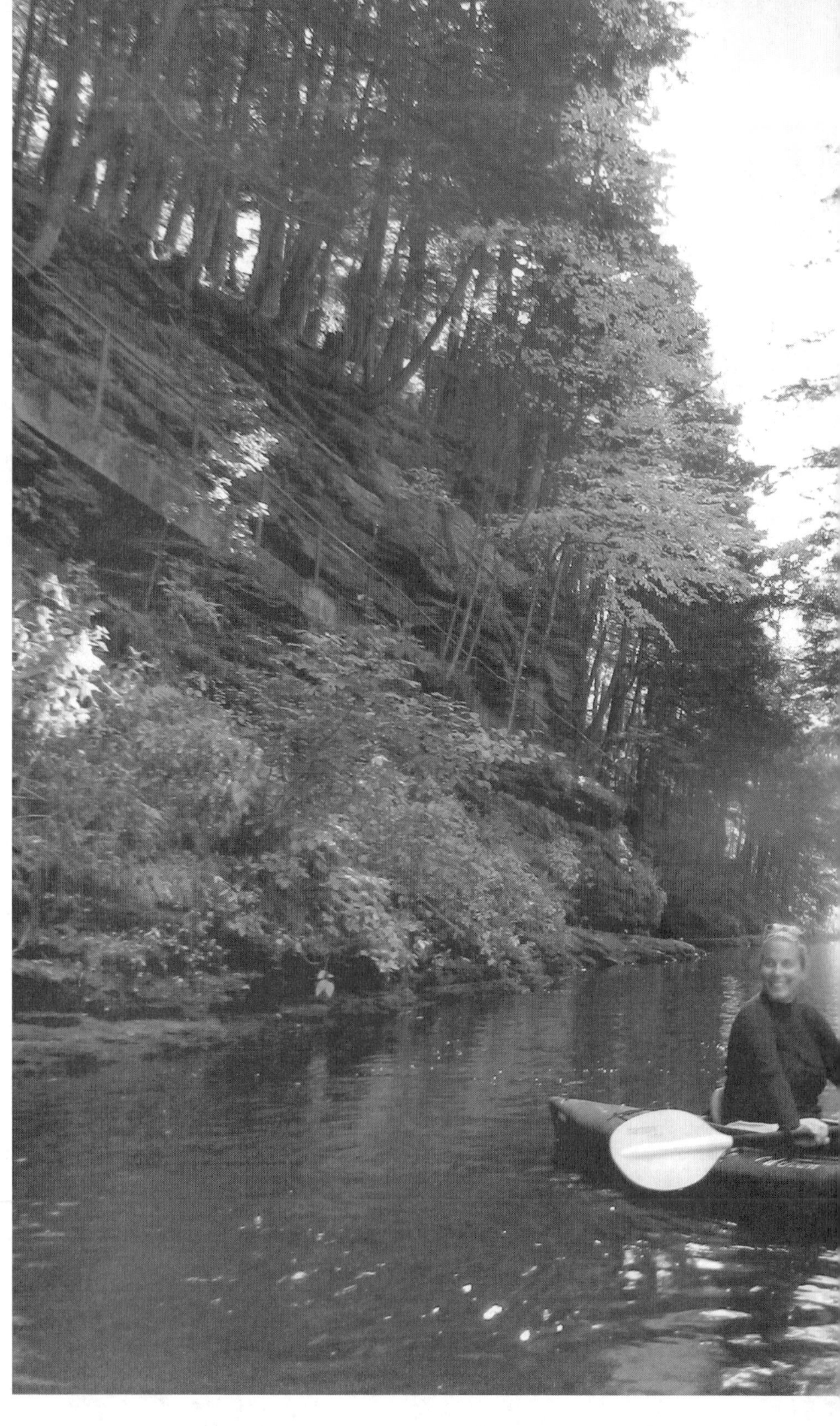

CANOEING & KAYAKING

SOUTH CENTRAL WISCONSIN

60 Paddling Adventures Within 60 Miles of Madison

Timothy Bauer

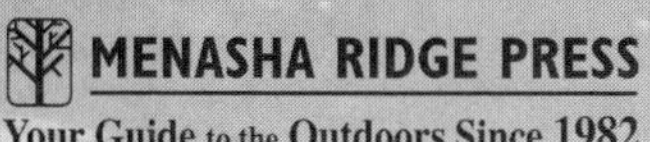

MENASHA RIDGE PRESS

Your Guide to the Outdoors Since 1982

Canoeing & Kayaking South Central Wisconsin: 60 Paddling Adventures Within 60 Miles of Madison

Published by Menasha Ridge Press
Distributed by Publishers Group West
Printed in the United States of America
First edition, third printing 2022

Editor: Carolyn Acree Jones
Project editor: Ritchey Halphen
Cover design: Scott McGrew
Cartography: Scott McGrew, Tommy Hertzel, and Timothy Bauer
Text design: Annie Long
Cover and interior photographs: Timothy Bauer, except where noted
Copyeditor: Kerry Smith
Proofreaders: Rebecca Henderson, L. Amanda Owens, Vanessa Lynn Rusch
Indexer: Rich Carlson

Frontispiece: Paddling Coldwater Canyon in the Upper Dells will put a smile on anyone's face.
(See Trip 58, Wisconsin River A: Upper and Lower Dells, page 292.)

Library of Congress Cataloging-in-Publication Data

Names: Bauer, Timothy.
Title: Canoeing & kayaking south central Wisconsin : 60 paddling adventures within 60 miles of Madison / Timothy Bauer.
Description: First edition. | Birmingham, AL : Menasha Ridge Press, [2016] | Series: Canoeing & kayaking "Distributed by Publishers Group West"—T.p. verso.
Identifiers: LCCN 2016017897 (print) | LCCN 2016025327 (e-book) | ISBN 978-1-63404-020-4 (paperback) | ISBN 978-1-63404-021-1 (ebook) | ISBN 978-1-63404-210-9 (hardcover)
Subjects: LCSH: Canoes and canoeing—Wisconsin—Guidebooks. | Kayaking—Wisconsin—Guidebooks. Wisconsin—Guidebooks.
Classification: LCC GV776.W6 B38 2016 (print) | LCC GV776.W6 (e-book) | DDC 797.12209775—dc23
LOC record available at lccn.loc.gov/2016017897

MENASHA RIDGE PRESS
An imprint of AdventureKEEN
2204 First Ave. S., Suite 102
Birmingham, Alabama 35233

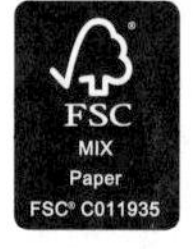

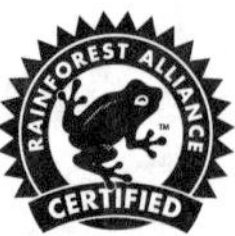

Visit menasharidge.com for a complete listing of our books and for ordering information. Contact us at our website, at facebook.com/menasharidge, or at twitter.com/menasharidge with questions or comments. To find out more about who we are and what we're doing, visit blog.menasharidge.com.

Disclaimer This book is meant only as a guide to select paddles in south central Wisconsin and does not guarantee your safety in any way—you paddle at your own risk. Neither Menasha Ridge Press nor Timothy Bauer is liable in any way for property loss or damage, personal injury, or death that may result from accessing or paddling the waterways described in the following pages. Please read carefully the introduction to this book as well as safety information from other sources. Familiarize yourself with current weather reports, maps of the areas you intend to visit (in addition to the maps in this guidebook), and any relevant public-land regulations. While every effort has been made to ensure the accuracy of this guidebook, water, land, and road conditions can change greatly from year to year.

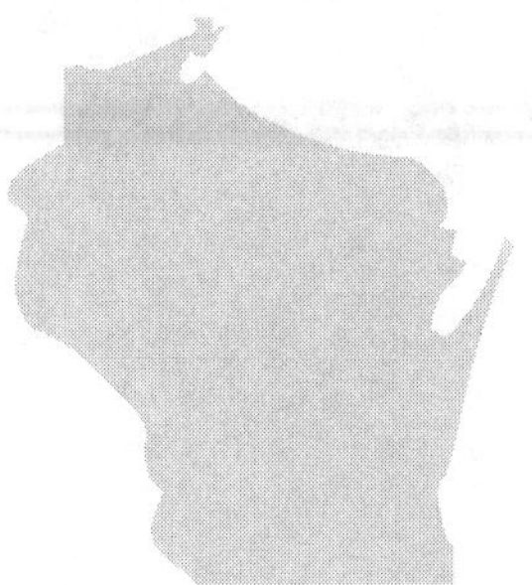

Believe me, my young friend, there is nothing—absolutely nothing—half so much worth doing as simply messing about in boats.

—Kenneth Grahame

When a man is part of his canoe, he is part of all that canoes have ever known.

—Sigurd Olson

Fish
    fowl
        flood
    Water lily mud
My life

in the leaves and on water
. . .
                  born
in swale and swamp and sworn
to water

—Lorine Niedecker, "Paean to Place"

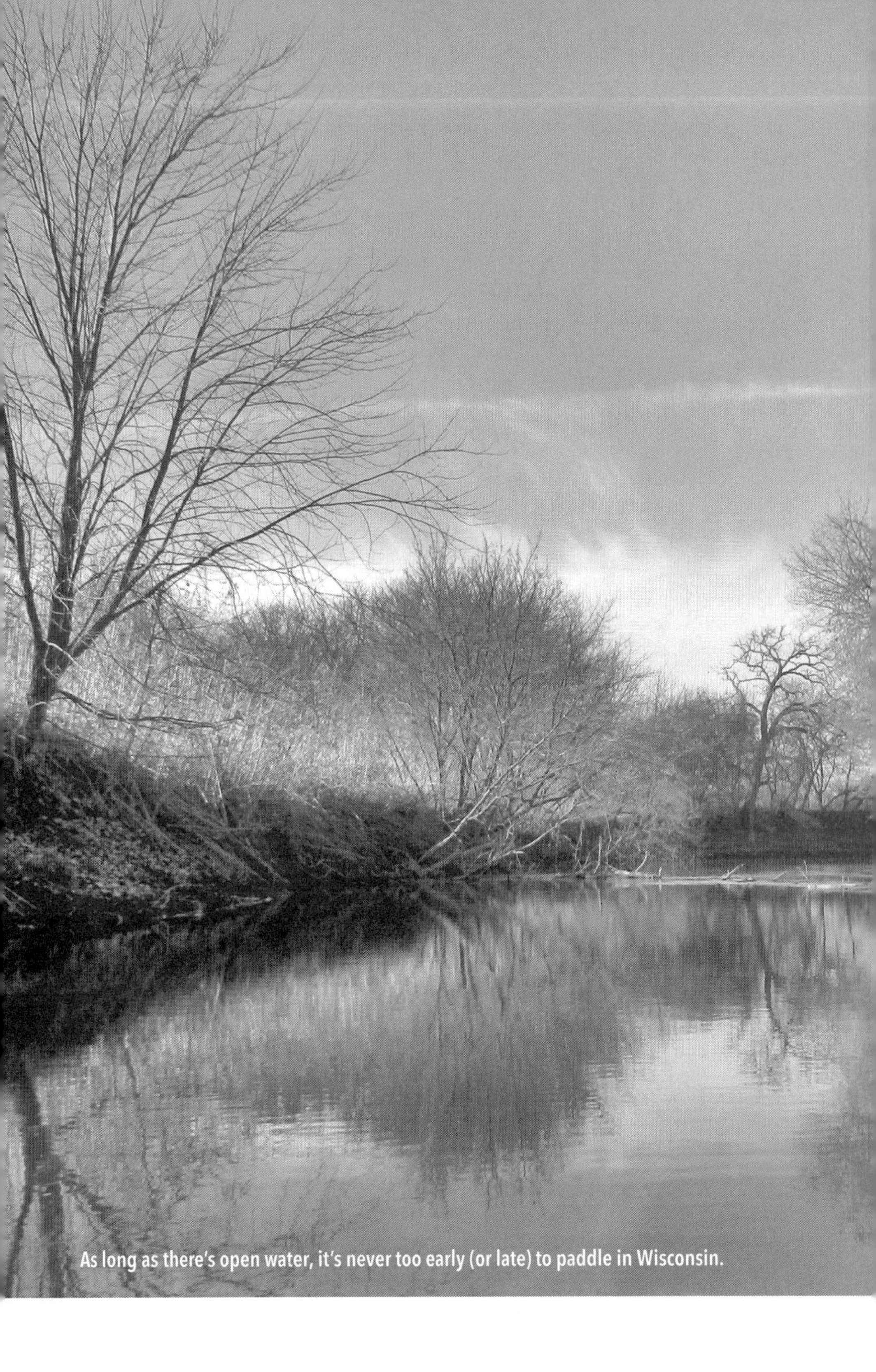
As long as there's open water, it's never too early (or late) to paddle in Wisconsin.

table of contents

PART FOUR NORTHWEST OF MADISON 225

APPENDIXES 315

Acknowledgments

THIS AUTHOR IS INDEBTED to friends and strangers alike who have in some humble or humongous way shaped my paddling sensibilities. Innumerable websites, clubs, organizations, outfitters, nonprofits, private campgrounds, tourism bureaus, and local historical societies have contributed to the effort of writing this book.

Among the individuals to whom I am ever beholden are my soulmates Ken Baun, who first sat me in a kayak back in the summer of 2008 and still teaches me a thing or two, and Jeff Kjos (a.k.a. "Kayak Guru"), who helped cultivate a sense of paddling wanderlust and DYI "bushyaking." Tim Carlisle helped me foster the concept of this book from its inception, and Rachel Friedman has always been there with a meal, a beer, and a listening ear. There are many other good folks who have championed this book through conversation and encouragement, chief among them Dennis Harrison-Noonan and Maury Smith. Yet no one has supported me more with stupefying optimism and positive reinforcement than David Sandoval, who lives a thousand miles away and has never stepped in either a canoe or kayak.

I cannot thank loudly enough Barry Kalpinski, the brain, brawn, and beauty behind the website I am proud to partner with and to which I contribute my writing: **Miles Paddled** (milespaddled.com). I never would have thought of writing a paddling book without first cutting my teeth on his stylistic considerations and then emulating his enthusiasm for sharing a love of paddling with others.

Finally, this book is dedicated to Sue DeBuhr, without whose saintly patience and unconditional support I never could have researched these trips nor written a manuscript in the first place.

—*Timothy Bauer*

Introduction

YOU ARE HOLDING IN YOUR HANDS a book borne of an indefatigable love for paddling in general and in Wisconsin specifically. Despite the state's long winters of frozen water, short exclamations of spring thaw and autumn foliage, and summers ridden with mosquitoes and ticks, Wisconsin is blessed with many gorgeous streams and lakes. Our state has further benefited from forward-thinking lawmakers who years ago set in place commendable policies granting virtually unlimited public access to all navigable waters. As a result, plenty of guides have expounded upon the more popular paddling trips our state offers. This book strives to be both a part of that guidebook tradition as well as *apart from* it by detailing trip ideas for a surprisingly rich paddling territory that has previously been forgotten or ignored.

The premise of this book is simple: 60 trips within 60 miles of Madison. Why Madison? For one, it's where I live, plus it's the state's capital. For another, it's centrally located in southern Wisconsin, which, while not as abundant as the state's northern portion in opportunities to "get away from it all," is nonetheless rich in outdoor offerings—they just take a little more time and inclination to find. In addition to convenience, Madison provides a tidy geological demarcation: Everything to the east was glaciated in the last ice age some 13,000 years ago, while everything to the west wasn't. With Madison at the center, the 60-mile circumference extends to Platteville to the southwest, Horicon to the northeast, Lake Geneva to the southeast, and Wonewoc to the northwest.

Purists might disregard the premise of a paddling guidebook whose target area is south central Wisconsin, due to the urban sprawl associated with the Madison and Milwaukee suburbs, not to mention the agriculture in between. Yet not everyone has the time or means to spend a week up in the Boundary Waters or even Sylvania. Not everyone can or wants to spend a week down the Flambeau River. Wilderness areas are spectacular, to be sure, but they're often impractical for most of us who seek some communion with the outdoors on a more regular basis. This book is intended for folks who can't feasibly work in those types of adventures with regularity but nonetheless yearn for paddling excursions.

Nature is all around us; we do not need to venture far to find it. Being "in touch with nature" should not be the exclusive privilege of those with the means to leave their own homes in hopes of some kind of exotic escapism. Nature is outside and outdoors, you bet, but not necessarily "out there" in some metaphysical landscape off the grid requiring a long drive and a full tank of gas. My backyard doesn't look like the backdrop to an REI ad, but I can drive 20 minutes and find a Class I trout stream with Class I rapids surrounded by an ancient valley of glacial hills—and still make it home in time for the Packers game.

This book primarily offers single-day outings, with the exception of a few trips that require a one-night minimum campout on a river (or two nights, depending on your pace and water levels). The landscapes these rivers and creeks course through are as varied as the streams themselves: Driftless cliffs and glacier-deposited drumlin hills, gentle prairies and wind-swept marshes, oak savannas and floodplain swamps, just to name a few. You won't see bears or wolves down here, but otters and yellow-crowned night herons are good bets.

No trip in this book requires expert skills, though I have distinguished those who are new to paddling ("Beginners") from those who have many miles under their belts ("Experienced"). Because of the broad range of this guide, some of the trips here are bound to disappoint one kind of paddler as "not enough" while intimidating another paddler as "too much." Duck Creek in Columbia County might be too dull for some but is perfect for beginners, kids, and bird-watchers. The Little Platte River in Grant County is a jubilation for experienced paddlers but too dangerous for newbies.

Just the same, it is my hope that this book inspires an appreciation for our local landscape through water, whatever one's paddling experience.

What Is and Isn't Included

Just as no one part represents the whole, the story of Wisconsin's streams is told big and wide as well as small and meandering. I have presented here the bustling Dells, together with the solitude of the Montello River and the literal circus and calliope of the Baraboo River, alongside the quiet rustle of Badfish Creek.

This book encompasses some 11,000 square miles in territory. More than 560 miles of rivers and lakes are covered here, not including another 240 that I personally paddled but did not pass muster.

In selecting which trips to profile for this guide, I have tried to be as inclusive as possible while advocating for those places about which there is not already plenty of information. But I decided it would be quixotic to the point of preposterous not to include certain popular trips, too, however well known and elsewhere covered. (I will be the first to wax poetic about the incomparable Wisconsin Dells. In much the same way that Todd Snider still loves to sing "Beer Run" at every concert so many years later and after a million times performed, I will defend paddling down the Dells to my dying breath. The area now caters to tourists and has become distractingly tacky, yet there simply is nowhere else in the state with such exquisite riverside geology.) Where I have recapitulated certain sections of rivers that are covered in other guides, I have furnished new information or added my own twist. Even seasoned veterans of our rivers can find something new to discover in this book.

Another of my guiding principles in sharing the trips featured here has been a sense of balance: Do the pros outweigh the cons? Some trips in this book require putting up with an impediment or two. Ducking underneath low-hanging branches or bridges and riding over the occasional log is par for the course. It is my belief that portaging, while seldom welcome, is part of the paddling experience. When deadfall and logjams are a likely albeit infrequent occurrence on a trip, I will point them out. But I have opted not to include trips whose nuisances and obstructions are so prominent as to undermine the whole reason for being outdoors in the first place. Mill Creek in Iowa County and Honey Creek in Sauk County, for example, are both rich in potential but poor in reward due to their many frustrations.

Just as I sought a departure from the conventional wisdom of most paddling guidebooks by featuring lesser-touted trips, I have also distinguished this guide by including lakes. (Of the five lake trips in the book, four are on lakes that prohibit all but electric boat motors; Red Cedar Lake is in a designated state natural area where *all* motors are prohibited.) I prefer moving rivers to staid lakes, but there's a lot to like in a lake. A lake is a great place to get one's feet wet in a canoe or kayak. Plus, there are no shuttling logistics to work out when paddling lakes, there are typically no obstacles, and there is something downright majestic about letting yourself drift on a calm lake at sunrise or sunset. But moving water is a dynamic all its own, so it's wise to learn some basics of boat control, even on still water.

While lakes are pretty lazy, on a windy day they are suddenly awoken from their slumber and aroused, heaving waves one after another. Here in the Upper Midwest, the closest proxy to sea kayaking is the Great Lakes; alas, neither Lake Michigan nor Lake Superior falls within a 60-mile range of Madison. But when the wind is whipping at 20 miles per hour and up, splashy whitecaps as high as 2 feet can form on Lakes Koshkonong and Mendota, the largest two lakes in south central Wisconsin. Bobbing up and down and riding these modest waves make for a fun rodeo-type outing, provided that you have the right gear and know how to roll a kayak or perform a wet entry.

As for the streams featured in this book, they are purposefully varied. They range from 15 feet to more than 500 feet wide; some are only a few inches deep, others seemingly infinite. There are streams with gradients of 10 feet per mile (fpm) or more, with the effect of frisky riffles and fun rapids, and those that give tortoises a run for their money. There are streams that meander and those so straight you can set a rudder on automatic pilot. Some streams can be run all year long, and some are more fickle, requiring a delicate balance between just enough rain to run without scraping and so much rain that the stream becomes pushy and unsafe. Some of these trips are entirely urban (but still highly desirable), such as Turtle Creek in Beloit, while others are a true getaway, such as the White River in Neshkoro. Regardless, most of the trips here begin and/or end near a town for ease of access and practicality.

Cue the Violin: Trips That Didn't Make the Cut

In addition to excluding trips whose cons outweighed their pros, I did not include trips within the city of Madison or any in north central Illinois. Why didn't either of these regions make the cut? Let me address that question in two parts.

Madison is heavy on lakes but light on rivers. The lakes themselves are pretty and quintessentially Madison, but they don't make for the most exciting paddling in my opinion—especially when one considers the volume of motorboats and Jet Skis. One exception to this is Lake Wingra, which is almost entirely surrounded by the University of Wisconsin Arboretum and upon which all motors are prohibited. It's a pretty sanctuary in the heart of the city, but it's unlikely that anyone from out of town would purposefully come to Madison just to paddle it. But if you're already here, it's worth a couple hours of your time. Altogether, there are a handful of places like this in the Madison area that aren't so notable as to warrant their own chapters in a guidebook like this but are pleasant enough as asides.

Illinois, our neighboring state to the south, is another matter. Illinois suffers from a self-inflicted curse of antiquated bylaws that are unfriendly to the public (to put it mildly). In Wisconsin, virtually all streams that can reasonably float a boat are considered public right-of-ways; more on this below. In Illinois, the opposite is predominantly the case. That said, Stephenson and Winnebago Counties in north central Illinois are the progressive exceptions to the reactionary rule, offering some of the relatively few public waters in the state, so I want to at least recognize these streams. But limiting myself to 60 trips was difficult enough without blurring the line of a porous border where the climate for paddlers is less than welcoming. (Sorry, Kishwaukee!)

Nonetheless, you will find suggestions for paddles in Madison in Appendix A at the back of this book. In Appendixes B and C, I have listed additional destinations in metro Madison and north central Illinois that did not merit detailed paddling-trip profiles but are otherwise worth consideration.

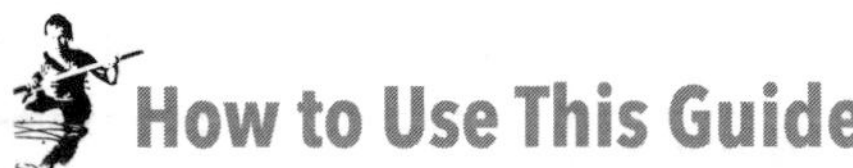

How to Use This Guide

Before launching into the specifics of each trip, you can use the Trips at a Glance section (page 16) following this introduction to pinpoint excursions based on factors of interest other than geography. Feeling skittish about tipping over or triumphant after handling your first rapids while staying dry? Then scan the Trips by Skill Level list (page 18) to see the list of trips best suited for beginners and those for more experienced paddlers, respectively. Planning to take the kids this time? Check out the Best Trips for Kids list (page 16). Feel the need to commune with the water but only have time for a short jaunt? Peruse the Trips by Distance list (page 17).

Be sure as well to reference the glossaries in the back (pages 337–340) to learn more about paddling terms and how they're used specifically in this guide.

The Overview Map, Overview Map Key, and Legend

The overview map on the inside front cover shows the primary locations for all 60 trips. The numbers on the overview map pair with the map key on the facing page. A legend explaining the map symbols used appears on the inside back cover.

Regional Maps

Prefacing each regional chapter is an overview map. The regional maps provide more detail than the overview map, bringing you closer to the trips.

Trip Maps

Each trip also includes a detailed map showing the route, the put-in and take-out, and landmarks/points of interest such as bridges, parks, and boat landings.

Trip Profiles

These are organized according to their geographic relation to Madison: northeast, southeast, southwest, and northwest. Each profile begins with "The Facts" of the trip at a glance, followed by a brief overview of the trip and shuttle directions for getting to and from the water, which include GPS coordinates for the take-out and put-in in degree–decimal minute format (first latitude, then longitude).

Next comes "The Flavor," the trip description itself. This detailed narrative shows you what to expect while you're on the water.

The final portion of the profile is "The Fudge," where, when relevant, I've tried to describe any possible additional trips you might want to consider (or were wondering about) in close proximity to the trip being profiled. In many cases, this entails a description of what you might encounter if you'd paddled farther up- or downstream. Also in "The Fudge" are mentions of nearby curiosities, spots to enjoy a post-paddle bite to eat, nearby campgrounds, rental outfitters, and so on.

"The Facts" lists the following information:

Put-in/take-out Where to begin and end

Distance/time Length of trip in miles and hours

Gradient/water level Slope of water bed (measured in feet per mile [fpm]) and measurement of water flow (in cubic feet per second [cfs])

Water type Typical motion associated with the trip's waters

Canoe or kayak Type of boat better suited for the trip

Skill level Beginner or experienced

Time of year to paddle Seasonal preference (if any)

Landscape Prairie, marsh, hardwood forest, bluffs, sandbars, and the like

---

Allow me to explain aspects of these in more detail:

PUT-IN/TAKE-OUT Only a few streams and lakes offer dedicated boat launches, so usually getting in and out of the water is done where the banks are most convenient. Most often, these will be at bridges, sometimes at dams. As such, there are no street addresses per se.

Instead, you can translate the GPS coordinates provided in the shuttle directions into driving directions quite easily using **Google Maps.** To do so, go to maps.google.com and then type the latitude and longitude, with a comma between, into the search box, and click "Search" (magnifying-glass icon). Next, click on the blue arrow in the search box to "Get Directions." Now enter the address of your starting point—Google will fill in the coordinates you typed earlier and the return directions, which you can then have sent to your phone.

DISTANCE/TIME Most of these trips will take the casual paddler anywhere between 2 and 6 hours to complete. There is no golden rule for how long it takes to paddle a river, since all rivers are different and everyone paddles at different paces. Width, water volume, wind, curves, obstructions—all determine how long it takes to get from point A to point B. Plus, sometimes you'll want to take a break to picnic, and sometimes you'll need to pause to let cows cross the stream. Keep my time frame in mind, and then allow for your own preferences within that range.

GRADIENT/WATER LEVEL The term *gradient* refers to how many feet a river drops per mile between two points. It's also a way of determining how fast a river will flow. For instance, a gradient of 10 fpm will mean a peppy stream featuring a lot of riffles and probably some light rapids as well. By contrast, a gradient of 1 fpm will be pretty slow (and if you're paddling against a strong wind, you might even go backwards!).

Water level (or *streamflow*)—a catch-all term for data collected about the flow and height of water in a stream or river at any given time—can be an essential element of planning a paddling trip. In many cases, water levels determine whether it's a good time to go as well as whether *the skill levels of the paddlers involved are appropriate* to the trip being considered.

Sometimes a stream has to be caught at just the right time in order to paddle it—after a hard rain or snowmelt, for example. It's almost always a bad idea to paddle a river when the water is very high; the current can be pushy, and there probably will be deadfall in the water. (And then, it could affect your plans when not on the water, as in the case of camping on a sandbar; if the river is too high, you might not even find a sandbar.) On the other hand, it's impractical to paddle a river when it's too low, as you will frequently scrape the bottom of the boat and sometimes have to get out and walk your boat.

That said, many of the trips suggested in this book are on waters that maintain consistently reliable levels and are relatively safe for paddlers of any skill level. See, for example, among the first few trips in Part One, Northeast of Madison. The Crawfish River B and Duck Creek trips are almost always prime for paddling, while I've recommended that you investigate levels further if considering the Beaver Dam River and Crawfish River A trips.

Profiles for such trips include additional information to help you determine whether levels are right. Sometimes, a quick phone call to an outfitter in the know is all you need; in other cases, it's a good practice to seek out water-level tracking information from the websites of the government agencies that provide this service: the United States Geological Survey (USGS) or the National Oceanic and Atmospheric

Administration (NOAA), both of which use gages to measure water height and flow. (USGS uses one spelling, *gage,* while NOAA uses *gauge.*) Even though the USGS website acknowledges that the agency "has been measuring streamflow on thousands of rivers and streams for many decades," deciphering those measurements in terms of making paddling plans can still be challenging, so stay with me here!

The first important point to note is that rivers and streams are long, and the trips I'm recommending compose very specific stretches of those ever-changing waterways. Likewise, the agencies' tracking gages have specific locations, which don't always correlate to the trips as suggested in this guide or with my recommended put-in/take-out points. Remember, though, that my goal is to suggest trips based on the criteria in Trips at a Glance, not the locations of measuring devices.

Another seeming discrepancy involves GPS coordinates. Those I provide in the shuttle directions identify put-in and take-out locations for making your trip plans; the GPS coordinates on the government websites identify the location of the gage that provides the measurements you're observing. Where the USGS is involved, each gage is assigned a number, while the NOAA identifier is the name of the town or area in closest proximity.

So, to continue with our example of the first few trips in Part One: We see from my notations in "The Facts" that water levels for a possible Beaver Dam River trip are not reliable for every paddle jaunt, so here is my notation for it:

Gradient/water level 10 fpm/See USGS gage 05425912. The ideal level is at or above 200 cfs. At 300 cfs or higher, the river will be pushy and should be considered only by paddlers with good boat control.

We see already that there is a fairly steep gradient—10 fpm—which could suggest the presence of ledges or drops that create rapids; we also see that there is a recommended range of water flow—200–300 cfs—that paddlers need to target. As such, we definitely need to go online to determine whether the river's levels fall within that range before heading out—in this case, to the USGS gage site (because I've already checked to see if the USGS provides information for that particular trip and provided the gage number where it exists). For trips where there is no corresponding USGS gage but there is one placed by the NOAA, I've prompted you to seek out the NOAA data instead.

Now you know to be alert to water levels whenever you are planning a paddling trip, and you know to make sure you seek out *current water-level data* before heading out. For a detailed explanation of how to read the online data provided by the USGS and NOAA sites (because it can be confusing at first), turn to Appendix D: How to Read USGS and NOAA Water Level (Gage) Data Online, on page 322.

WATER TYPE The three types of water motion you'll encounter on these trips are *quietwater* (or, in context of a lake trip, *flatwater*), *riffles*, and *rapids* (or *whitewater*). Whereas flatwater contains no current, quietwater hosts a gentle current that moves you downstream but nothing more; most of the trips in this book are on quietwater.

Riffles are little more than flickers on the surface—fun to be sure, but nothing to worry about.

American Whitewater's International Scale of River Difficulty (see Appendix F, page 335) establishes a six-classification standard for rating how challenging a stream or river's rapids will be for paddlers. **Class I** rapids are the easiest to maneuver, even for beginners, while **Class VI** rapids can be impossible or suicidal to run (think Niagara Falls). A **Class I** rapid, as opposed to flatwater, will feature swiftly moving water and small waves. A **Class II** rapid has more force, with waves as high as 2 or 3 feet. **Class II** rapids are appropriate for experienced paddlers or beginners who are paddling with others who can assist in a rescue if a run goes awry.

Only a few streams in southern Wisconsin possess continual runs of rapids. Therefore, most of the trips feature calm water punctuated by occasional manageable (Class I) rapids, and only one trip contains Class II rapids (Little Platte River). Often, the only rapids are "one and done" drops at isolated ledges or below bridges. Almost always, these can be portaged around. You will find several trips with Class I rapids but only a few that have sustained stretches of this kind of light whitewater (the Beaver Dam River and Baraboo River D trips, for instance). Keep in mind that water levels fluctuate daily, sometimes hourly. So, during high-water conditions, a normally Class I rapid could be technically considered a Class II.

CANOE OR KAYAK Due to the narrow and meandering nature of some of the streams included in this book, I have offered suggestions on which type of boat is better suited for a specific trip, canoe or kayak. With few exceptions, a canoe can go wherever a kayak can, but sometimes it's easier in a kayak (as when low-hanging branches, low-clearance bridges, or slim pass-through situations are involved).

SKILL LEVEL As I've mentioned, this book strives to be all-inclusive, with some trips more suited for beginners and others for more experienced paddlers. I have made a recommendation for one or the other under skill level, although in most cases a trip will appeal to both types of paddler. For example, a beginner should not try her luck on the Mecan River on account of its meandering nature and occasional obstacles. Or a stream may simply be too long for beginners to attempt in one day. (Most folks new to running wouldn't sign up for a marathon.)

Some streams in this book (such as Badfish Creek) will require good boat control and knowledge of reading a river, meaning you're not merely at the mercy of the current like a runaway train without brakes *and* you can discern what obstacles lie ahead before encountering them. It simply takes experience (and maybe taking a lesson) to develop these skills. But just because some trips have skill levels rated as "Beginner" does not mean that experienced paddlers will be bored. Most of the trips in this book will appeal to both types of paddler simply on account of the opportunity they offer to witness natural beauty.

TIME OF YEAR TO PADDLE Recommendations for the best time of year to paddle for each trip are based upon a variety of factors. A high-gradient stream, for example, will be more runnable after the snow and ice melt or after a hard rain falls. Some recommendations are based on the likelihood of witnessing a surge of dazzling wildflowers in late spring or a brilliant blaze of foliage in early autumn. Sometimes it's preferable to paddle a stream when the trees are bare to better appreciate the landscape and hills. Sometimes you'll want to time a trip in accordance with flight migrations of birds. Conversely, there are times to avoid a place because of unbecoming algae blooms or mucky duckweed, mosquitoes, ticks, tourists, or the high heat of summer. *These are simply tips based on my own experience, not advisories.* Just because I've recommended a spring trip doesn't mean a summer trip won't work for you.

LANDSCAPE A smorgasbord of paddling environments within 60 miles of Madison awaits exploration, ranging from urban water trails to prairie streams, recreational lakes to floodplain swamps, flat pastureland to towering bluffs, and it is these types of environments that are listed alongside the landscape descriptor.

Finally, in the freestanding Shuttle section of each trip profile, you will find directions in reverse—since, of course, you want to drop a vehicle at the take-out (so it will be there waiting for you at trip's end), then drive a separate vehicle to the put-in. All of these trips can be shuttled by bicycle, and several even offer dedicated bike-trail shuttle options. Personally, I love the paddle-and-pedal combo (and there is a list of these in Trips at a Glance, on page 17). It's a great workout, good for the environment, and a means of experiencing the landscape from a different perspective. I have noted when there is a distinct difference between bike-shuttle and car-shuttle routes. Otherwise, they are the same.

Trips Requiring Special Passes

At least two trips in this book require a **Wisconsin State Parks** vehicle-admission sticker ($28 annually or $8 daily): **Devil's Lake State Park** (Trip 50, page 258) and **Governor Dodge**

State Park (Trip 33, page 176). If you leave a vehicle within the boundaries of **Mirror Lake State** Park (Trip 49, page 252), you'll need a sticker here, too.

Furthermore, if you do a bike shuttle on a dedicated trail, you will need a **Wisconsin State Trail** sticker ($25 annually or $5 daily). Visit tinyurl.com/witrailpassfees for details. If you do a bike shuttle on the two Pecatonica River trips (Trips 36 and 37, pages 190 and 195), you will need a separate **Cheese Country Trail** sticker ($15 annually); for details, visit tricountytrails.com and click "Trail Stickers" on the left.

Planning for a Safe Trip

Preparing for Rapids and Obstructions (and Wind)

Keep the following in mind: An empty boat stays afloat, even in rapids; it's when humans get involved that all bets are off. As in most situations that trigger adrenaline, when paddling it's in your best interest to always stay calm while remaining mindful of your environment. Adapting to the changing dynamics of the current as well as to "suddenly appearing" boulders or tree branches is critical to keeping safe and dry.

Rapids (explained in more detail in the discussion earlier in this introduction regarding water type, on page 9) are exhilarating but can pose certain dangers, not the least of which are the unexpected objects in water that change its flow. In a certain sense, and for the purposes of the paddling environments you'll find in this book, paddling in rapids is all about the *V*s—from upstream, an obstruction in water creates two angles of deflected current that resemble the letter *V*. Think of these as signals that you're coming to a possible barrier to avoid. By contrast, your best friend is the inverted *V*. That's usually where there is the most water and the least chance of collision. Think of it as an arrow pointing you in the right direction for billowy fun.

Obstacles are a big part of paddling, so it's important to consider how they can affect your trip. Sometimes, a strong current can broach (pin) the boat sideways against an obstacle such as a downed tree, which can damage the boat and trap the paddler. If this happens, always lean toward the object the boat is pressed against, never toward the current. When leaning into the obstruction, one can reasonably free oneself by scooting/rocking back and forth or by getting out of the boat and pulling it over the obstruction. (By contrast, if you lean into the current, it will immediately fill up your boat, spin you upside down, and drag the boat beneath the obstruction. This can be extremely dangerous.)

Because there are potential dangers to any paddling excursion, take time to practice the techniques (such as forward and reverse strokes, sweeps and low braces) that enable you to easily maneuver your canoe or kayak. This will help you learn how to maximize your efficiency and not waste energy. Practice your rescue skills as well; this is imperative. Learning how to safely roll or reenter your kayak from the water should you submerge is paramount (see below).

A note about wind: When you're on the water, especially in flat environments with sparse trees that are highly susceptible to vast sweeps of wind, wind can mean the difference between a pleasant, tranquil outing and a teeth-clenched workout. Windy days usually diminish wildlife sightings as well. When planning for a trip in environments where wind is a factor, I've tried to remind you to check the wind forecast early in "The Flavor."

For further general safety information, see Appendix F: Safety Code of American Whitewater (page 328).

What to Do When (Not If) You Do Get Dumped

It happens to all of us, at least once: Whether you see it coming before it occurs or it blindsides you, at some point you and your boat will go separate ways. So, what do you do? First and foremost, stay calm and relax. Seriously. Overreacting makes it worse.

What you do next depends on the current and the environment. If the water is deep and slow and the river wide and straight, you'll probably want to swim to your boat and collect anything that fell out (as long as it floats). If the stream is shallow and the current relatively gentle, chances are pretty good you'll be able to just stand up.

But if the current is strong and the river rocky and deep, do not stand up and try to walk. Your foot could get stuck underneath a submerged rock or tree root, but the current from behind will knock you over—and a combination of current and confinement could be deadly. Instead, make your way over to the shore with your feet out in front of you, your back flat and belly up. Try as well to keep upstream of your boat, so that it doesn't run into you or pin you against an object.

In the event that you and your boat are pinned against an object in a river, such as a fallen tree or a boulder, *always lean toward the object against which you are pinned.* The bottom of your boat will act as a buttress against the current; you will be stuck but safe. If you lean into the current, it will drag you beneath the surface and under the obstruction, which can be lethal.

It bears repeating: Stay calm. Don't let a couple seconds of panic cost a lifetime.

Baby, It's Cold Outside: How to Avoid Hypothermia

Generally, if the outside temperature and the water temperature add up to less than 100, hypothermia is possible. The easiest prevention method, of course, is to stay off the water, but I paddle year-round. In general, when paddling in cold water/weather, it's wise to keep to the nearby streams that you know already, and save the explorations of more exotic places for warmer conditions.

Keep your cold-weather trips modest in length and time, and try to find another romantic fool who wants to be on the water, so that you're not paddling alone. Like any cold-weather activity outdoors, you'll want to dress in layers, and choose clothing made from moisture-resistant materials. It's always a good idea to pack a change of clothes inside a dry bag stowed inside your boat. When it comes to cold-weather paddling, this is critical. I've been dumped a couple times on wintertime trips, and having a new outfit to change into was the best thing since bread got sliced—and it probably saved my life.

Paddles and PFDs

In Wisconsin, you are not legally required to wear a personal flotation device (PFD), but you must have one with you while on the water, whether stowed inside the boat or tied down on top. Especially in rapids or sandbars with sudden drops, wearing a PFD can save your life.

Also, it's not a bad idea to have a spare paddle with you. Investing in a cheap backup could be the difference between a great day on the river and a terrible one. No one wants to be that person up the creek without a paddle! Many rental outfitters will sell you a basic paddle for next to nothing.

Other Helpful Tips

- Carefully review the map before and during your paddle, being mindful of take-outs and potential portages. Sometimes it's a good idea to mark a branch on a tree or a bridge by the take-out with a bandana, colorful cloth, or surveyor's tape to help signal that this is where to pull into. You don't want to miss your take-out! (Just don't forget to remove your reminder.)
- Whenever you know you'll be running a sudden drop or continuous rapids, it's a good idea to scout the river from dry land first so as to avoid unpleasant surprises while on the water, when it could be too late.
- When on lakes or large rivers, always paddle defensively when motorboats and Jet Skiers are around. Make yourself visible and keep a wide berth of their wake. Always point the front end of your boat (the bow) into the direction of an oncoming wave to avoid capsizing or getting swamped.
- Always bring extra water and plenty of sunscreen, and be sure to include safety equipment, such as a weather radio, first-aid kit, throw rope or rescue line, a bilge

pump or sponge, dry bags, snacks, and rain gear. Don't forget a hat and sunglasses, too. Expect the best, but prepare for the worst.

Public Access and Trespassing

NAVIGABLE PUBLIC WATERWAYS IN WISCONSIN ARE DEFINED, according to the Wisconsin Department of Natural Resources, as "lakes, rivers, and streams [that] have a bottom (bed) and side (bank), and enough water to float any boat, skiff, or canoe of the shallowest draft on a reoccurring basis." In addition, "barriers such as wood or plant debris may impede actual navigation but waters are public even when multiple portages are required to get around obstructions." And, finally, "a waterway does not need to be regularly used for recreational or other general purposes, but is a public waterway based on its capacity to be navigable and public." For more on this, see tinyurl.com/wiwaterwayandwetlandpermits and tinyurl.com/wipublictrustdoctrine.

Paddlers are not allowed to go beyond the ordinary high-water mark on private land (this is usually the top of a riverbank) but do have reasonable access to shoreline (which will often be private land) "only if it is necessary to exit the body of water to bypass an obstruction." It's never unwise to have something in writing, so here's the actual statuary language you can print out and have ready in case an ornery landowner shakes his cane at you in a "Get off my lawn, you kids!" kind of way: tinyurl.com/wisconsinriparianrights.

On the whole, it's best for all involved if paddlers are mindful of private landowners and as unobtrusive as possible. Remember: How you conduct yourself on the river impacts other canoeists and kayakers. Like it or not, we're all paddling ambassadors. The cooperation between landowners and paddlers will ensure river access for future generations.

Leave No Trace

The guidelines below are derived from the Seven Principles promoted and copyrighted by the Leave No Trace Center for Outdoor Ethics (lnt.org):

1. Plan ahead and prepare.
2. Travel and camp on durable surfaces to minimize disturbance of natural areas.
3. Dispose of waste properly.
4. Leave what you find (unless it's trash!).
5. Minimize campfire impacts.

6. Respect wildlife.
7. Be considerate of others.

Respect private property and publicly owned property along the water. For your own safety, the well-being of livestock, and as a courtesy to landowners, always yield to cattle and other critters in the water. When you encounter wire strung along a river, gently thread your way under or through it; do not tamper with it. (Keep in mind that wire almost always comes in pairs, and it's strung not to injure you but to keep farm animals from escaping.)

Please park only in designated areas and lots. If there is no parking explicitly denoted on the trip map, please pull off the road as safely as possible and park in compliance with local ordinances.

Do not ever bring glass on the water—period. Make sure that your beverages are either in aluminum cans or plastic bottles. There's nothing better than a tasty drink on a hot day while paddling, but be responsible and don't litter.

Finally, *dispose of waste properly.* That includes human waste. If you are camping in a site without facilities, dig a hole at least 1 foot deep and as far away from the water as possible, deposit waste, and cover.

Trips at a Glance

Best Trips for Camping

Best Trips for Geology

Best Trips for Kids

Best Trips for Paddle-and-Pedal Combos

Best Trips for Riffles/Rapids

Best Trips for Wildlife

Trips by Distance

4 TO 9 MILES

TRIPS BY DISTANCE *(CONTINUED)*

4 TO 9 MILES *(continued)*

9+ TO 12 MILES

12+ MILES OR LONGER

Trips by Skill Level

BEGINNERS

EXPERIENCED PADDLERS

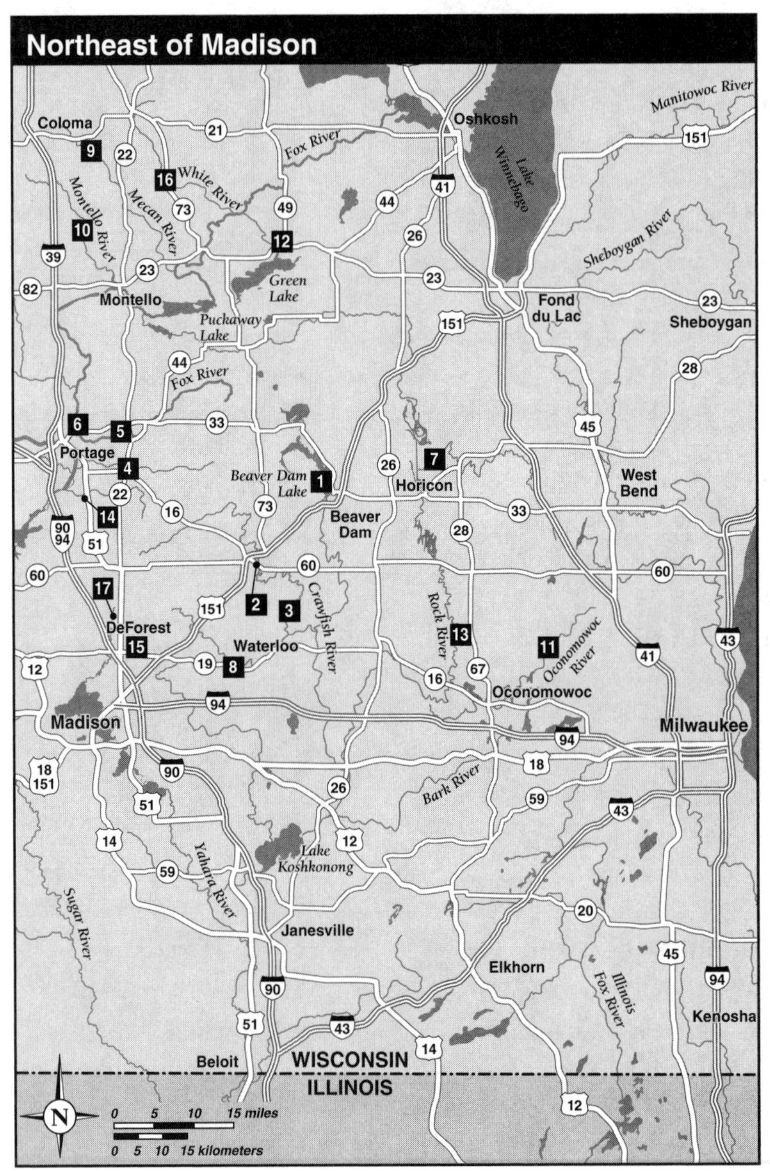

Northeast of Madison
Coloma
Oshkosh
Montello
Green Lake
Puckaway Lake
Fox River
White River
Mecan River
Montello River
Manitowoc River
Sheboygan River
Lake Winnebago
Fond du Lac
Sheboygan
Portage
Beaver Dam Lake
Beaver Dam
Horicon
West Bend
DeForest
Waterloo
Crawfish River
Rock River
Oconomowoc River
Oconomowoc
Madison
Milwaukee
Bark River
Lake Koshkonong
Yahara River
Sugar River
Janesville
Elkhorn
Illinois Fox River
Kenosha
Beloit
WISCONSIN
ILLINOIS
0 5 10 15 miles
0 5 10 15 kilometers

part one

Northeast of Madison

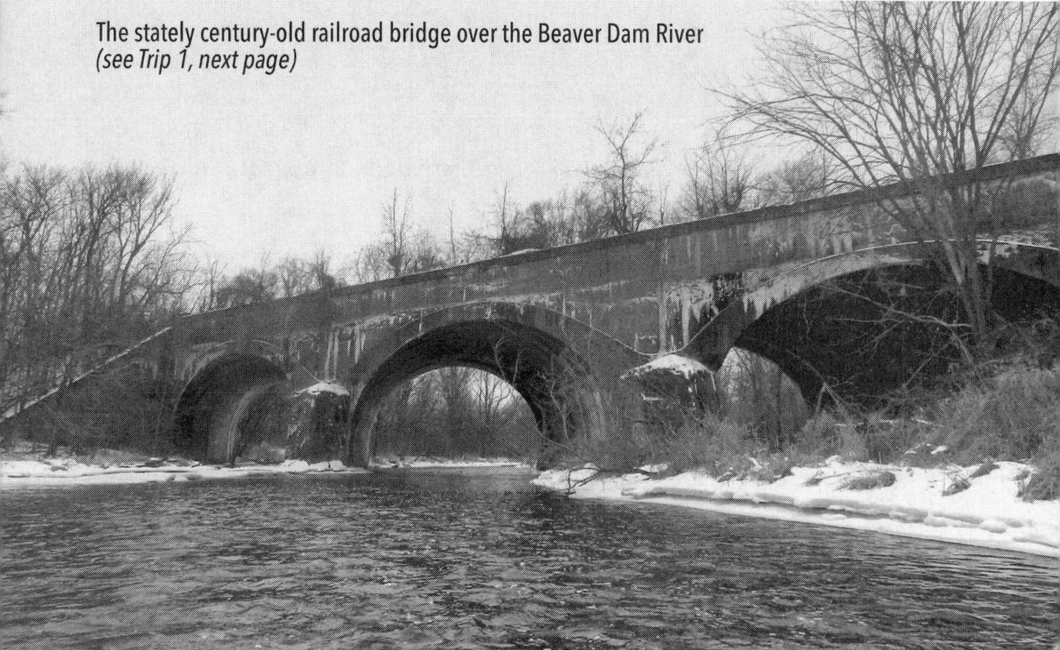

The stately century-old railroad bridge over the Beaver Dam River *(see Trip 1, next page)*

1 Beaver Dam River: BEAVER DAM TO COUNTY ROAD J

•THE•FACTS•

Put-in/take-out Cotton Mill Park/County Road J

Distance/time 5.5 mi/Allow for 2.5 hrs

Gradient/water level 10 fpm/See USGS gage 05425912. The ideal level is at or above 200 cfs. At 300 cfs or higher, the river will be pushy and should be considered only by paddlers with good boat control.

Water type Several Class I rapids, riffles, and quietwater

Canoe or kayak Kayak

Skill level Experienced

Time of year to paddle Anytime

Landscape Urban in first half, secluded woods with hills in second half

---

OVERVIEW This exhilarating trip begins in an urban downtown but ends in the country, with constant riffles and a dozen Class I rapids along the way. A wooded corridor between the put-in and take-out adds to the variety of this trip. You might spot pelicans at the lake above the dam, but expect to see ducks, geese, muskrats, fish, and great blue herons below US 151.

SHUTTLE **5.1 miles.** From the take-out, head northeast on CR J. Turn left onto CR G and take it into town. Turn left onto Mill Street. Turn right onto Madison Street, then left into the parking lot at the dam.

TAKE-OUT N43° 23.640' W88° 52.132' **PUT-IN** N43° 27.278' W88° 50.570'

•THE•FLAVOR•

PUT IN AT COTTON MILL PARK on the north bank of the river below the dam, opposite the large brick building that used to be a mill but now is rehabbed apartments. Cotton Mill Park is little more than a strip of land in the backyards of residential houses. It is open to the public, though, and parking is permitted in a lot contiguous with the apartment building. Launching here is via rocky riprap, where you will be sharing space with those who come here to fish.

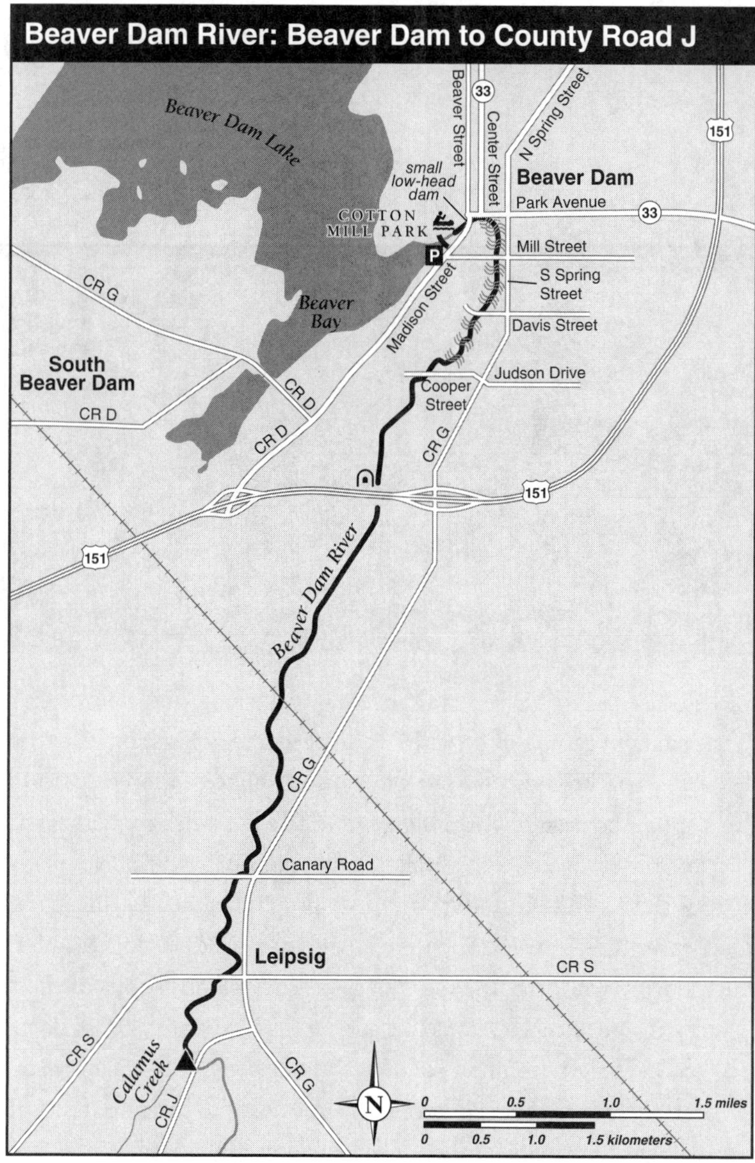

Only 50 yards ahead is the Beaver Street bridge, beneath which is a small low-head dam. Normally, you should not entertain the notion of running low-head dams, but this one is an exception to the rule. There is enough clearance between the top lip of the dam and the water surface to run without scraping, and the drop itself is only 18 inches or so.

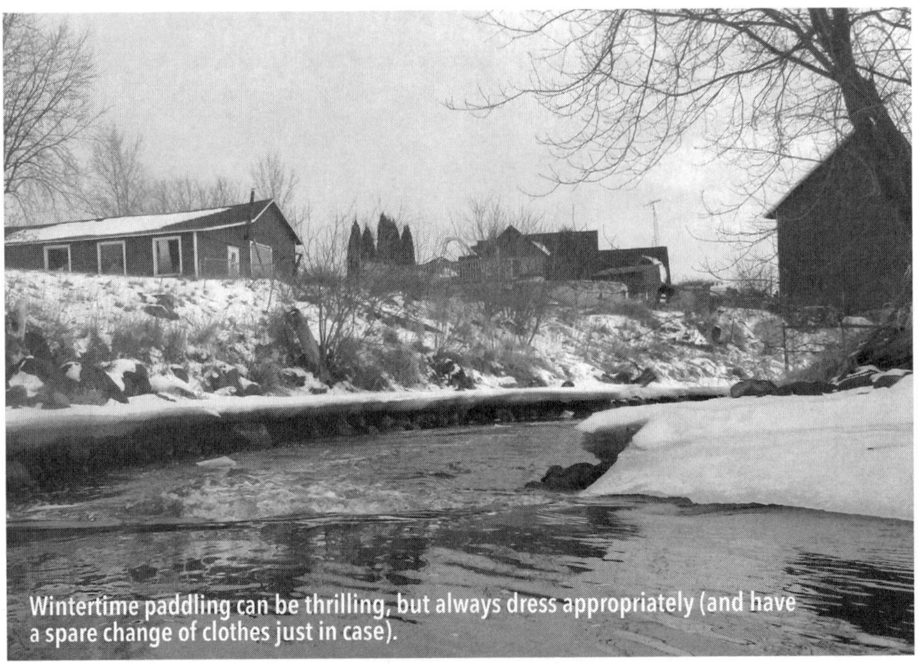
Wintertime paddling can be thrilling, but always dress appropriately (and have a spare change of clothes just in case).

If you run the dam, it's best to do so with some speed and not just inch up to the edge. That said, there is a backroller at the bottom of the drop, so caution is critical. You can portage the dam at the far left where there is an eddy as well as some rocks along the concrete wall of the bridge; use this wall to dock, get out, and pull your boat below the drop. Scout this before you run it, and steer away from the I-beams in the water.

Below Beaver Street, the rapids begin as the river makes a clockwise 180-degree turn through downtown. After the Center Street bridge, both banks of the river are lined with attractive rock rubble, no doubt adding to the stream's riffles. Approaching the water tower on the left be mindful and keep a wide berth of remnant posts sticking out of the water; the current here is fast, so you don't want to run into these. (In higher water, these will be submerged.) On your left will be a high, flat wall creating a canal feeling—and again adding to the swiftness of the current. A fun drop lies just below the wall. This in turn is followed by an even better drop just below the Mill Street bridge.

A long, narrow straightaway announces the gigantic Kraft factory on your right. Light rapids and riffles will continue through a series of pleasant city parks around which the river meanders. At Cooper Street, you'll come upon four culverts. They look intimidating because they lie on a diagonal, so you can't see proverbial light at the other end of the tunnel. You can easily portage around these, but rest assured it's totally safe. Choose the rightmost culvert, as there's a fun small rapid just below the clearance. Consider this short-but-lively stretch part one of this trip.

Part two consists of Cooper Street to just downstream of the US 151 underpass. This stretch is a little dull, to be frank. The river widens and thus gets quite shallow and slow. Notwithstanding the clarity of the water, there's a considerable amount of trash in this section—mostly tires. The culprit is no doubt the large landfill you'll see in the form of a hill on the right. Fortunately, all of this is quickly passed through. Another tunnel, this time concrete-lined, the US 151 underpass is pretty fun to paddle through. Since the current here is virtually nonexistent, there are no safety concerns. On the downstream side of US 151, you'll see a new housing development off to the right. The general dullness of this section resumes for a quarter of a mile more before the river again narrows, woods enclose, and the best part of the trip begins—indeed, the best portion of the entire Beaver Dam River!

Past the barn on the right and then a set of power lines lies a wonderfully easy 1-foot drop—you'll see a modest horizon line and hear the rapid. The river flows fairly straight through a woodsy corridor for the next few miles, and riffles are everywhere, occasionally punctuated with small rapids. The left bank will rise about 20 feet high, and then the right bank as well. You'll pass only two houses here, side by side on the right above a series of concrete terraces. After these, the river zigzags through more charged riffles leading to a magnificent and colossal railroad bridge seemingly in the middle of nowhere and more or less resembling a Roman aqueduct. At least 50 feet high, it was built in 1910 and straddles the tall banks. Be careful though: On the downstream side of the bridge is a wire, not barbed, but you don't want to become entangled.

After the bridge, the river is shallower, so in low water you will need to pay attention for the deepest channels. There are a number of small boulders and a few strainers to watch out for and maneuver around. It's not necessarily dangerous, but you must be mindful and on-game—but in a fun way, not a dangerous one. Leading up to and following Canary Road, the woods thin out and you're in farmland. The riffles continue, the water is still clear, and the river meanders more here, so the paddling remains a delight.

Immediately upstream of a charming red barn is one last super-fun rapid at a right-hand bend. As usual, you'll hear the sound of it before seeing it. The rapid peters out to a riffle leading to CR S. The current will remain lively for the next 0.5 mile, to the bridge at CR J, where you'll see a small stream enter on the right. Take out on the right bank on the upstream side of the bridge, where there is a convenient flat spot for ease of access.

•THE•FUDGE•

ADDITIONAL TRIPS There's a pretty stretch a few miles downstream beginning at Meadow Road to the dam in Lowell. Except for one random stretch with riffles, it's slow and becomes somewhat monotonous, but the beginning meadow is especially lovely in spring. A couple hundred yards of Class I rapids and riffles lie below the dam, but there's no good spot to take out. It's slow and agrarian downstream of Reeseville, and eventually the river splits around two huge islands studded with subdued quartz. The area is interesting but very marshy and often frequented by motorboats.

Beaver Dam Lake itself is not recommended for paddling due to the motorboat traffic it receives.

CAMPING **Derge Park** (N8379 CR W, Beaver Dam; 920-386-3700)

FOOD FOR THOUGHT For a great cup of coffee as well as sweet and savory treats, head over to **Black Waters Coffee** (308 S. Center St., Beaver Dam; 920-887-8100), two blocks from the put-in.

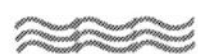

2 Crawfish River A: COLUMBUS TO ASTICO PARK

•THE•FACTS•

Put-in/take-out Columbus Dam off Campbell Street/Astico Park near Danville Dam

Distance/time 8.6 mi/Allow for 4 hrs

Gradient/water level 0.5 fpm except for the riffles section/Use USGS gage 05425912 (Beaver Dam River) since the official Crawfish River gage is too far downstream to correlate. Look for a minimum of 60 cfs to avoid scraping.

Water type Quietwater with a section of riffles

Canoe or kayak Either

Skill level Beginner

Time of year to paddle Anytime

Landscape Urban, agrarian, hardwood forest

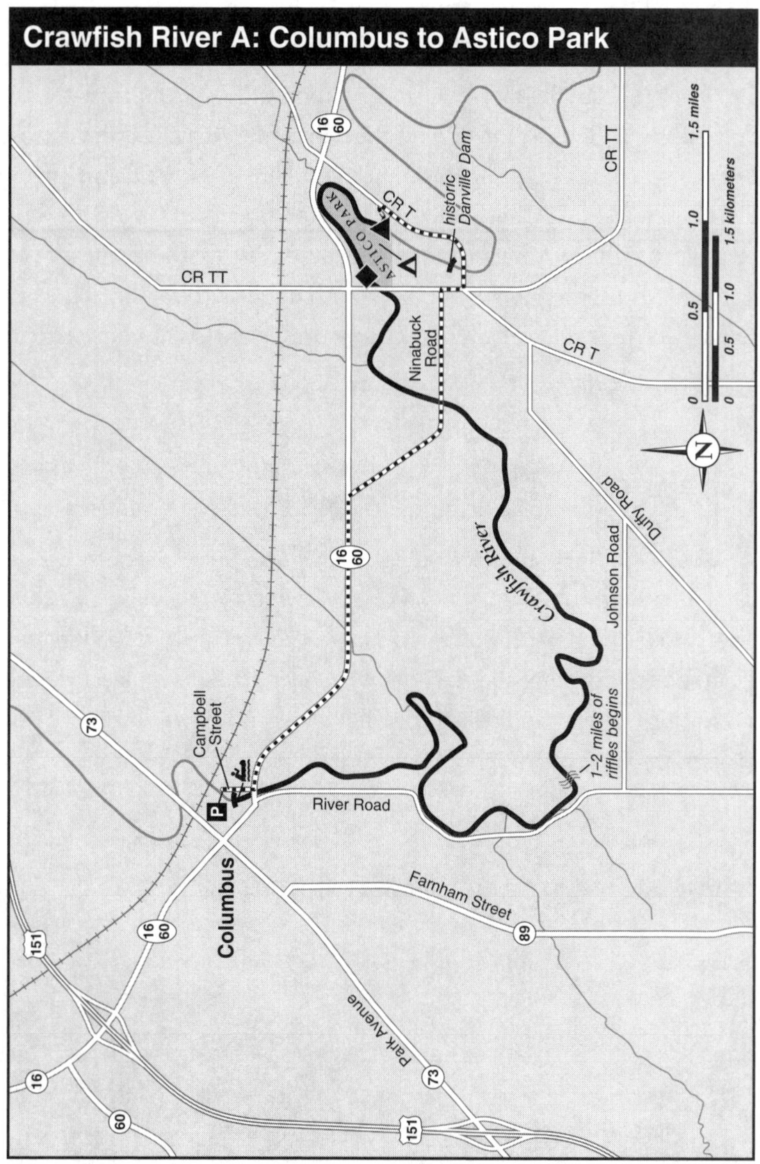

OVERVIEW A pleasant trip offering a surprising amount of diversity, this upper stretch of the Crawfish has a lot to like. While never far from town or farms, the river nonetheless retains a secluded feel. An unexpected boulder garden with riffles and light rapids adds a spike of fun to an otherwise lazy float trip. The county park at the take-out offers pretty campsites and hiking trails on a peninsular hill, as well as a beautiful old powerhouse next to a dam. Expect to see great blue herons, muskrats, ducks, kingfishers, turkey vultures, hawks, and turtles—maybe even egrets and owls.

SHUTTLE 4.3 miles. From the take-out, turn right on CR T. As you cross the bridge, be sure to slow down and look to the right at the handsome Danville Dam. (Also, you can anticipate the water level by seeing how much is spilling over the dam.) Turn right on CR TT, then turn left on Ninabuck Road. At the stop sign, turn left on WI 60 and take it into town. Turn right on Campbell Street; if you cross the river again, you've missed Campbell. At the end of Campbell, you'll see a path on the left leading to the base of the dam. Park roadside near the path and walk the short distance to the bottom of the dam.

TAKE-OUT N43° 19.565' W88° 56.950' **PUT-IN** N43° 20.250' W89° 00.608'

•THE•FLAVOR•

PUT IN BELOW THE DAM. Immediately there will be large rocks to dodge in the streambed, some hard to see due to the clouded water. You will be able to tell right away if the river is shallow: If you're scraping here, you will be walking your boat downstream. Below the dam, the river is unusually narrow; with trees flanking both banks, the setting is pretty and relaxing. As it widens and slows down, you'll see some buildings on both banks and a set of power lines overhead.

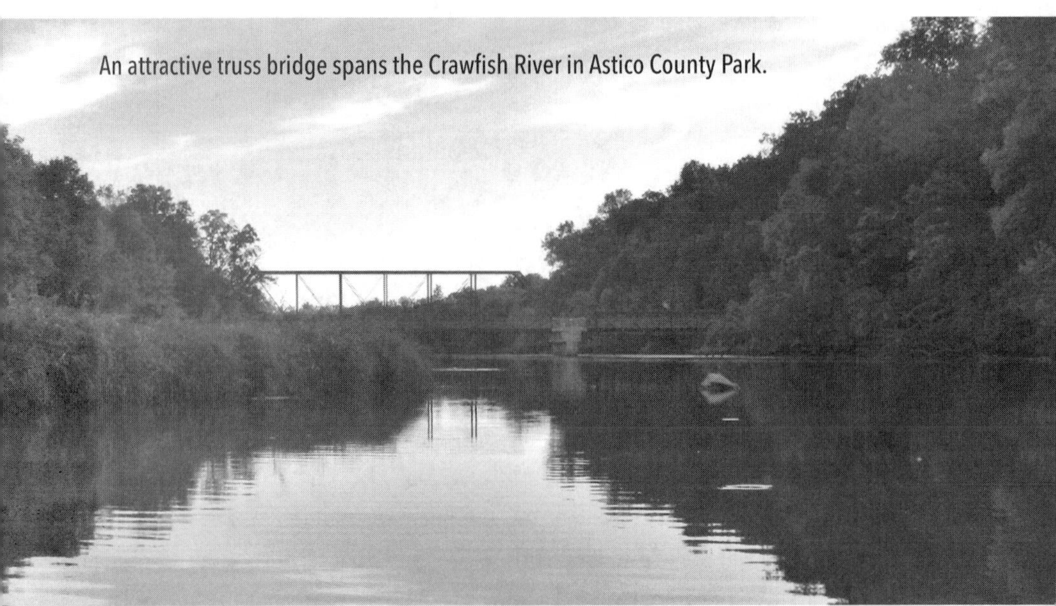

An attractive truss bridge spans the Crawfish River in Astico County Park.

After a long straightaway, the river bends to the left to begin a bizarre loop. It's a welcome aberration though, as a pretty set of deep woods lines the left bank. A series of three sharp right-hand turns follows. After the third, you'll come upon a humongous logjam on the left; fortunately, there's plenty of clearance on the right to pass it by. It's an impressive pile up of wood and debris 5 feet high. After this is a random footbridge spanning the entire river, succeeded by another power line.

For a short way, there will be woods on the left and an 8-foot-tall bank on the right. Here, the Crawfish runs parallel to aptly named River Road, but cars are rare. Soon you'll see an isolated farm on the right up a gentle hill followed by the same power line crossing the river a third time. This signals an unexpected but entirely welcome increase in the gradient, where boulders add to the velocity.

What follows for the next 2 miles are riffles and, in higher water, light rapids through a boulder garden where the river is narrow and the woods deep. Considering how ordinarily slow the Crawfish—a.k.a. "Crawl-fish"—is, this exceptional section is a real treat. The muddy water becomes clear, and even the banks rise to add to the woodsy feel. A mix of hardwoods predominates. If the river is low, this already shallow section will not be runnable. It's too fun and unusual to forfeit due to bad timing, so be sure to check the water levels before you go.

Alas, the river will widen again, and where there's a clearance of trees on the left, you'll see a large house. Immediately after is the restored Ninabuck Road bridge. From here, the river makes a child's crude letter *N* to the northeast, passing under the stately CR TT bridge as it does so. You will see a dock for canoes and kayaks on the right just below the bridge; it's one of two landings in Astico County Park. Just after this, you'll see a wayside park on the left parallel to WI 60.

The river will then make a bend to the right, following the curve of a hill in the park. You'll see some attractive—and secluded—campsites, some with their own private access to the river. There's even an artesian spring well. The Crawfish becomes wider yet as it straightens out. A beautiful truss bridge for hikers in the park lies before you. On the left, you'll see a pier and dock, but wait! There's one last thing to see before taking out.

Paddle downstream less than half a mile to the Danville Dam. Rising 4 stories above the river, its wood handsomely weathered and resembling an old mill from New England, the house on the right is so photogenic that the lake-like impoundment hardly matters. Unfortunately, it's private property, so the right bank is off-limits. But there's a portage trail to the left if you want to get out for a better view. Or simply turn around and paddle back to the bridge.

•THE•FUDGE•

ADDITIONAL TRIPS Continuing downstream from Astico County Park is rather dull, due to the monotony of agricultural fields and development. Putting in upstream of Columbus also is not recommended on account of the many logjams, even though the river here is pretty.

CAMPING AND RENTALS **Astico County Park** (just south of WI 60 at N3620 CR TT; 920-386-3700)

SHOUT-OUT If you've never been to Columbus, check it out. There's impressive architecture, including the city hall and the ornate **Farmers & Merchants Union Bank,** designed by Louis Sullivan.

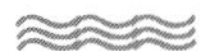

3 Crawfish River B: COUNTY ROAD I TO COUNTY ROAD G

•THE•FACTS•

Put-in/take-out County Road I/County Road G

Distance/time 6.8 mi/Allow for 3 hrs

Gradient/water level Under 1 fpm/There should always be enough water to paddle this trip.

Water type Quietwater

Canoe or kayak Either

Skill level Beginner

Time of year to paddle Anytime

Landscape Marsh, sedge meadow, glacial drumlins, hardwoods, prairie

---

OVERVIEW This a perfectly delightful jaunt, half of which lies within a protected wildlife area, so encounters with critters are excellent here. Expect to see bald eagles, great blue herons, sandhill cranes, hawks, snowy egrets, deer, turkey, turtles, pheasants—maybe even mink and beaver. On a sunny day in autumn when the colors are peaking and migrating birds are a-wing, this trip can be truly blissful.

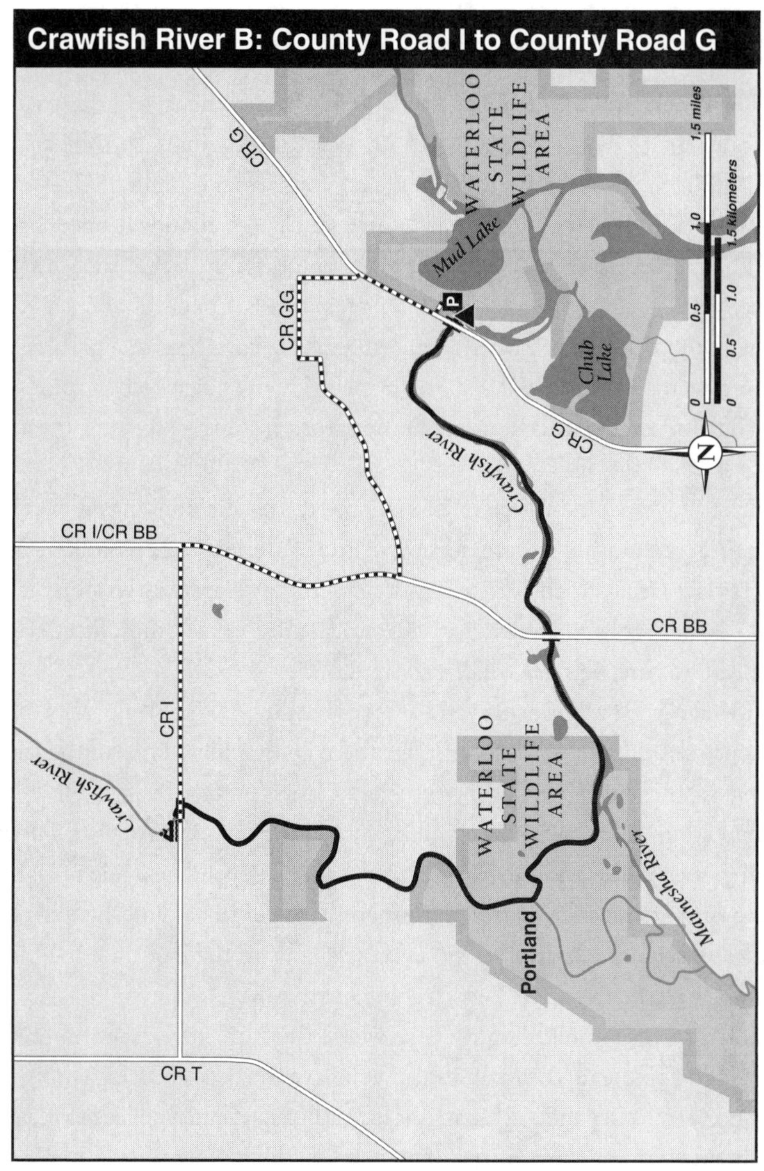

SHUTTLE **5.4 miles.** From the take-out, turn right onto CR G, then bear left on CR GG. (CR GG is quite a pretty drive in its own right as it passes over a drumlin.) Turn right on CR BB, then left on CR I. The put-in is on the upstream side of the bridge, on river right. Park roadside.

TAKE-OUT N43° 14.058' W88° 53.192' **PUT-IN** N43° 15.374' W88° 56.366'

•THE•FLAVOR•

THE CRAWFISH IS ABOUT 80 FEET WIDE HERE, but in this stretch in particular it retains its intimacy. For what it's worth, the width does diminish the likelihood of deadfall. Off in the near distance, you'll see one of several drumlins. After an abrupt right-hand turn followed by a left-hand turn, you'll see an undeveloped landing on the right at the mouth of a slough. You can't go too far upstream the slough, but it is a pretty little nook worth a look-see. This trip offers a handful of such backwater diversions, any of which are worth exploring if you have the time and inclination. The main stream then briefly flows past a row of houses signaled by some weeping willows. But for a few farms and one home across from the take-out, these are the only houses you'll see on this trip.

As you leave behind the signs of settlement, the surroundings grow with wild abandon. You're entering a main section of the Waterloo State Wildlife Area some 4,000 acres large that supports a variety of habitats, such as open-water marsh, sedge meadows, ferns, hardwood forest, native prairie, and shrub swamps. Ready your camera when you're here, because wildlife abounds.

Ringing much of the background are more drumlins. The scene lacks the immediate drama of rock outcrops or bluffs, but there is a graduated rise to the landscape, which makes the entire setting nonetheless rather pretty. Additionally, there are numerous old or dead trees still standing in solitude in contrast to the flourish of leafy living ones in the backdrop for stunning relief. Beyond a couple of tight twists where the river is unusually narrow is the confluence of the Maunesha River, but in a rather inconspicuous spot that's easy to miss. Strangely, the mouth of the Maunesha is narrower than the river itself, which subdues the effect.

Look for a break on the right banks where there are large rocks on the left. It's worth paddling upstream the Maunesha if you have the time and inclination—there's virtually no current to paddle against. About 1 mile upstream, you'll see a gigantic and seemingly surreal rock quarry so out of place it looks like a tornado randomly dropped it there. The huge mounds of crushed stone, gleaming white and beige, could be mistaken for cliffs of clay if you didn't know it was a quarry.

Back in the main stream again, the Crawfish widens out as it approaches the bridge at CR BB. On the right is a lovely farm field on a hill that, with a little imagination, could be a runner-up for Little House on the Prairie. Just upstream from the bridge you'll find the decrepit remains of foundation supports adjoined by a very tiny island with a tree growing out of it. There's a good chance you'll happen upon folks

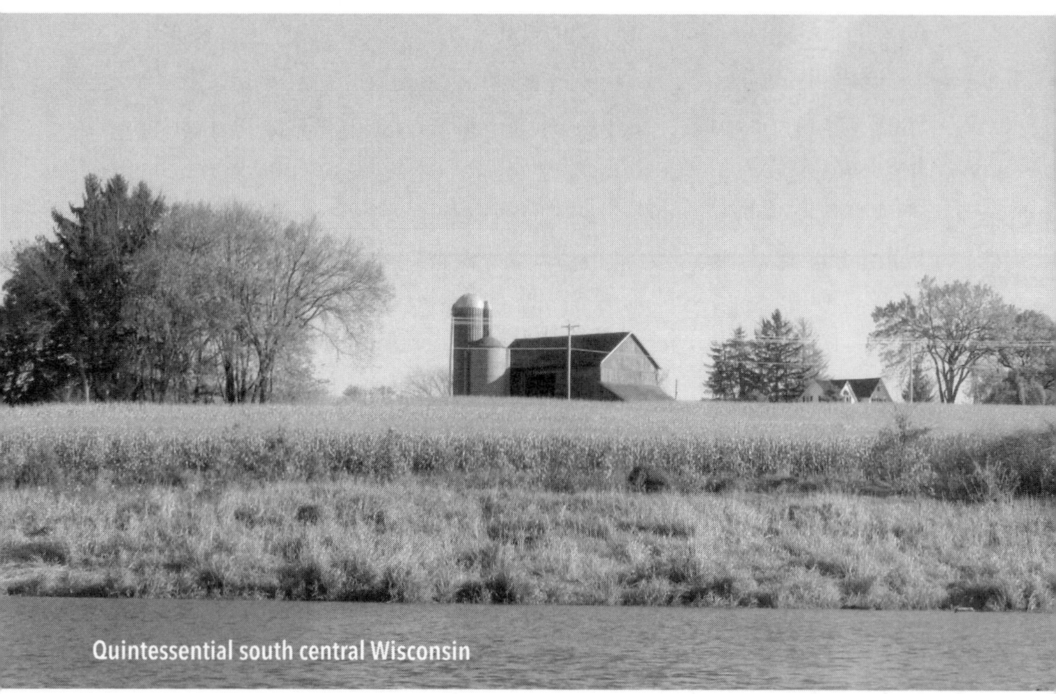
Quintessential south central Wisconsin

on the banks here casting fishing lines. On the downstream side of the bridge are a few boulders to dodge, maybe a small riffle, and a few more attractive tree islands. The river slowly glides past a hill on the right, where you'll see more boulders both on the bank and tucked into the earth. In autumn, the colors here simply blaze.

The end of the trip comes quickly: Turn right and suddenly the take-out bridge is before you. The landing is on the downstream side on the left, an official parking lot for the Waterloo State Wildlife Area. Look for the GLACIAL HERITAGE AREA WATER TRAILS sign for the most convenient spot to take out.

•THE•FUDGE•

ADDITIONAL TRIPS Downstream of CR G, within half a mile, you enter a sprawling marsh near the confluence of the Beaver Dam River and Mud Lake. After Mud Lake, the Crawfish is humongous—more than 400 feet wide most of the time. Added to that, it's slow and muddy, and most of the surroundings are large farms.

CAMPING AND RENTALS **Astico County Park** (just south of WI 60 at N3620 CR TT; 920-386-3700)

FOOD FOR THOUGHT Located in the one-block burg of Millville, **Crawfish Junction** (W6376 CR A, just north of I-94; 920-648-3550) caters to Cajun tastes, offering andouille sausage and deep-fried gator.

SHOUT-OUT Both the put-in and take-out are dedicated (though undeveloped) landings thanks in large part to the **Glacial Heritage Area (GHA),** an organization whose mission is "to reconnect people to the land through recreation, conservation and tourism," mostly but not exclusively in Jefferson County areas where glaciers left their marks. A number of trips in this book have been inspired by the GHA's work. For a map of the lakes and streams in the GHA, a guide, and lots of great info in general, see glacialheritagearea.org.

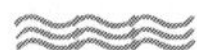

4 Duck Creek: WYOCENA TO DUCK CREEK ROAD

•THE•FACTS•

Put-in/take-out Lovers Lane in downtown Wyocena/Duck Creek Road off US 51. See "The Flavor" for an alternative put-in.

Distance/time 9 mi/Allow for 5 hrs

Gradient/water level 2 fpm/Water levels should always be reliable, but wind can be a factor, so try to pick a still day.

Water type Quietwater

Canoe or kayak Either

Skill level Beginner

Time of year to paddle Spring and autumn

Landscape Marsh, woods, savanna

OVERVIEW A mix of woods and marsh, Duck Creek is a mostly isolated stream with very little development along the banks. It's not the best trip to paddle if the wind is against you, but it's an awesome spot in spring and autumn during migration—for

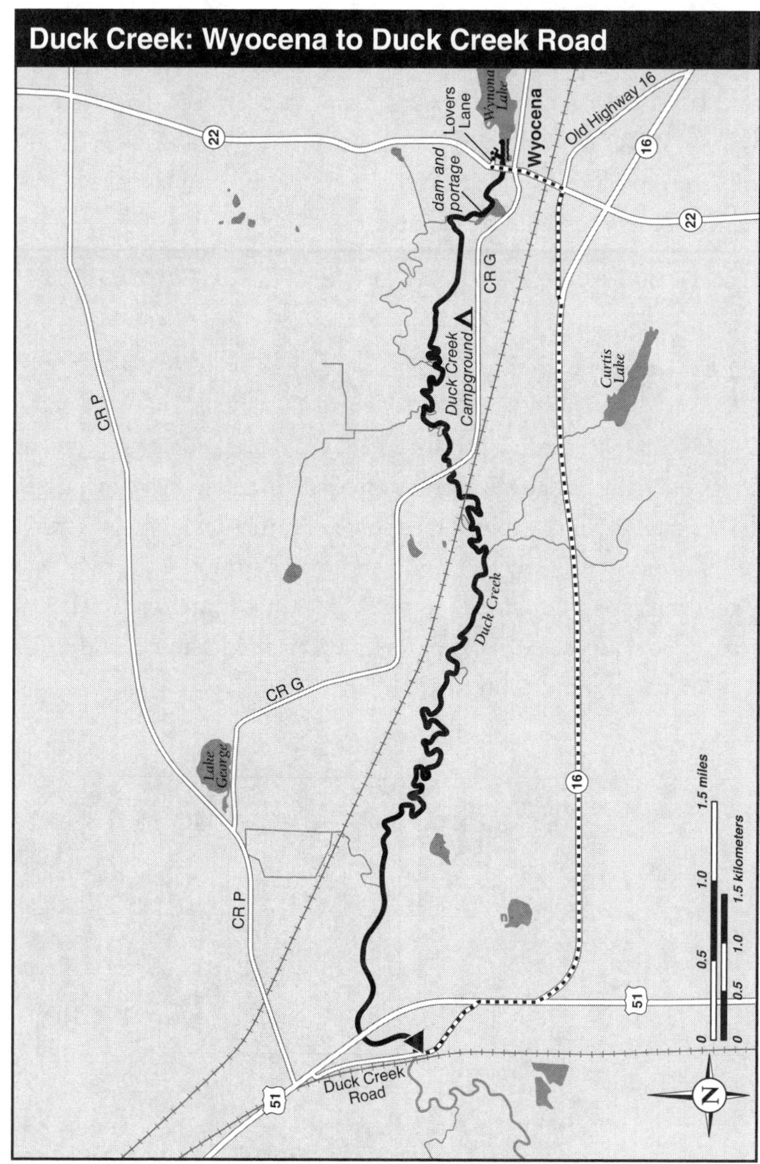

sandhill cranes especially, but you can expect to see various birds as well as deer and muskrats. This trip can easily be broken into two segments.

SHUTTLE **6.3 miles.** The take-out is along Duck Creek Road, which is less a road than a snowmobile trail. Whatever you call it, it's rough and rutty. You may want to park your vehicle or bicycle before the road gets dodgy. (A kayak caddy is great for such occasions.) From the take-out, head south on Duck Creek Road, then turn right on US 51. Turn left on WI 16 and head east. Coming into Wyocena, bear left on Old WI 16. Turn left on WI 22, cross the river, and then turn right onto Lovers Lane. The boat launch will be on your right. Put in at the semi-developed boat launch at Lovers Lane. There's plenty of room for roadside parking.

TAKE-OUT N43° 30.240' W89° 24.900' **PUT-IN** N43° 29.820' W89° 18.540'

•THE•FLAVOR•

FOR THE FIRST 0.5 MILE, you'll paddle on a flowage past some Wyocena buildings. There's a cool old truss bridge followed by an iconic barn on the right. Depending on how high the water is, you'll probably see some branches and roots of scrub partially submerged. The dam will be on your right, and you'll portage to the right of the dam; there's a sign indicating this, too. The creek jackknifes northward below the dam. There are a couple sloughs you can explore for up-close encounters of the old dam, of which there are three components.

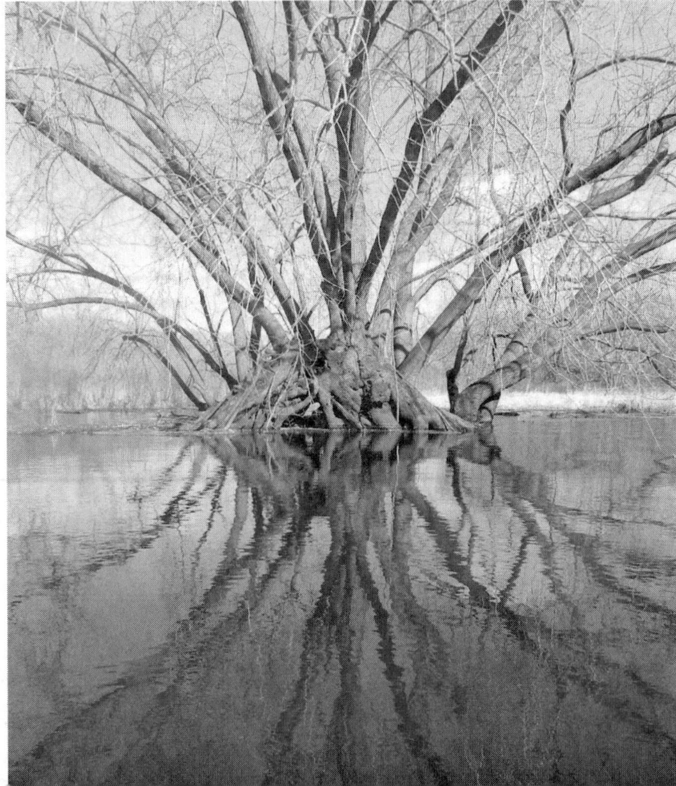

"Treeflection" in the backwaters of the Duck Creek confluence at the Wisconsin River

The creek then heads west along straightaways, where you will need to duck (no pun intended) and maneuver around some obstructions. It's a pretty scene back here tucked away from development. The creek is wide and the water usually deep. Where it's on the shallow side, it's clear and the bottom sandy. The banks alternate between very low and 8 feet high. As the creek begins to meander in earnest, the banks will gently rise—some sandy, some supporting tall stands of pine. After a right-hand bend comes the CR G bridge (**N43° 30.090' W89° 20.711'**), a solid access point for a shorter trip.

Below the bridge, Duck Creek is almost entirely marsh, but the current remains surprisingly steady. A railroad bridge, power lines off in the distance, and two separate farm buildings are the only signs of civilization you'll see for the next 5 miles. The sense of isolation is surprising and special. Expect to see—and hear—majestic sandhill cranes, especially in spring and fall. While this second stretch is mostly marsh, the creek does meander quite a bit, narrowing around bends as it does so. And there are some hills in the distance, with a periphery of pine. Still though, avoid paddling here on a windy day since the creek is essentially flat for the last few miles.

Eventually the meandering will slacken, and as the creek straightens out, it becomes wider, too. Off to the left you'll see the twin smokestacks of the Alliant Energy Plant above Lake Columbia. Next comes the US 51 bridge, below which the creek will gently curve to the left and then to the right leading up to the take-out. There are two parallel bridges: one at the take-out at Duck Creek Road, the other a railroad bridge. The take-out is on the upstream side of Duck Creek Road on the left.

•THE•FUDGE•

ADDITIONAL TRIPS From the take-out to the Wisconsin River and back is another 5 miles through floodplains and various channels (some leading to dead ends, others leading to Lake Columbia). This no-man's-land (or -river) is certainly fun and interesting, but it can be disorienting. There is a time and a place for purposefully getting lost, at least temporarily losing one's way—how else are discoveries made?—but make sure you plan and prepare for such sojourning. The current here is next to nothing, so you can do a there-and-back trip using the Duck Creek Road bridge as your put-in and take-out.

An alternative upstream trip on the middle branch of Duck Creek is quite pretty and can be added to this trip or done on its own. Put in at Schliesmann Road east of Wyocena and take out either at Wyona County Park off CR GG (4.2 miles) or at the Lovers Lane boat launch (5.5 miles).

The water is terrifically clear and the current is peppy. There is a dam to portage around midway.

CAMPING **Duck Creek Campground** is located along the banks of this trip (W6560 CR G; 608-429-2425). **Indian Trails Campground** is situated on a small lake in Pardeeville, a few miles east of Portage (W6445 Haynes Road; 608-429-3244).

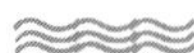

5 Fox River A: INDIAN HILLS CAMPGROUND TO PORTAGE CANAL

•THE•FACTS•

Put-in/take-out Indian Trails Campground/Portage Canal on Agency House Road

Distance/time 8.7 mi/Allow for 4–5 hrs

Gradient/water level 1 fpm/See the NOAA gage in Pardeeville. Look for a minimum height of 7 feet. Call Indian Trails Campground (608-429-3244) for real-time water levels. Higher water is better for paddling up the canal. Also, check the wind forecast to try to avoid high winds from the north or west when paddling across Swan Lake.

Water type Quietwater and flatwater

Canoe or kayak Either

Skill level Beginner

Time of year to paddle Anytime

Landscape Sedge meadows, oak savanna, prairie remnants, tamarack swamp, historic lock and canal through urban downtown

---

OVERVIEW This day journey for the adventurous type explores the historic Fox River, where it begins as a narrow, meandering creek through woodsy meadows, empties into a lake, quietly exits the lake amid a pristine setting of tamaracks and barrens in a protected wildlife area, and finally becomes a river as it takes up its long trek to Green Bay. Passing through an unspoiled landscape as it enters the city of Portage, the river is linked to a famous canal that once connected to the Wisconsin River. Expect to see sandhill cranes, great blue herons, deer, wood ducks, fish, and lots of turtles, including the cool spiny softshell.

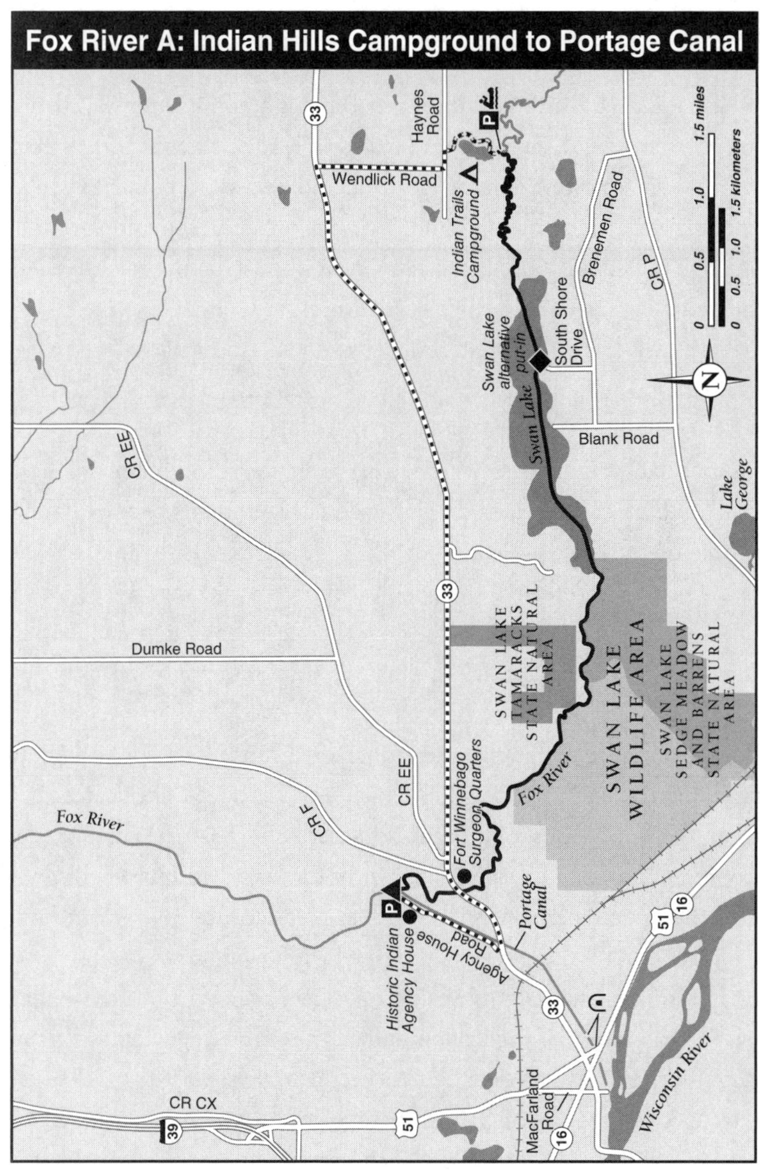

SHUTTLE 9 miles. From the take-out, head south on Agency House Road, then turn left onto Cook Street/WI 33. Stay on WI 33 for approximately 6 miles, then turn right onto Wendlick Road. Turn left onto Haynes Road and then turn right into Indian Trails Campground.

TAKE-OUT N43° 33.544' W89° 26.217' **PUT-IN** N43° 32.940' W89° 19.380'

•THE•FLAVOR•

PUT IN AT THE PRIVATE CAMPGROUND, where there is a nominal fee ($6) to access the river. There is a free public boat launch at the lake in Pardeeville, but I don't recommend using it as a put-in, due to the many logjams and necessary portages you'd endure from the boat launch to the campground. Plus, the owner of the campground does an outstanding job of keeping the narrow river clear of obstructions, so think of the fee as gasoline money to keep those chainsaws running.

The Fox here is sweetly intimate, only 20 feet wide and shallow. The water is clear, the bottom sandy. The landscape is marshy, but not flat; tall grass and alders in the foreground contrast with the slopes of pine behind. The river does meander quite a bit, with ubiquitous oxbows, so expect a small workout if you're in a canoe or longer kayak.

After a mile or so, you'll pass under the derelict remnants of a bridge and then a beautiful cabin on the left. A welcome straightaway announces the inlet to Swan Lake, 407 acres large and 80 feet deep. The opening upon the lake reveals sections that are wild, undeveloped, and lovely. Alas, it's more than 2 miles of lake paddling from the inlet to the outlet, so you may wish to preserve your stamina by not tooling around the outskirts too long.

From the outlet to the public boat launch on Swan Lake, off South Shore Drive, is less than a mile; houses and docks line the shore. (The boat launch can be used as an alternative put-in or take-out for those looking for a shorter trip.) Fortunately, there's less development in the far southwest corner of the lake, which is where you want to head to find the outlet back to the river proper. Look for the yellow Fox River canoe signs. It's a pretty cool feeling to leave the lake by following a river trail.

Back in the river, the water is wonderfully clear again, the bottom a mix of sand and gravel. You can essentially relax now and let the surprisingly reputable current do some of the work. Besides, the river here is twice as wide as upstream, so there should be no obstacles to dodge. The next 2 miles take you through the Swan Lake Wildlife Area, an undeveloped 2,400 acres of wetlands, grassland, and wooded habitats, including sedge meadows, cattail marshes, oak barrens, and tamarack swamps. It's a truly beautiful place hidden in the shadow of historic Portage. Also, as you make your way northwest, you'll begin to see the big beautiful Baraboo Range off to your left, a rather dramatic contrast to the lowlands of the marsh. (See Baraboo River C, page 236, for more information on the range.)

After a longish straightaway, the river will begin to meander gently as trees come closer to the banks; there are billowy weeping willows in one particularly pretty

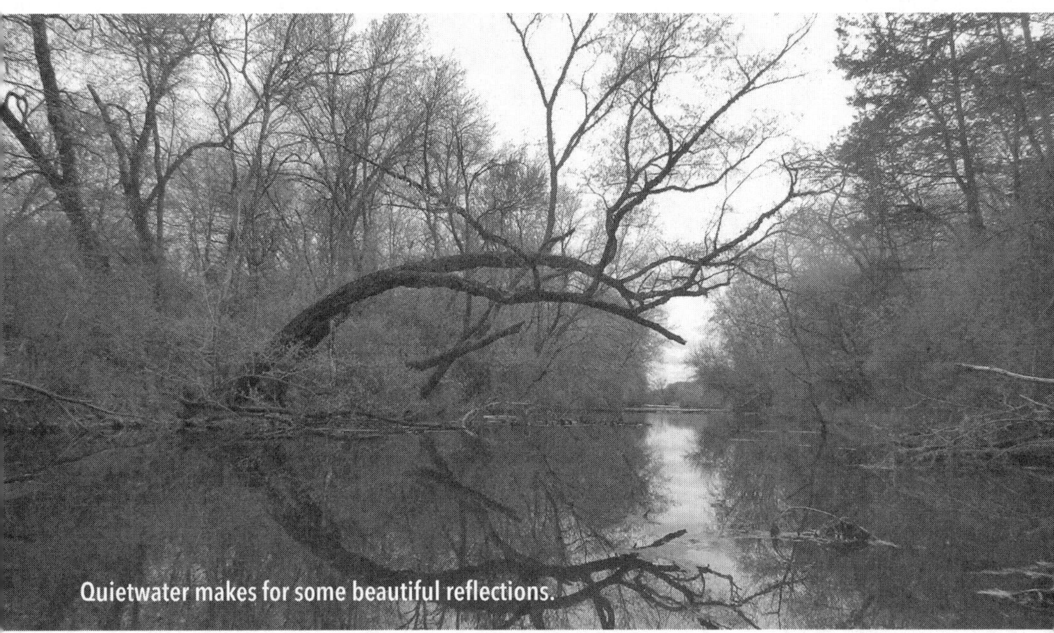
Quietwater makes for some beautiful reflections.

bend. A few more meanders lead to a tight right turn immediately followed by one to the left, where you'll find five foundation pylons in the water supporting a nonexistent bridge, a sort of Fox River Stonehenge.

A few more gradual bends follow as you'll begin to hear the sound of traffic coming from the bridge across WI 33. On the right bank, upstream of the bridge, is the Surgeons' Quarters, the only surviving building of Fort Winnebago, one of three such forts protecting the trade route between the Fox and Wisconsin Rivers. Built in 1828, the handsome old building is open to the public. (Fun fact: For a brief spell, some 30 years before going on to become the president of the Confederacy, Jefferson Davis was stationed here.)

Below the bridge is a wayside on the right (see Fox River B, page 43), but you'll paddle past this for close to a mile before the river heads north, then east, through shallow, sandy shoals. After a quick succession of left–right–left turns, you'll come upon the Portage Canal, technically an outlet from the Wisconsin River to the Fox River (more on that following).

Turn left into the canal, paddle 300 feet up to the derelict lock and dam, and take out on the right at the grass. Just down the road is the Historic Indian Agency House, a home first built in 1832 by the US government to house the Indian agent John Kinzie and his wife for the purposes of "negotiating" with the Ho-Chunk (a.k.a. Winnebago). Today, it can be toured for a fee between May 15 and October 15.

•THE•FUDGE•

ADDITIONAL TRIPS You might consider paddling the canal itself, about 2.3 miles from end to end. There is an imperceptible gradient from the Wisconsin River side to the Fox River, so paddling from the latter to the former is pretty easy. It's stagnant water, however, prone to some pretty funky algae sludge in warm weather, and the canal tends to be very shallow. But the tunnels, tall old mill buildings, concrete walls, and medieval fortress–looking gate, all closer to the Wisconsin River end, make for a fun and scenic side trip.

There is no direct access to the Wisconsin River anymore. That said, it's a short 300-foot walk to the big river over the levee. Consider this: If a raindrop falls to the south of the levee, it eventually makes its way down to the Mississippi River via the Wisconsin River, past St. Louis and Memphis and New Orleans, and into the Gulf of Mexico. If that same raindrop fell to the north of the levee, it would end up in the canal, travel down the Fox River, into Lake Michigan, through Lakes Huron, Erie, and Ontario (tumbling down Niagara Falls in the meantime), past Montreal and Quebec along the St. Lawrence River, and into the Atlantic Ocean.

CAMPING AND RENTALS **Indian Trails Campground** is situated on a small lake a few miles east of Portage (W6445 Haynes Road, Pardeeville; 608-429-3244).

FOOD FOR THOUGHT For a savory meal or sweet treat, stop by **Le Croissant Bakery and Restaurant** (235 W. Pleasant St., Portage; 608-742-5466).

SHOUT-OUTS For **Historic Indian Agency House** tour information, call 608-742-6362 or go to agencyhouse.org.

Special thanks to the **Friends of the Fox** and the **Fox Wisconsin Heritage Parkway,** advocacy groups working to preserve and promote the river's heritage. And for a fascinating read, check your public library or antiquarian bookseller for a copy of Reuben Gold Thwaites's ***Historic Waterways: 600 Miles of Canoeing Down the Rock, Fox, and Wisconsin Rivers,*** published in 1888.

Two blocks west of the canal take-out, on West Edgewater Street, is a Greek Revival home built by **Zona Gale**—writer, activist, and the first woman to receive the Pulitzer Prize for drama—as a gift to her parents.

6 Fox River B: PORTAGE TO BUFFALO IN COLUMBIA AND MARQUETTE COUNTIES

•THE•FACTS•

Put-in/take-out WI 33 at Wayside Park/County Road O

Distance/time 10.5 mi/Allow for 4 hrs

Gradient/water level 2 fpm/See the NOAA gage at Pardeeville, but there's usually plenty of water to paddle this trip.

Water type Quietwater with one Class I rapid from a ledge at a removed dam

Canoe or kayak Either

Skill level Beginner

Time of year to paddle Anytime

Landscape A pretty mix of marsh, drumlins, and hardwood forest

---

OVERVIEW A trip steeped in history, human and geologic. Here,s you will mimic the ghosts of commercial barges and paddle-wheel boats of a bygone age, when the city of Portage was the link between the Great Lakes–St. Lawrence Seaway and the Mississippi River–Gulf of Mexico, while the Fox River itself threads its way through glacial deposits left in the last ice age. Expect to see sandhill cranes, great blue herons, sandpipers, and lots of turtles.

SHUTTLE **9 miles.** From the take-out, head east on WI 33, then turn left onto CR F. Turn left again onto CR O to reach the bridge.

TAKE-OUT N43° 40.320' W89° 23.760' **PUT-IN** N43° 33.300' W89° 26.100'

•THE•FLAVOR•

PUT IN AT WAYSIDE PARK ON WI 33,just east of downtown Portage. For the first 0.5 mile, the river is unusually narrow and shallow, 40 feet wide and 1 foot deep (or less). If you happen to get stuck on the bottom, don't be discouraged or deduce that it will be like this for the remainder of the trip; it won't. Just butt-scoot your way to deeper parts, or take your boat for a short walk. The water is clear, with a mostly sandy bottom, and the river has a slow current.

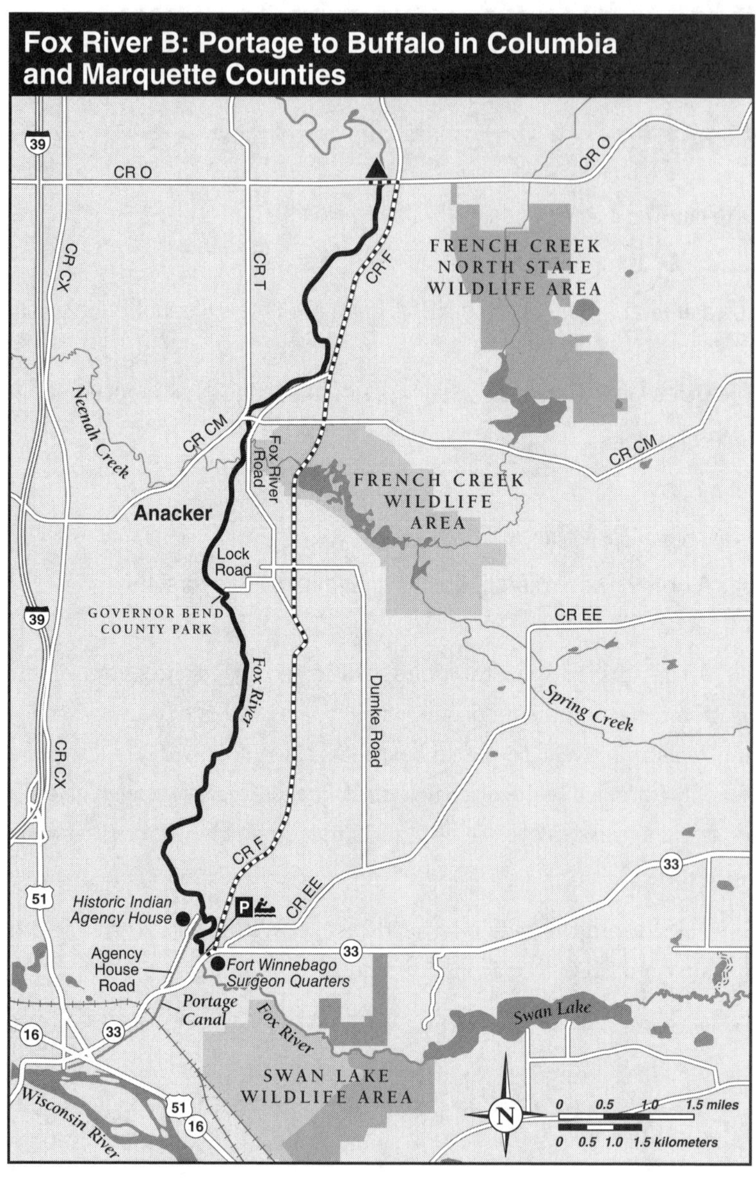

After 1 mile the river widens out to 60 feet (and it is wider still in other parts downstream), so deadfall and obstructions should not ordinarily be problematic. Soon, on the left, you'll see the channel of the old canal, upstream from which lie the ramshackle remains of the lock and dam. It's a popular spot for fishing. After the canal, a series of straightaways with gentle bends takes you through an attractive environment of 10-foot-tall banks topped with tall grass waving in the breeze and stands of pines lined behind.

The river here widens out even more, and there are no signs of development anywhere. In fact, the Ice Age National Scenic Trail—which follows the path of the last glacial advance 12,000 years ago—is on your left for half of this entire trip. Also to your left, in the distance, you'll begin seeing drumlins. You'll pass under a low-clearance wooden footbridge; portage around it if it is impassable. The first road bridge you'll come upon is at Clark Road, preceded by the remains of concrete abutments.

Another long straightaway continues below the bridge. The landscape is especially pretty where the river is cleft a few hundred yards downstream from Clark Road. The main channel is to the left, a slough is on the right, and in between is a soft hill about 30–40 feet high with a variety of trees. On your left, the drumlins come closer into focus. The river will make an abrupt right-hand turn followed by a small 1-foot drop and Class I rapid where an old dam used to be. This marks Governor Bend County Park, a very pleasant spot to picnic and fish.

Before you approach the rapid, it's best to scout it. A wooden pier surrounded by a rubble of boulders makes this easy and approachable. There is an obvious "tongue" of water with which you want to line up to run the drop safely, essentially in the

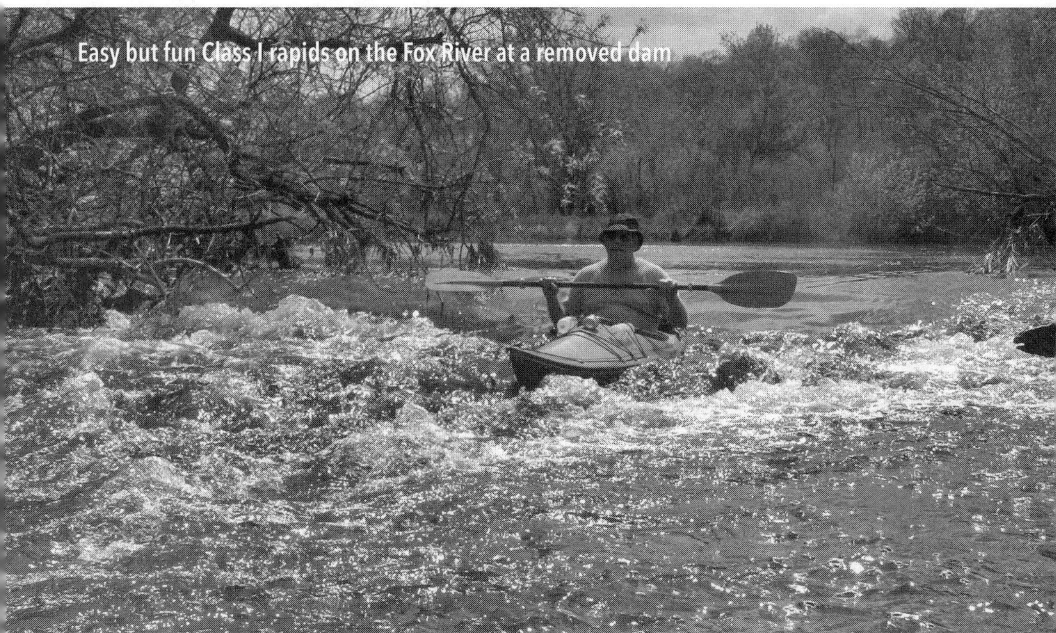
Easy but fun Class I rapids on the Fox River at a removed dam

middle (look for the inverted *V*). Conversely, this can be portaged by taking out by the pier on the left and putting in again below the rapid. It's a fun little drop though, both running it and then surfing upstream in it. Shortly after the rapid, there is a wooden pedestrian bridge with a convenient alternative landing on the downstream river-right side (**N43° 36.595' W89° 25.834'**); you could take out here for a short after-work paddle of 4.5 miles. There's an outhouse in the park, too, should nature call.

Drumlins continue on your left, while the landscape in general remains open, pretty, and undeveloped. A little more than 1 mile later, on your left, is the mouth of Neenah Creek (see Neenah Creek C, page 275), the first big tributary of the Fox River. About 100 yards later, French Creek will appear on your right—blink and you'll miss it. Here, the surroundings flatten out momentarily. Paralleling the aptly named Fox River Road, the river takes a couple of subtle left and right bends followed by long straightaways nestled in a narrow corridor of trees and high sandbanks.

Take your time here to appreciate the seclusion and sanctuary; this is an especially pretty little nook before the first signs of town encroach upon the shores. The river will begin veering east in earnest, widening as it does. After Good Earth Creek appears on the left, you will begin seeing signs of settlement. The good news is this announces the end of the trip anyway, so it's hardly a spoiler. The CR O bridge is impossible to miss. The landing is on the left, on the downstream side at a gravel easement.

•THE•FUDGE•

ADDITIONAL TRIPS Downstream from CR O, the river will begin to widen and slow to a crawl due to a dam in Packwaukee. There's a pleasant 5.5-mile

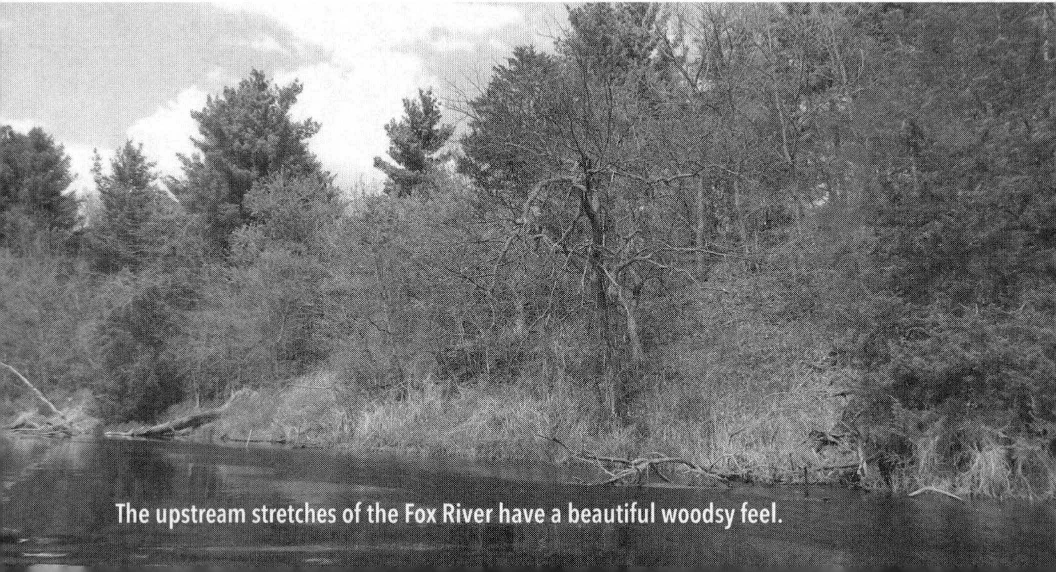

The upstream stretches of the Fox River have a beautiful woodsy feel.

trip from CR O to an inconspicuous public landing off Island Drive that shies away from the worst of the lake effect. Virtually this entire trip falls within the **Fox River National Wildlife Refuge,** comprising more than 1,000 acres of federally protected wetland and upland habitat primarily for sandhill cranes. During spring and fall migrations particularly, this makes a lovely late-afternoon trip, especially if you don't have to paddle against wind.

While not a paddling trip, it's well worth your time to stop and walk around two protected areas accessible from the shuttle route: **French Creek State Natural Area** and **French Creek Wildlife Area.** Mostly marshy, both are respites for wildlife.

About 1.5 miles north of the CR O intersection, off CR F, is the boyhood home of **John Muir,** one of the fathers of our national parks and patron saint of the environment. Today, the land around the lake where he grew up (after his family emigrated from Scotland) is preserved as **John Muir Memorial County Park.** There's a beautiful 1.5-mile hiking trail around the lake that is part of the Ice Age Trail. See tinyurl.com/johnmuirmemorialpark for more information.

CAMPING AND RENTALS **Indian Trails Campground** is situated on a small lake a few miles east of Portage (W6445 Haynes Road, Pardeeville; 608-429-3244).

FOOD FOR THOUGHT For a savory meal or sweet treat, stop by **Le Croissant Bakery and Restaurant** (235 W. Pleasant St., Portage; 608-742-5466).

SHOUT-OUT At the put-in is a state historical sign that tells you how the city of Portage received its name. Also, while exploring the Upper Midwest, in June 1673, the French priest and missionary Jacques Marquette, together with the French Canadian Louis Jolliet, did what Native Americans had done for thousands of years: disembark from the Fox River, carry their boats—or, as they say in French, *portage*—over the terra firma between it and the Wisconsin River (a narrow 1.3 miles), and continue all the way downstream to Prairie du Chien, where they "discovered" its confluence at the Mississippi River. In doing so, the two established a major trading route. Marquette is also credited with coming up with the name *Meskousing*—his adaptation of an Algonquian word meaning "where the waters gather"—to refer to the river. Later French explorers modified the spelling to *Ouisconsin,* which finally got Anglicized to *Wisconsin.*

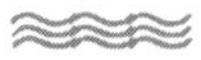

7 Horicon Marsh:
GREENHEAD LANDING TO BOWLING GREEN PARK

•THE•FACTS•

Put-in/take-out Greenhead Road boat launch/Legion Auxiliary Park

Distance/time 7.2 mi (longer if you paddle down ditches or around islands)/ Allow for 3 hrs (longer if you wish to linger)

Gradient/water level 1 fpm/minimum of 100 cfs at USGS gage 05424057

Water type Flatwater

Canoe or kayak Either

Skill level Beginner

Time of year to paddle Spring and autumn during the migrations; early morning is best. (See Planning Advisory following.)

Landscape Huge marsh with some hills in the background

OVERVIEW A vast wetlands complex that is home to the largest freshwater cattail marsh in the country, Horicon Marsh is a truly intriguing and special place. Each spring and autumn, it's a junction for tens of thousands of migrating birds, and paddling the marsh during these times, with a spectacular number of birds coming and going overhead, crouched in trees, and on the water, is truly a treat. The marsh is home to seemingly every variety of goose and duck, not to mention herons, egrets, pelicans, bald eagles, turtles, deer, and otters.

PLANNING ADVISORY You don't want to paddle the marsh when the water's low—it's a mucky mess from which to dislodge your boat—and you definitely don't want to paddle against the wind in this huge open space. This may sound counterintuitive, but trust me: If the wind is coming from the south, even at 10 miles per hour, you should *reverse the put-in and take-out points* and begin this trip at the Legion Auxiliary Park, then paddle upstream to the Greenhead Road boat lot, to avoid a lot of strenuous paddling and splashy whitecaps. Additionally, pack a lot of water, sunscreen, and a hat—especially on a sunny day, as there's essentially no shade.

SHUTTLE 5.8 miles; *see planning advisory above to decide the order of put-in and take-out for this trip.* To shuttle from the Legion Auxiliary Park take-out, turn right onto

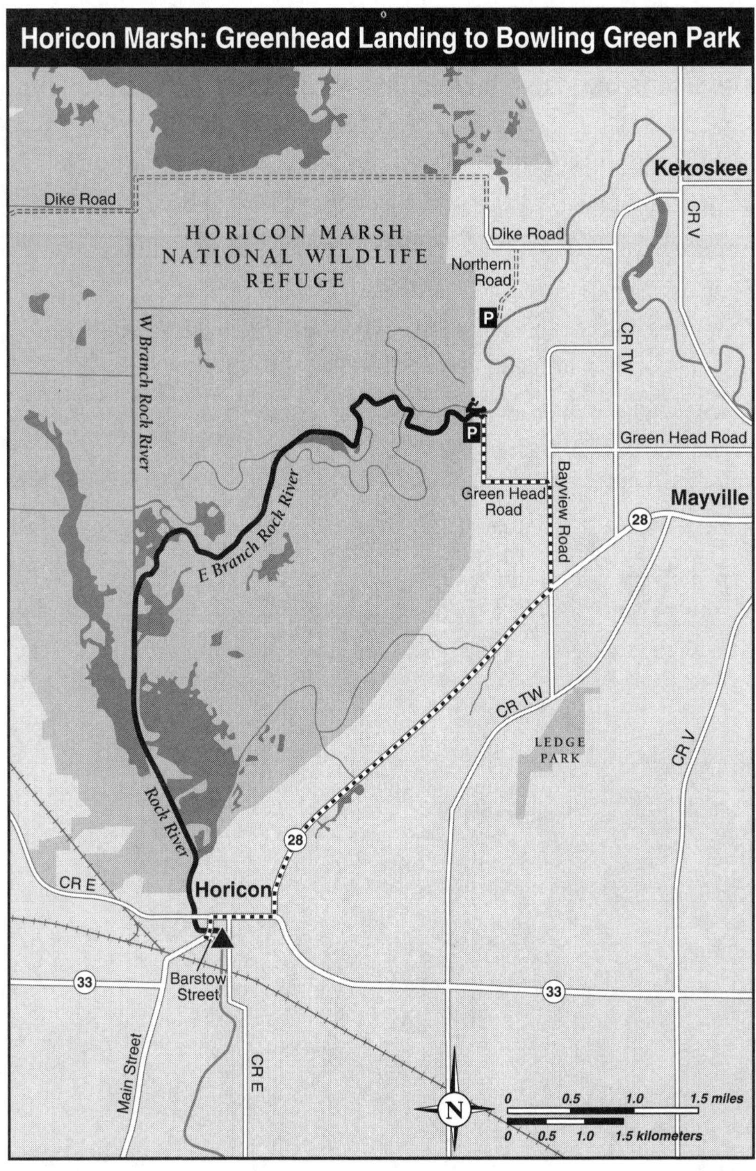

Barstow Street/WI 33 and cross the Rock River. Turn right onto Lake Street, following the signs for WI 33. Before WI 33 veers to the right and southward, turn left onto WI 28. Turn left onto Bayview Road, then left onto Greenhead Road. Bear right on Greenhead Road to the boat launch.

TAKE-OUT N43° 26.940' W88° 37.860' **PUT-IN** N43° 30.300' W88° 35.520'

•THE•FLAVOR•

LOCATED IN DODGE AND FOND DU LAC COUNTIES, Horicon Marsh is a shallow, peat-filled lake bed that was created some 12,000 years ago after a glacial lobe from Green Bay receded and filled in the basin it had earlier scoured. Today, at 33,000 acres total, Horicon is the largest freshwater cattail marsh in the United States. The northern two-thirds comprise a US National Wildlife Refuge and are off-limits to visitors (that is, the bipedal, wingless type). The southern third is overseen by the Wisconsin Department of Natural Resources and is open to the public. It's here where our trip begins.

Put in at the official boat launch off of Greenhead Road, where there's plenty of room for parking, easy access to the water, and even a bathroom. At this point, you will be on the East Branch of the Rock River. You may wish first to paddle to the opposite shore to the Greenhead Impoundment, get out, and hike up the berm to take in an impressive view of the marsh. Once you're on the water, this perspective of the complex landscape shrinks, and it's easy to forget just how vast it is.

Back on the water, you'll begin seeing the official canoe-trail signs (denoted by an orange square on a green post), but take these with a grain of salt; they're not

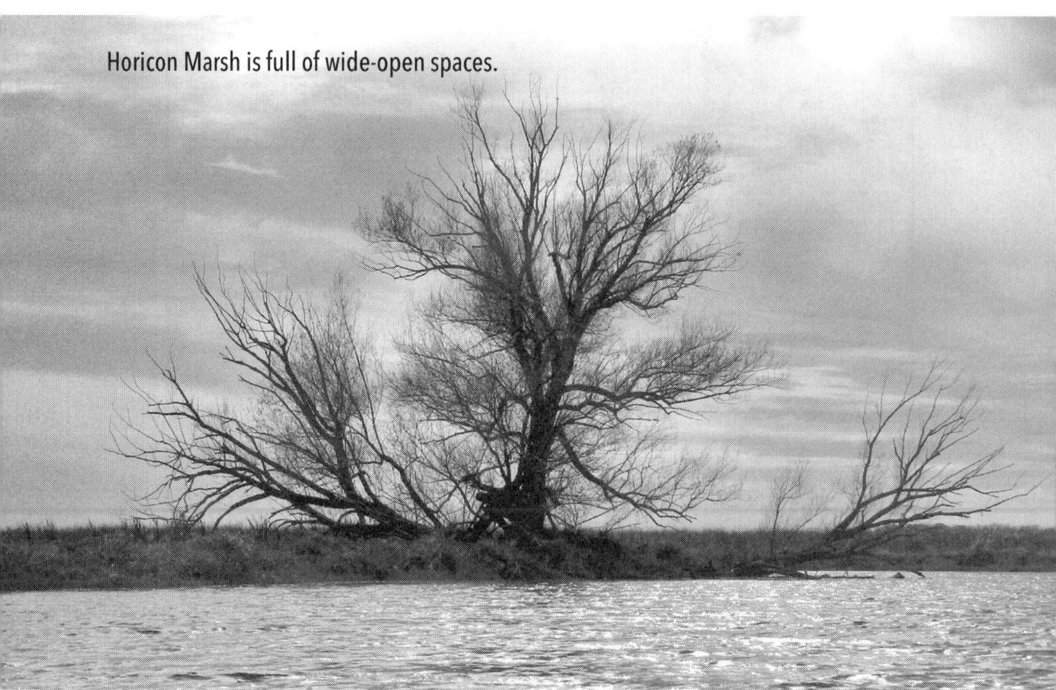

Horicon Marsh is full of wide-open spaces.

terribly instructive, for they seem to be posted only in obvious segments when you already know where you are, not when facing a dilemma of which channel to take. The river will bend here and there, but mostly in broad strokes.

Only half a mile or so from the put-in, you'll be facing east for a moment (a rarity on this trip) and will see the Niagara Escarpment, a huge layer of raised rock, locally known as "The Ledge," that arches from northwest of Chicago through Door County and Lakes Michigan and Huron into southern Ontario, and then eventually reaches out to form the rock formations (and plunge) at Niagara Falls. (You can camp in the county park connected with The Ledge.)

Soon, the turns will diminish and yield to long straightaways, but side channels appear. Together with innumerable ditches, these side channels provide for opportunities of welcome intimacy. This trip mainly goes west then due south, for the sake of simplicity. But there are several diversions north, far west, and even southeast, all off of the main channel. If and how many of these side channels you choose to explore is entirely up to your own curiosity and the time you have to be on the water. They're certainly fun and interesting, and your chances of rousting some hidden wildlife are quite good. If you do choose to veer off the main channel, I recommend having a map of the marsh with you. It's not likely that you'd get lost without one, but the sheer size of the marsh can be disorienting. Think of it like straying off the trail when hiking in the woods.

After you find yourself on the first long straightaway, begin looking to your left. Soon you'll see Fourmile Island, a protected state natural area and one of the largest heron rookeries in the Midwest. It's off-limits from April to September, so you may have to appreciate it through your binoculars. It's one of many islands in the complex of the marsh (with names like Apple, Cotton, Gardener, Strawberry, and Steamboat). After Fourmile, the main channel will bend to the right and then left before opening out to a wide expanse. Here, as elsewhere, there are many nooks and crannies by way of side channels and ditches you can explore. Otherwise, follow the main channel south. Off in the faraway distance you'll see the Horicon water tower and some grain elevators, a seeming mirage of buildings in the midst of this wildlife refuge.

Once you paddle through a narrow cattail corridor, the marsh will open out to its widest. If you wish to explore the eastern side of the marsh, you would want to turn left and paddle half a mile. Or if you wish to explore the northern backwaters, you'd make a 180 to your right. But if you prefer to take the most direct route, then continue paddling straight south, keeping closer to the western shore (on your right). After some wide water, you'll discern a narrow channel on your right that looks like a long, straight corridor into town. Here, it feels like you're on a river again, with banks on each side beneath attractive tree canopy. Off to your right will be Onemile Island, the last notable landmark in the marsh.

As you approach town, you'll paddle past a huge John Deere factory on the left, followed by an attractive bridge at Lake Street. The river will make a sharp bend to the left at a city park, after which you'll pass under the bridge at WI 33. Immediately after a right-hand bend, you'll come upon the concrete rubble of the boat launch and take-out at Legion Auxiliary Park, on the right.

•THE•FUDGE•

ADDITIONAL TRIPS If you want to add more river miles onto this trip, put in below the dam in the town of Kekoskee, off Valley Street, 4 miles upstream of Greenhead Road. It's a pleasant stretch of the Rock River's east branch, where there's actual current and even some woodsy segments before the huge sprawl of the marsh. Alternatively, there's a pleasant trip on the south branch of the Rock River (which, confusingly, is northwest of the marsh) through the small city of Waupun. It's a narrow and riffly stream amidst a mix of woods, backyards, and farmland. Put in at Waupun Park and take out at the wayside park off WI 49 for a 7-mile trip.

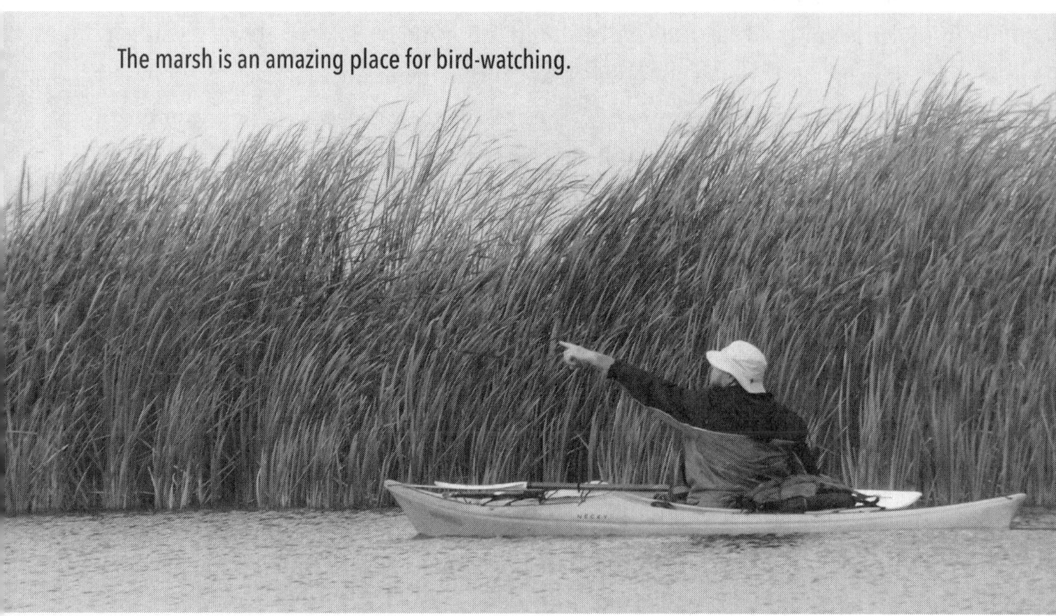
The marsh is an amazing place for bird-watching.

CAMPING Ledge Park (N7403 Park Road, Horicon; 920-386-3700)

RENTALS Horicon Marsh Boat Tours (305 Mill St., Horicon; 920-485-4663)

SHOUT-OUT The best way to fully appreciate the rich history and incredible vastness of the marsh is to spend at the very least an entire day here, and combine this paddling trip with a bike ride, hike, car tour, visitor-center tour, and/or camping overnight, including an exploration of the **Friends of Horicon Marsh Education and Visitor Center,** at N7725 WI 28 in Horicon. For more information, call 920-387-7890 or visit horiconmarsh.org.

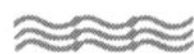

8 Maunesha River:
MARSHALL TO WATERLOO

•THE•FACTS•

Put-in/take-out Access road off Waterloo Road/Firemen's Park in Waterloo. See "The Flavor" for an alternative put-in.

Distance/time 8.2 mi/Allow for 4 hrs

Gradient/water level 6 fpm/There is no gage for the Maunesha. For the best run of the rapids, do this early in spring or after a hard rain. In downtown Waterloo, two bridges cross the river on Madison Street/WI 19; scout the water at the bridges, and if it is high enough here to paddle without scraping, you will be fine upstream, too.

Water type Riffles, several Class I–II ledges, and 1 mile of Class I rapids

Canoe or kayak Kayak

Skill level Experienced

Time of year to paddle Early spring, after a hard rain, or anytime there's enough water

Landscape Woods, farms, drumlin hills, marsh, urban downtown

OVERVIEW This fun and scenic trip offers considerable diversity in only 8 miles, including a scenic mill, a hometown amusement park, rustic railroad bridges, old oaks, drumlins, and several small but reputable rapids. It's well worth the occasional tree to dodge or portage, which you will definitely encounter. Expect to see deer, turtles, hawks, sandhill cranes, geese, clams, and fish.

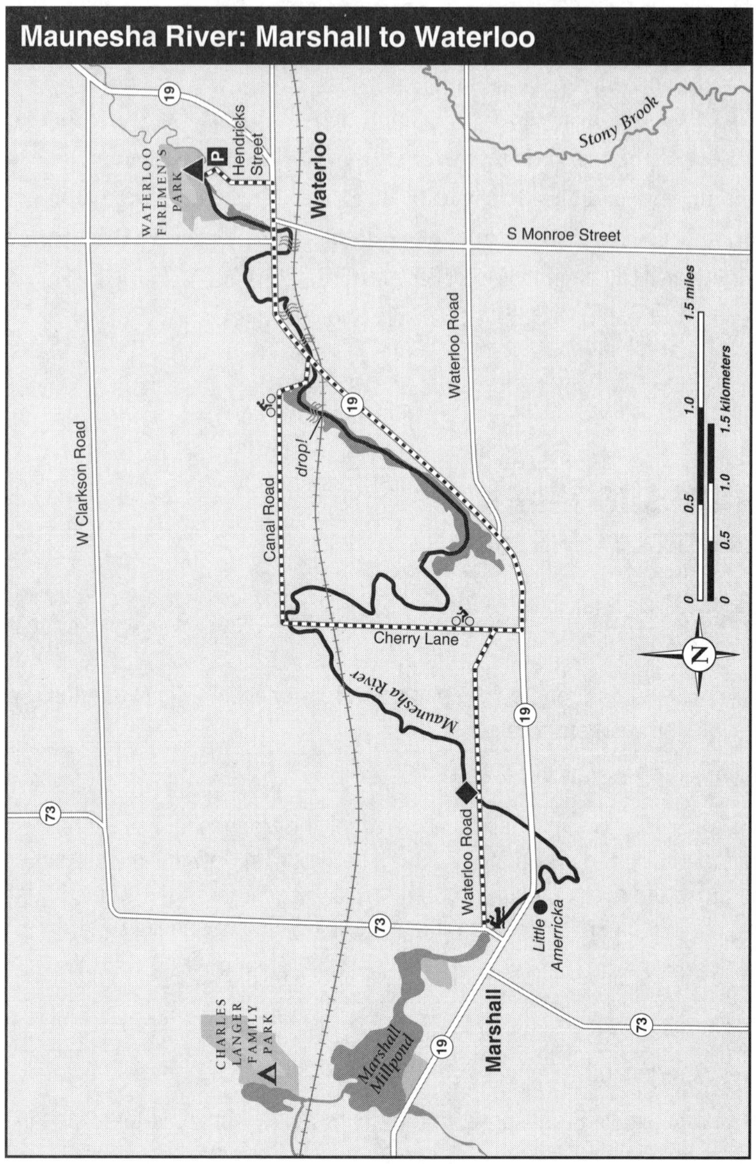

CAR SHUTTLE **4.2 miles.** From the take-out, head south on Hendricks Street, then turn right onto East Madison Street/WI 19. (Leaving downtown Waterloo, you'll cross the river four times on WI 19. Any of these bridges is a good place to scout the river for water level.) Stay on WI 19 until you enter Marshall. Turn right on Cherry Lane, then left on Waterloo Road. Cross the river once. Just before the stop sign at Hubbell Street and WI 73, turn left onto the dirt road or park on Waterloo Road.

BIKE SHUTTLE 5.5 miles. Follow the directions above, but turn right off of WI 19 onto Canal Road as you leave the town of Waterloo; then turn left onto Cherry Lane, then right onto Waterloo Road.

TAKE-OUT N43° 11.359' W88° 58.999' **PUT-IN** N43° 10.027' W89° 03.607'

•THE•FLAVOR•

PUT IN AT THE END OF AN INCONSPICUOUS ACCESS ROAD off of Waterloo Road near the bridge and dam. This will be on the north bank of the river, or river left, below the dam. The road here is muddy and rutty. If it's impassable, you'll have to schlep your boat and gear to the water (a very short walk) or put in at the other Waterloo Road bridge on the downstream side, river right, where a gravel area leads to the river (N43° 10.093′ W89° 02.803′).

The current here is swift as the water comes out of the dam. On the opposite bank is a scenic old mill. Only 200 feet downstream, a concrete ledge offers the first of several light rapids on this trip. Run the ledge toward the left side. The river is usually muddy and about 50 feet wide. Shortly downstream, you'll probably be treated to the sights and sounds of a quaint amusement park called Little Amerricka, depending on the time of year. A straightaway leads you to the first of six times you'll paddle under WI 19. After a few meanders, you'll see a small bridge on your right. If you follow this detour only 25 yards, you'll end up at an adorable tyke-sized railroad bridge that's part of the park above a fun spillway.

An occasional set of riffles will lead you to the next two bridges at WI 19 and Koch Drive, respectively. There will be obstructions to avoid here and there, but none that should require portaging. Just after the next bridge at Waterloo Road, you'll see a couple of huge old bur oak trees at water's edge on the left. These sentinels are particularly attractive in spring and late fall. As the river then bends to the left, a gentle drumlin appears on the right. For a moment, you'll paddle parallel to but then cross under a set of power lines.

After the power lines, the river will narrow, the gradient will increase, and the current will pick up some speed. A tall bank with pine trees lines the left as you approach the first railroad bridge, 20 feet tall on wooden piers. Be careful passing underneath. Below the bridge is a fallen tree with little clearance. You can relax for a moment as the current slackens and the landscape flattens out. You'll see a few farms on the left-hand side as the Maunesha heads north. Just after the modest bridge at the intersection of Canal Street and Cherry Lane, the Maunesha changes its directional mind and now heads south. Here, you will encounter some downed trees, most of which can usually be negotiated without your having to portage. A second railroad bridge soon appears, this one supported by attractive limestone foundations.

Following an abrupt left-hand bend, the river can be obstructed by deadfall where again the current will quicken. Depending on water levels, there may be some ledges. Portage if the conditions feel unsafe. Soon the left bank rises 40 feet high; the setting is woodsy and remote, almost wild-feeling. For a moment, the woods on the right will clear and you'll see an old red barn, but then the river will veer to the left and back into the woods. WI 19 will appear on your right and run parallel to the river for a short while. At this point, the landscape is all marsh. If water conditions allow and you're feeling adventurous, you can portage around a beaver's nest and explore the backwaters in between the mainstream and WI 19, a fun and unique diversion.

A relaxed current and a straightaway take you to the third and final railroad bridge. This one is the most prominent but also the most intimidating. Roughly 30 feet high and supported by a system of wooden piers, it affords only one open slot between piers to paddle through, followed by a 2- to 3-foot drop. Furthermore, old piers remain just below the drop on both left and right. You need to have solid boat control and line up for this just right. If in doubt, portage on the left or right.

After the bridge, the river passes a large malt factory on the right, signaling the beginning of Waterloo. One of the best rapids lies on the left side of the river, just

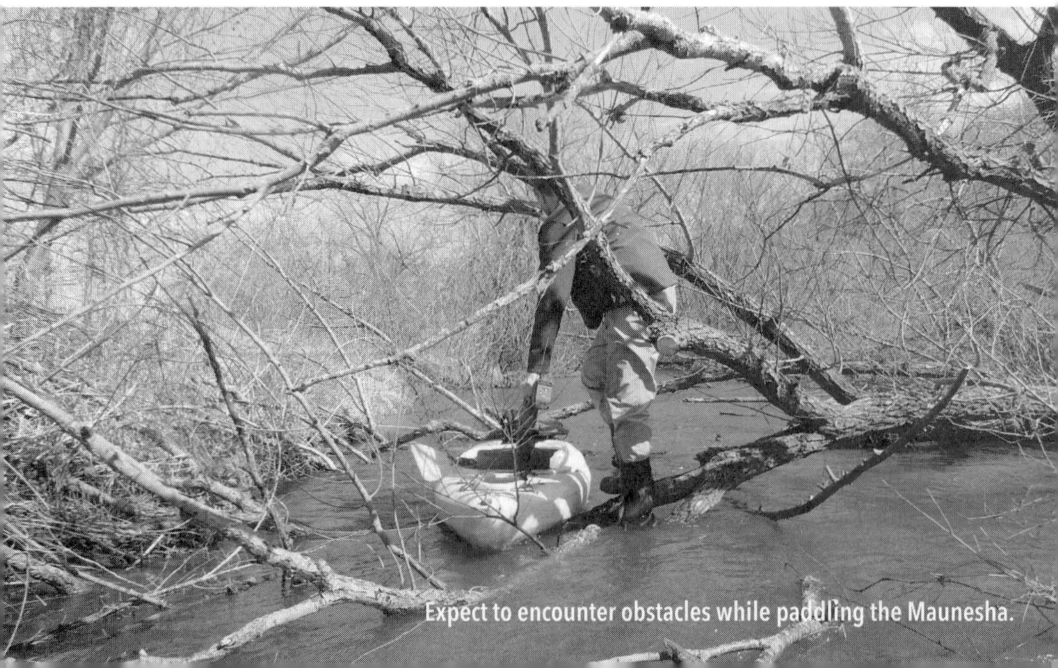
Expect to encounter obstacles while paddling the Maunesha.

after the factory. The river takes a sharp left and runs parallel to the train tracks before passing underneath WI 19 and another set of power lines. In a little more than 100 yards, another set of fun rapids appears, where an old dam had been removed.

What might be the most exhilarating part of this trip is saved for last as the gradient steepens near downtown Waterloo. You'll pass under WI 19 again, immediately followed by a pedestrian footbridge and then a second footbridge during a southward horseshoe bend. Another WI 19 bridge comes next, followed by another horseshoe bend, this one going north eventually. Positively delightful riffles, light Class I rapids, and even some humble standing waves await you in this downtown stretch.

On the way to yet one last bridge at WI 19, you'll see a few houses on the right; then, immediately below the bridge, are some handsome late-1800s brick buildings with rough-hewn facades lining the river. A stretch of easy riffles passes along backyards, one last footbridge, and then some parks. After a couple of baseball diamonds on the left and the wastewater-treatment facility on the right, you'll see a bridge shortly downstream. Look for the parking lot on the right-hand side and take out wherever is convenient and/or closest to your car or bike. (You don't want to go as far down as the bridge for this take-out, as there's no practical place on the banks of the river to do so, and the parking lot is on the upstream side of the bridge.)

•THE•FUDGE•

ADDITIONAL TRIPS If you're interested in exploring the Maunesha but you don't yet possess the experience for the rapids of the trip described above, consider instead the final leg of the Maunesha River, from Waterloo to the town of Portland, where it feeds the Crawfish River (see Crawfish River B, page 30). It's a pretty section, but deadfall is problematic. Protected public land is abundant, but it lacks the diversity and swift current of the trip as described above. Upstream, the river runs as straight as a channelized arrow through Deansville State Wildlife Area; to run it, you can put in at CR TT and paddle upstream and back down as far as conditions allow (there will be some maneuvering and portaging), as there is virtually no current. Additionally, see Appendix B (page 319) for a short but unique trip on the upper Maunesha . . . in the middle of US 151!

CAMPING **Charles Langer Family Park** (860 Canal Road, Marshall; 608-655-4017)

RENTALS Rutabaga Paddlesports (220 W. Broadway, Madison; 608-223-9300)

FOOD FOR THOUGHT For a great bite to eat in a cool restaurant, check out Soular Pizza Grill (1003 N. Monroe St., Waterloo; 920-478-4441).

SHOUT-OUT Little Amerricka amusement park (700 E. Main St., Marshall; 608-620-5224, littleamerricka.com) offers 26 rides and attractions and features "restored rides from classic amusement parks of a bygone era."

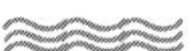

9 Mecan River: 11TH ROAD TO DIXIE AVENUE

•THE•FACTS•

Put-in/take-out 11th Road/Dixie Avenue. See "The Flavor" for an alternative take-out.

Distance/time 9.5 mi/Allow for 5 hrs

Gradient/water level 3 fpm/There is no gage, but levels are almost always sufficient since the river is spring-fed. However, it's worth a phone call to Mecan River Outfitters (920-295-3439) to ask for current conditions, because if the river is high, low-clearance bridges and fallen trees will require portaging and the current can be pushy, making for challenging moments at obstructions.

Water type Quietwater with riffles and light rapids

Canoe or kayak Kayak preferred

Skill level Experienced

Time of year to paddle Anytime, but exceptionally lovely in autumn

Landscape Upland forest, bogs, and grasslands

OVERVIEW A virtual mecca for paddlers in southern Wisconsin, the Mecan features crystal-clear water with a peppy current surrounded by vast tracts of sparsely developed land. Enhancing that allure is the river's narrow width and meandering path through soggy bogs, spongy fens, and small boulders in the streambed, flanked by gnarled oaks, birch, and pine trees atop the banks.

It's impossible to overestimate the enchantment of such an environment in contrast to development elsewhere in the southern part of the state. There are also

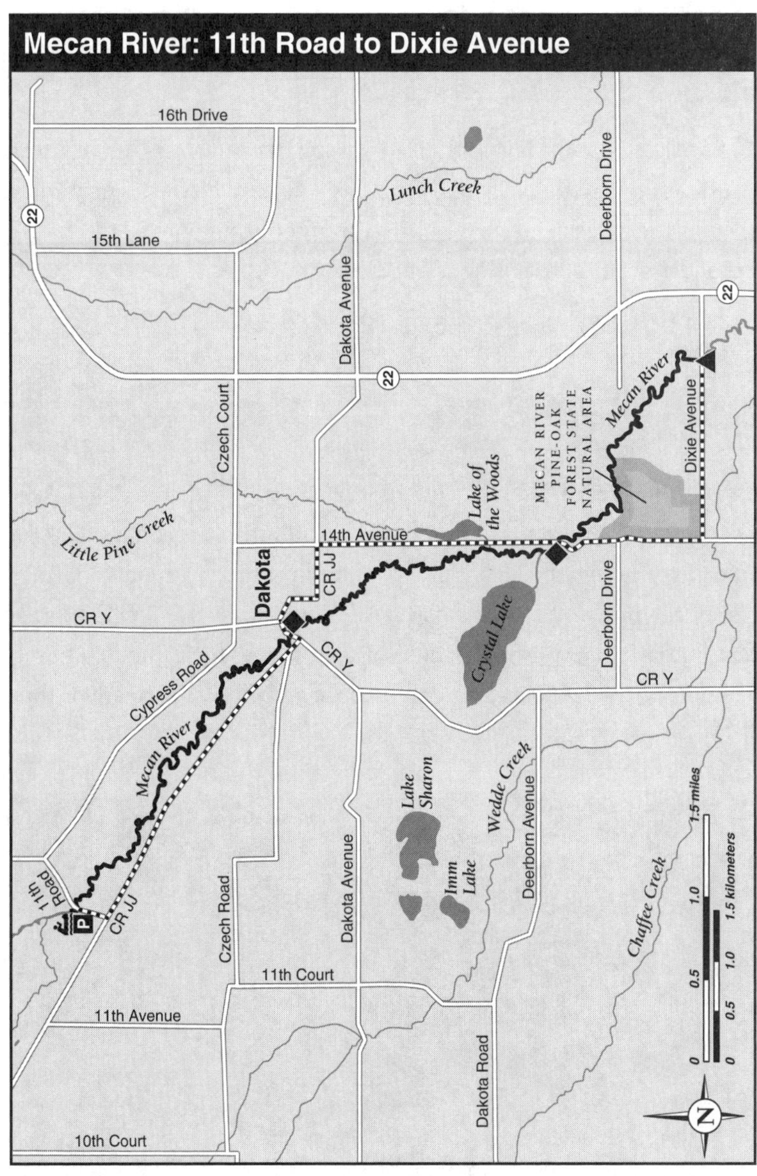

lots of kettles in the forest here, as well as trout, great blue herons, sandhill cranes, kingfishers, turtles, wood ducks, deer, beaver, wild turkey, and owls.

Planning Advisory While the Mecan River is a popular paddling area, don't underestimate the current, the need to maneuver around obstructions, or the meandering nature of the stream (I like to call it the "Mecander"). Make sure you pack a dry bag of extra clothes, food, and water, and that you are physically and mentally prepared for a long day on the river. It's a truly beautiful stream that I highly recommend; just plan accordingly.

SHUTTLE **6.5 miles.** From the take-out, head west on Dixie Avenue. Turn right onto 14th Avenue. Turn left onto CR JJ. Stay on CR JJ as you turn left at the next intersection, and then cross the bridge and turn right. Turn right again onto 11th Road. There's a parking area just north of the bridge.

TAKE-OUT N43° 57.120' W89° 19.560' **PUT-IN** N44° 00.420' W89° 23.520'

•THE•FLAVOR•

PUT IN ON THE UPSTREAM SIDE OF THE BRIDGE at 11th Road, river left. (You can park one or two vehicles here, but there's an additional area to accommodate more only 200 feet north.) The current here is swift as the river drops a foot, shooting into the left culvert of the bridge, so it is advised to paddle upstream 10 or 20 yards to get a better head start. The drop is fun! (Alternatively, if you don't mind paddling against the current some, the river environment is especially pretty upstream of the put-in.)

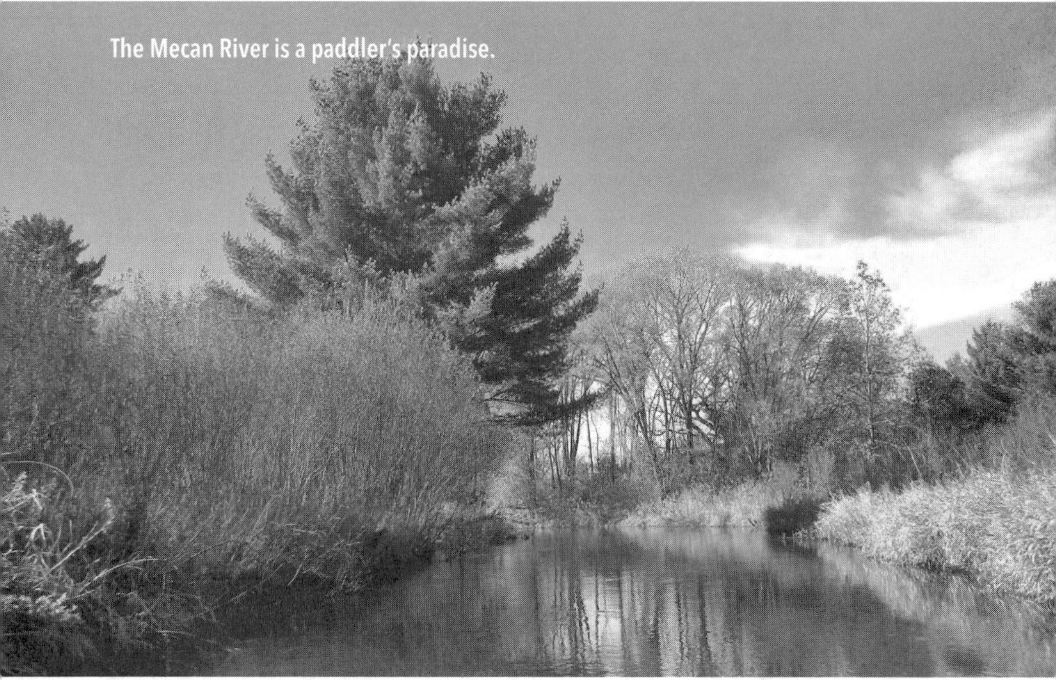

The Mecan River is a paddler's paradise.

Here and there, you'll come upon wooden pier remnants jutting just above the water line; some have improbably hosted enough grass to resemble a punk-rock hairdo. Complementing the natural feel of its surroundings, the river itself has a pleasant balance of obstructions to dodge, duck under, or ride over, but none so formidable as to require an actual portage. (That said, it behooves you, the paddler, to have the basic skills and boat control to experience this pleasant balance without getting frustrated—or wet!)

After a mile, you'll see a house or two (ranging from shabby cabins to country chic), but only briefly at the edges of bends. You'll pass under a rickety-looking wooden footbridge that belongs to one of them—the first of two in this stretch. The right bank rises some 15 feet, the current picks up, and the river zigzags around moss-strewn logs. The setting feels wild, even if you're never far from a road. Things will remain tranquil as the river meanders through secluded woods. An atypical straightaway precipitates the culvert at the CR Y bridge. As before, the current picks up as the river funnels through the culvert, and riffles prevail on the other side. Be careful not to get too close to the culvert walls to keep from tipping in the brisk current.

Many paddlers begin their trip on the Mecan at CR Y from the left, so don't be too surprised if you see someone at this point. (Indicative of this, you'll see more tree clearing and branch sawing here than upstream. Someone even thoughtfully cut out a notch for headspace on one large, bank-to-bank downed tree.) Downstream from CR Y, the river is very narrow along a corridor of rightward bends around a raised left bank. Soon you'll come upon a low-clearance farm bridge; if the river is high, it may be prudent to portage it. The river heads south in a low-lying area before heading east toward the 14th Avenue bridge (where the upstream side is notably lower than the downstream side). Paddlers can cut this trip to 7 miles by taking out on the downstream (right) side of this bridge (**N43° 57.889' W89 20.844'**).

After 14th Avenue, the river flows southeastward in one of the prettiest sections in the area. All along the river on the right lies the beautiful Mecan River Pine-Oak Forest, a Wisconsin natural area and the only known old-growth forest of white pines and black oaks in the Central Sand Hills Ecological Landscape. Some of these trees are as wide as 3 feet in diameter. The eye is beguiled by that which lies beyond as the stream nears, turns away, and then returns to the canopies of the right bank.

Eventually you'll see a stately log cabin atop a right bank, soon followed by another footbridge. Bends to the right and then left lead to a straightaway of some 500 feet before a final meander for good measure at the base of a 15-foot-tall right bank before the culvert bridge at Dixie Avenue. Take out here, on river right on the downstream side of the bridge. There's a parking area at the top of the small hill.

•THE•FUDGE•

ADDITIONAL TRIPS Upstream of the put-in, the river is quite beautiful, but poor accesses, shallow water, and deadfall should dissuade the casual paddler from exploring this section. However, there's an excellent boat launch at the headwaters of the Mecan at a spring-fed pond off Chicago Road, where most of the land is public and undeveloped. This is lake paddling, but the environs are pretty.

Downstream from this trip's take-out, the Mecan passes beneath several low-clearance farm bridges that are impassable when the water is high, and then the river slows to a crawl above the sprawl of Germania Marsh. Below the marsh lies a fun Class II drop at the CR N bridge. There's decent access on both sides of the bridge, allowing for play and multiple runs. Downstream from CR N to its confluence at the Fox River, the Mecan meanders 10.5 miles, but the landscape is a bit flatter and more monotonous, and obstructions can be quite a nuisance.

CAMPING AND RENTALS **Mecan River Outfitters & Lodge** (W720 WI 23, Princeton; 920-295-3439) offers log-cabin rentals and primitive tent sites along the river, as well as river-trip rentals.

FOOD FOR THOUGHT **Mecan River Outfitters & Lodge** serves food. Or, for a delicious vegetarian meal washed down with a local microbrew in a cute setting, stop by **MORE Healthy Foods and Cafe** (15 Main St., Montello; 608-297-8111), located at Marquette County's one and only stoplight. Also darling is **Once in a Blue Moon** (538 W. Water St., Princeton; 608-295-6100). In fact, there is much charm along Water Street in downtown Princeton.

SHOUT-OUT **Mecan River Outfitters & Lodge** is the kind of family-owned business that's almost too good to be true. They are good stewards of the land and lovers of the river, and they clear out the obstructions for the benefit of all. Whether you're renting, tenting, lodging, or dining, they're good folks to support.

The Mecan is simply radiant in autumn, bursting in yellows so crisp you'd think they were aspen cast against a blue sky or next to green pine. You'll have more solitude in autumn, too, especially on the second half of this trip.

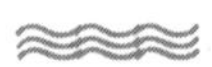

10 Montello River:
COUNTY ROAD J TO MONTELLO LAKE BOAT LANDING

•THE•FACTS•

Put-in/take-out County Road J/Lake Street public boat landing. See "The Flavor" for two intermediate access points.

Distance/time 11.7 mi/Allow for 5 hrs

Gradient/water level 2 fpm/There is no official gage, but levels are usually reliable. Call Rendezvous Paddle & Sports (608-297-2444) for current conditions.

Water type Quietwater and flatwater

Canoe or kayak Kayak only until 11th Road landing, then either to the take-out

Skill level Experienced

Time of year to paddle Anytime

Landscape Hardwood forest with tall sandy banks, lake paddling at the end

---

OVERVIEW This trip for the rugged adventurer offers a truly wild look and feel—the water is beautiful, clear, and surrounded by tall sandbanks, in a lush forest full of spectacular wildlife—and offers alternatives for access. Expect to see fish, deer, turtles, turkeys, turkey vultures, wood ducks, mergansers, ruffed grouses, woodpeckers, great blue herons, sandhill cranes, minks, and barred owls.

PADDLING ADVISORY The river has innumerable obstacles to paddle under, over, and around, plus a handful of inevitable portages, which is why this trip is appropriate only for experienced paddlers seeking a fun, out-of-the-way challenge on an intimate stream. If bending, ducking, twisting, contorting, plowing over, and occasionally portaging over downed trees in a meandering river are not your cup of tea, this trip isn't for you.

SHUTTLE **7.6 miles.** From the take-out, head west on Lake Street, then turn right onto CR B. Follow B all the way north to the intersection of CR J, and turn right onto CR J. Turn right again to stay on CR J. The put-in bridge is just after Water Street. *Note:* Because Lake Montello is large and the boat landing fairly inconspicuous, make a mental note or leave an impermanent marker before you head to the put-in so you don't paddle past the take-out.

TAKE-OUT N43° 48.165' W89° 20.689' **PUT-IN** N43° 52.555' W89° 24.304'

Montello River: County Road J to Montello Lake Boat Landing

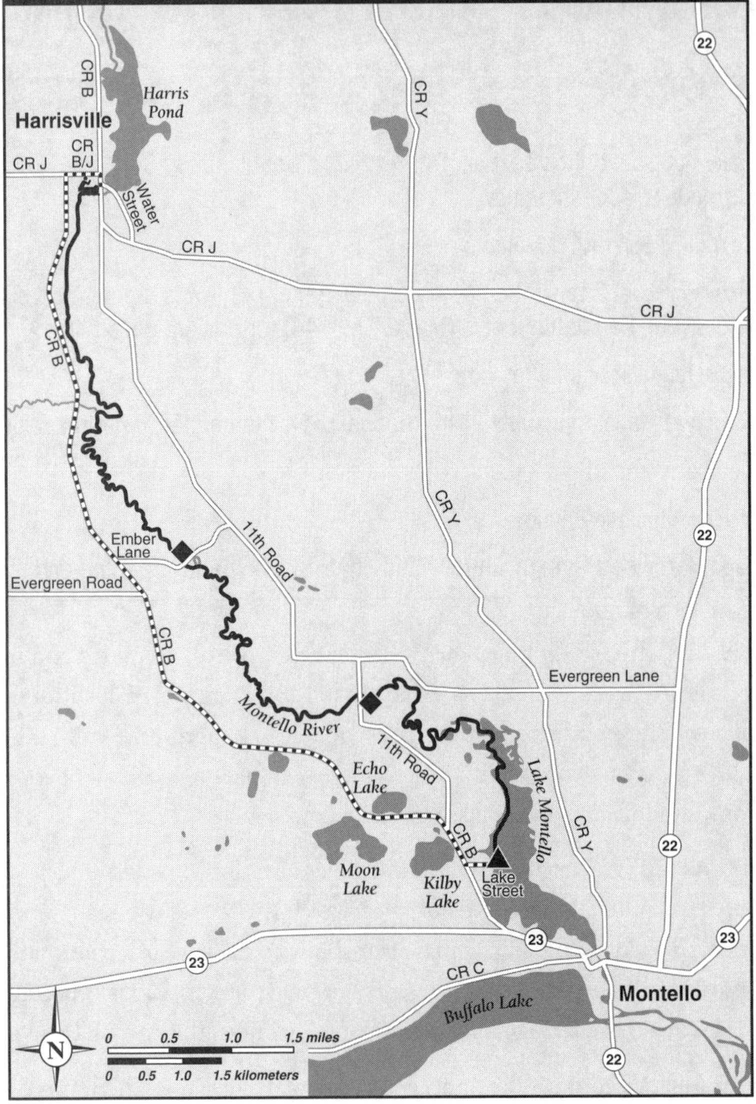

•THE•FLAVOR•

THE MONTELLO RIVER TRIP CAN BE BROKEN DOWN INTO FOUR SEGMENTS: (1) from the put-in to Ember Lane, where there are some houses early on, many tall sandbanks, and obstacles that don't require portage; (2) from Ember Lane to 11th Road, where the river is at its most isolated, but obstacles are at their worst and you'll have to portage; (3) from 11th Road to Lake Montello, where houses are sporadic and you'll pass a large and loud family campground, but the banks continue to rise again in gorgeous sweeps and the obstacles are the easiest to negotiate; and (4) from the lake inlet to the take-out, where the water becomes shallow and mucky (but it's only about half a mile). You can paddle all four segments or shorten the trip by using the take-out access points at the end of the second or third segments.

Put in at CR J on the downstream side of the bridge on river left. *Note:* This is a rugged access point with a steep slope leading down to the river. On the upstream side of the river is a spooky three-story building with just the right combination of grimy facade, broken windows, and detached wiring to make for a perfect horror-movie set. Also on the upstream side of the bridge is a raucous Class II+ rapid that can be run by climbing up the right bank.

Downstream from the put-in, the current from the rapid remains strong for 100 yards. If the water is low, you will likely need to portage around a partially submerged log; in average levels, you can ride over it easily enough. The river does reward the efforts it demands with clear water over a soft sand bottom, good current, lush forest surroundings, super-saturated green ferns, tall sand-and-clay banks, coniferous trees, outstanding wildlife opportunities, and almost certain solitude until the last few miles. The landscape could be easily mistaken for a national forest up north.

The only straightaways on the river are in the beginning, just after the put-in. At one, you'll pass under an iron-truss footbridge that looks absurdly disproportionate since it connects the backyard of a residential house to the left bank. (Farther downstream, you'll come upon another random truss bridge, this one partially submerged and slowly being swallowed by the river itself.)

The woods enclose you soon after that, and you won't see signs of human life again for a few miles—and then only briefly. A forest envelops the river and banks, lending to a welcome simplicity and isolation. If you're quiet and vigilant, the odds are pretty good you'll spot a barred owl or two. In spring, expect to see merganser mothers huddling their ducklings. And you'll lose count of how many deer you notice, whether leaping or lying on the grass in the shade. The banks will rise and fall, at times as high as 20 feet. Or sloughs going rogue will trickle off into the woods, never to be heard from again.

After Klawitter Creek enters from the right, the Montello River will begin meandering like it's the last thing it has left to do in this world. Obstructions typically follow, most if not all of which can be successfully resolved without portaging but with some creativity and curiosity. It behooves the paddler to be flexible in every sense of the word. Preceded by a tire swing and small cabin lined by attractive riprap, you'll pass a tall, sandy bank on the right just upstream from the Ember Lane bridge. There's rugged but adequate access on the upstream side, river left (**N43° 50.119' W89° 23.466'**).

One of the coolest visual effects on this trip is the number of submerged logs. Since the water is clear, they're all visible—like seeing an X-ray of an otherwise muddy river. And since the bottom is all sand, the river's depth varies, lending this trip additional exoticism. While you'll see a few more houses in this stretch (though not until you're close to the second bridge), the sand and clay banks are at their tallest and most beautiful here, many lined with pine trees. On the downstream side of the 11th Road bridge, there is an easy access on the right, made by much foot trampling from the nearby campground (**N43° 49.269' W89° 21.918'**). You'll hear before you see the queues of RVs. (The owners of Crooked River Campground do help maintain this segment of the Montello and deserve thanks for their efforts.) But only after half a mile from the bridge, the river feels wild and isolated again. Briefly.

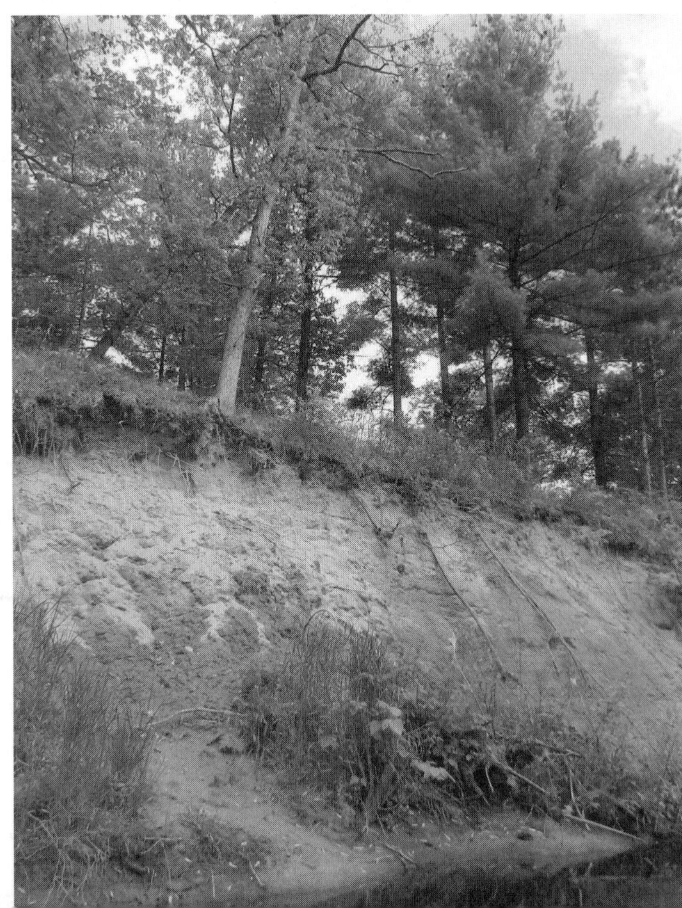

Tall sandbanks along the Montello

The river begins to widen and deepen, and the current slows to a crawl. Before houses dot the right shore in earnest, the river courses through a pretty terrain of tamaracks followed by telling cattail wetlands. Soon the river will yield to the lake, and finding the deepest channel at the inlet is not always obvious. The northeastern section of the lake is undisturbed. Alas, the boat launch is on the western shore, past a small peninsula. Look for the pier, your marker, or just your car.

•THE•FUDGE•

ADDITIONAL TRIPS Paddling upstream provides few inspiring options, most of which fall outside of the jurisprudence of this book. First, there's **Harris Pond,** which is a huge expanse of flatwater. Feeding the pond from the north are two streams, **Tagatz Creek** and **Westfield Creek** (also called Lawrence Creek), which combine magically to become the Montello River below the dam that creates Harris Pond.

Downstream from the lake, there's little left of the Montello River before it feeds the Fox River. Most of this is lake paddling, and accesses are next to nonexistent.

CAMPING AND RENTALS **Rendezvous Paddle & Sports** (201 Main St., Montello; 608-297-2444)

FOOD FOR THOUGHT For a delicious vegetarian meal washed down with a local microbrew in a cute setting, stop by **MORE Healthy Foods and Cafe,** at 15 Main St. in Montello (608-297-8111). **Rendezvous Paddle & Sports** also serves tasty home-cooked food.

SHOUT-OUT Take a moment in downtown Montello to stop by the quarry at **Daggett Park,** located at Marquette County's one and only stoplight intersection (WI 22 and WI 23). The granite excavated from the 150-foot-deep quarry was used for President Ulysses S. Grant's tomb—after 280 other samples from the world were rejected as inadequate. Four artificial waterfalls flow down the mineral-streaked rocks—a particularly pretty sight when lit up at night. Alas, several NO TRESPASSING signs are posted along the property, lest the paddler get a wild hair to paddle round the rocks.

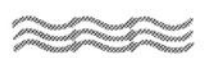

11 Oconomowoc River: LOEW LAKE

•THE•FACTS•

Put-in/take-out County Road Q

Distance/time 6–8 mi round-trip/Allow for 3 hrs

Gradient/water level Virtually no gradient/Water levels should always be reliable.

Water type Flatwater

Canoe or kayak Either

Skill level Beginner

Time of year to paddle Anytime, but exceptionally pretty in autumn

Landscape Cattail marsh, aquatic plants, sedge meadow, glacial hills, kettle lake

---

OVERVIEW Here is a there-and-back easy trip on a clear glacial river that winds through a beautiful valley of upland ridges and sedge meadows toward a hidden kettle lake in a nearly wild, undeveloped setting. Along the way, expect to see frogs, turtles, turkey vultures, great blue herons, redwing blackbirds, hawks, muskrats, mallards, geese, deer, and maybe even coyotes.

SHUTTLE N/A **PUT-IN/TAKE-OUT** N43° 11.591' W88° 20.281'

•THE•FLAVOR•

PUT IN AT THE SMALL BOAT LAUNCH at CR Q, at the northwest corner of the bridge. Aquatic plants like inverted columns of soft tulle and gossamer, green and glimmering, cast against the clear water, will surely catch your eye first. The river here is 60 feet wide, representative of this trip. You will be paddling upstream, technically speaking, but there is virtually no current, which is one of the two reasons why this there-and-back trip is popular; the other is its lovely landscape and lack of development. Cattails abound along both banks as you begin your way north, here and there punctuated with muskrat huts.

After a right-hand turn, a stand of attractive oak trees greets you on the left, while off to the right you'll see tamaracks marking a swamp. Soon you'll come upon a low-clearance footbridge, which can be portaged around on the right. The river will

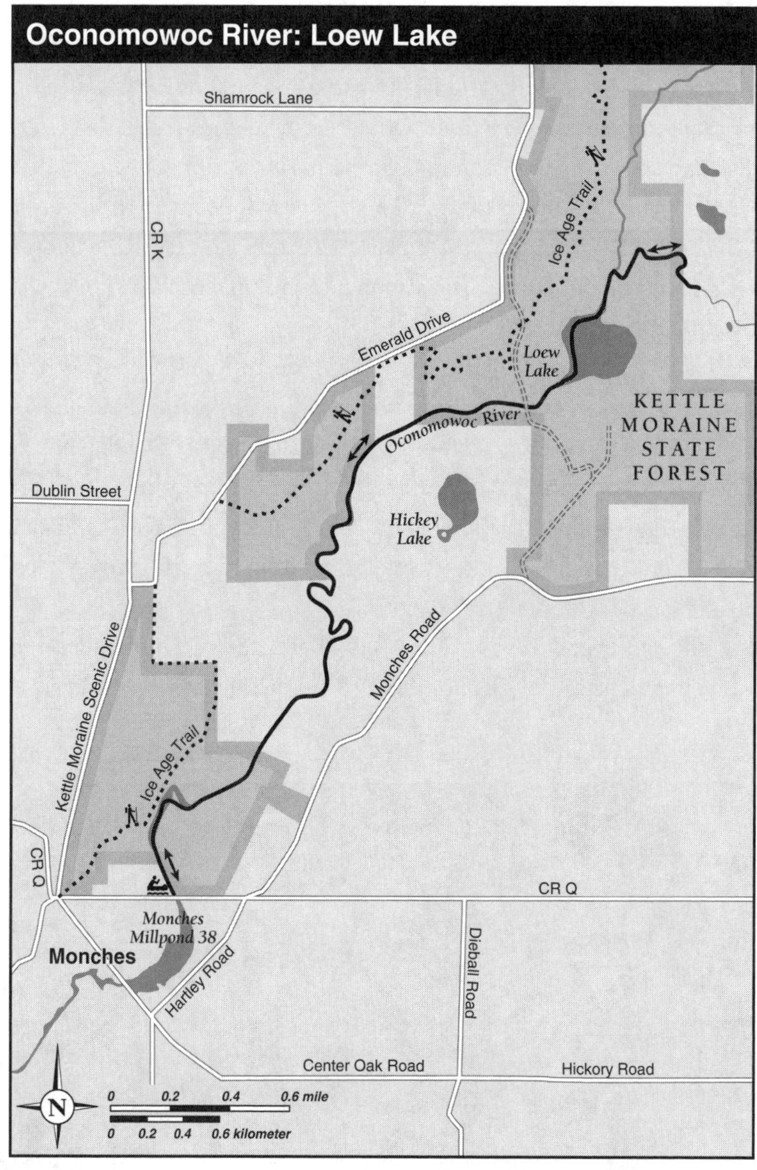

meander after this as the setting becomes increasingly isolated and pretty. A large hill comes into focus then disappears after a bend, only to return in sharper relief. (In glacial terminology, this is called a *kame*.) As the monstrously humongous sheets of ice began to melt, spectacular torrents of water flushed silt and sand, gravel and boulders, through paths of least resistance and deposited these materials—called *drift*—into rounded mounds not unlike sand through an hourglass. (Incidentally, this is why the area of Wisconsin unscathed by glaciers is called Driftless.) Surrounded by a lowland swamp girded still by cattails, the kame is even more pronounced.

A pleasant straightaway resumes with a teasing glimpse of an attractive pedestrian bridge and another kame looming behind it. As you come nearer, you'll see tall stands of pine to the right of a ruddy bridge, a popping contrast to the green trees and blue sky. The bridge is part of the Ice Age National Scenic Trail (see "The Fudge"); Loew Lake is a popular segment. The bridge also marks the entrance into Loew Lake itself, which is a slow, no-wake zone.

Loew Lake is as many acres large as it is feet deep: about 23. Long glacial ridges elegantly frame the west and north periphery, while the east is characterized more by woodsy pines and white birch. Reaching the lake itself is 3 miles one way, and paddling around it adds another 0.5 mile. If you wish to continue farther, you can paddle into the inlet on the north side of the lake (think of the lake as a clock face; the inlet is in between 11 and 12). A pretty knoll rises from the left bank with lush grass, abundant skunk cabbage, and attractive oaks.

At a right-hand bend, the stream seems to bifurcate: To the left is a creek with no name, to the right is the Oconomowoc River; either can be paddled as far as

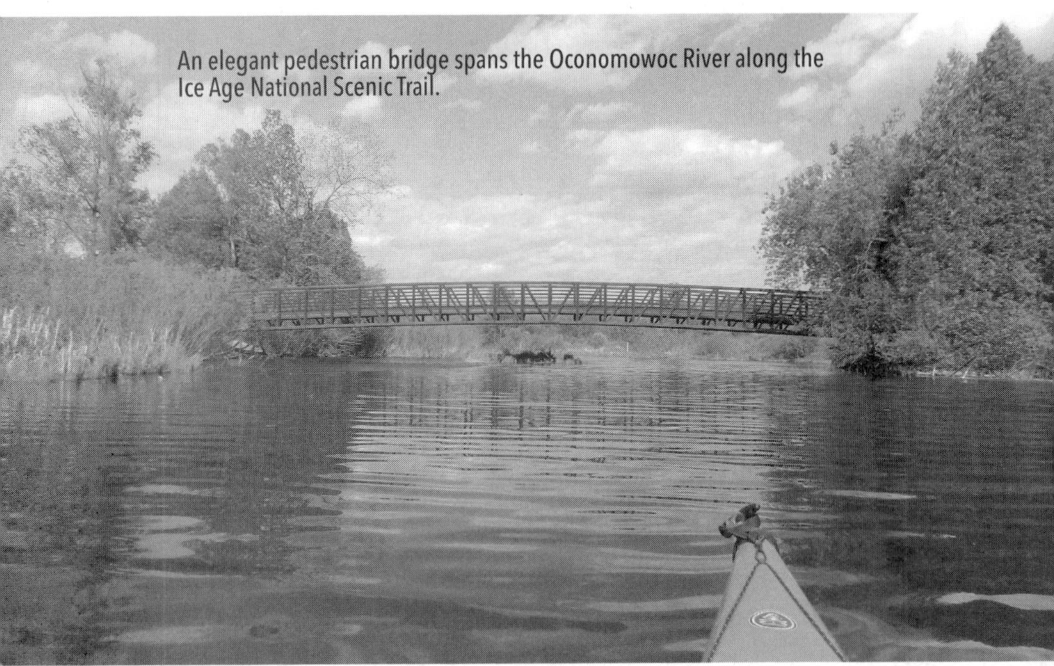

An elegant pedestrian bridge spans the Oconomowoc River along the Ice Age National Scenic Trail.

conditions allow, each about 1.3 miles forth and back. No-name creek is pleasant in an exploratory way, but doesn't show you anything you haven't seen already (or will see again on the return trip back to the boat launch).

Following the Oconomowoc River upstream, however, is gorgeous. The stream becomes shallow and rocky, the water clearer, and banks piney and boulder-lined—quintessential Kettle Moraine country. After a couple bends right and left, the river-bed will probably become too shallow and riffly to continue, unless the water is high. (The river does continue upstream for several more miles, but houses become prevalent and the current increases.) Rest here a moment, surrounded by the strewn rubble from a glacial lobe, and reflect that a sheet of ice a mile high left all of this around the time that nomads began gardening in the Tigris–Euphrates and woolly mammoths lumbered around the suburbs of Milwaukee.

Turn back around and experience the water trail anew now looking south. You'll see features you missed on the way up: a heron hidden in a glade, upended tree roots like giant elk antlers, maybe even the shadow of a mastodon cast by a setting sun on the dome of a kame.

•THE•FUDGE•

ADDITIONAL TRIPS Upstream of Loew Lake, the Oconomowoc River is too shallow to paddle most of the time, and accesses are scarce to nonexistent. Below CR Q, the river is drastically narrow, resembling more a babbling brook, before it begins to thread a concatenation of 17 lakes in the Oconomowoc area. However, putting in at South Concord Road below Lac La Belle and taking out above the fish barrier at North Side Drive makes for a very pleasant 12.5-mile trip (or even 16 miles, if continuing past the barrier into the Rock River to Pipersville).

CAMPING **Kettle Moraine State Forest-Pike Lake Unit** (3544 Kettle Moraine Road, Hartford; 262-670-3400)

RENTALS **Reef Point Resort** (3416 Lake Drive, Hartford; 262-673-9952)

FOOD FOR THOUGHT For a beer and sandwich in a beautiful indoors setting, head just north of Loew Lake to the **New Fox & Hounds Restaurant and Tavern** on Friess Lake Road (262-628-1111). Try it for lunch, as dinner gets pricey.

SHOUT-OUTS The **Ice Age National Scenic Trail** is the only national trail situated entirely within one state. With its western terminus at the St. Croix River, northeast of the Twin Cities, the trail follows the periphery of the last glacial advance some 13,000 years ago. The trail was the brainchild of a Milwaukee lawyer and avid outdoorsman named Raymond Zillmer, whose simple but subversive idea was to have a linear national park here in the state that would trace the effects of the last ice age close to people's backyards so that they could have a nearby sanctuary.

It took a lot of grit to fight for this idea and to coordinate private-land owners with conservationists; local, state, and federal politicians; and thousands of volunteers, particularly in the 1950s. Today, 60% of Wisconsin residents live within 20 miles of the Ice Age Trail. Millions do come to Wisconsin to use the trail, as nowhere else in North America did the glaciers bequeath such treasures in abundance; it's not for nothing that the last ice age is called the Wisconsinian.

You may not see it while on the water when the leaves are out, but at the put-in itself, off to the north 3.5 miles as the crow (or archangel) flies, you'll see a majestic cathedral ethereally shimmering up in the clouds: the **Basilica of the National Shrine of Mary, Help of Christians at Holy Hill** (or simply "Holy Hill"). It is a stunning sight in the quiet countryside of Washington County, standing nearly 300 feet above its base and 824 feet above the level of Lake Michigan.

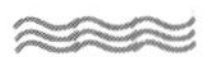

12 Puchyan River: GREEN LAKE DAM TO COUNTY ROAD J

•THE•FACTS•

Put-in Friday Club Park at Mill Street or along Water Street. See "The Flavor" for additional access points, including a mandatory portage.

Take-out County Road J

Distance/time 7.6 mi/Allow for 3 hrs

Gradient/water level 2.5 fpm/Look for 30–50 cfs on USGS gage 04073466 for nearby Silver Creek. A good visual gage is the modest rock garden at the take-out—if it looks low there, wait for some rain to do this trip. If only the peaks of the rocks show and the current is riffly, you'll have a wonderful time on this trip.

Water type Small Class I ledges, a short Class I–II rapids run, and quietwater

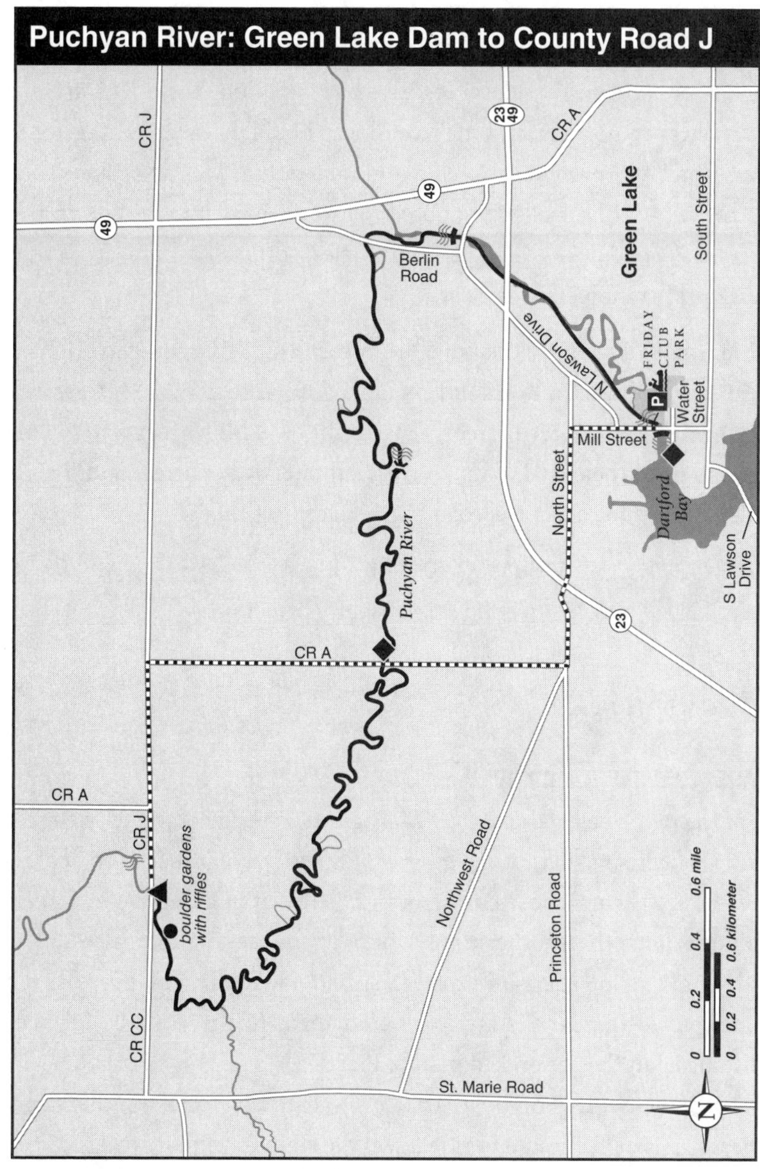

Canoe or kayak Kayak

Skill level Experienced

Time of year to paddle Anytime

Landscape Residential followed by pastures, cattail marsh, oak savanna, prairie, hardwoods with gentle hills, and boulder gardens

OVERVIEW An eclectic trip of contrasts—town and countryside, industrial and pastoral, rocky bottom with riffly rapids and sandy bottom with a slow meander—the "Puck" is a sweet stream that deserves better recognition. The only catches are that there is a spillway to portage, and the river doesn't hold its water volume for too long. There are several alternatives for put-in and take-out, as well as options to seek out some advanced paddling challenges, noted following. Expect to see great blue herons, sandhill cranes, wood ducks, fish, painted turtles, softshell turtles, snapping turtles, frogs, muskrats, sandpipers, and deer.

SHUTTLE 3.5 miles. From the take-out, head east on CR J, then turn right onto CR A. Turn left onto Princeton Road and stay straight past the WI 23 intersection (after which CR A will become North Street). Turn right onto Mill Street into town. Park on the street and put in below the dam, or turn left onto Water Street and then left onto Lake Street to the end of a gravel road to the river.

TAKE-OUT N43° 52.390' W88° 59.540' **PUT-INS** N43° 50.803' W88° 57.585' (Mill Street), N43° 50.775' W88° 57.638' (Water Street)

•THE•FLAVOR•

THERE ARE TWO PUT-IN OPTIONS in Green Lake (the town). The easier and more practical of the two is below the dam at Mill Street. The body of water on the other side of the dam is only a small bay of the otherwise huge Green Lake (the body of water).

The alternative and more daring option is to put in along Water Street, immediately plunge down the southernmost chute of the lake's 2-foot-high outlet, ride a fast rapid beneath a low-clearance tunnel, splash down a smaller drop, turn right on a dime, and proceed under the attractive bridge at Mill Street. This ride is only 340 feet in distance, but the action is nonstop. Practically speaking, this can be done only by skilled paddlers with good boat control. Realistically speaking, this can be done only if the water is high enough to ride down the chute—yet not so high as to prevent passing through the tunnel. Scout first and be smart.

Either way, below the dam, the river here is more like a creek at only 30 feet wide. It will expand along the way, especially toward the take-out, where it is 90 feet wide, but generally it's about 45 feet wide. Except for random deep pools, the river tends to run on the shallow side. You'll first paddle past tennis courts on the right and then an outlet from the lake on the left. The current here is quick, and the water clarity is excellent.

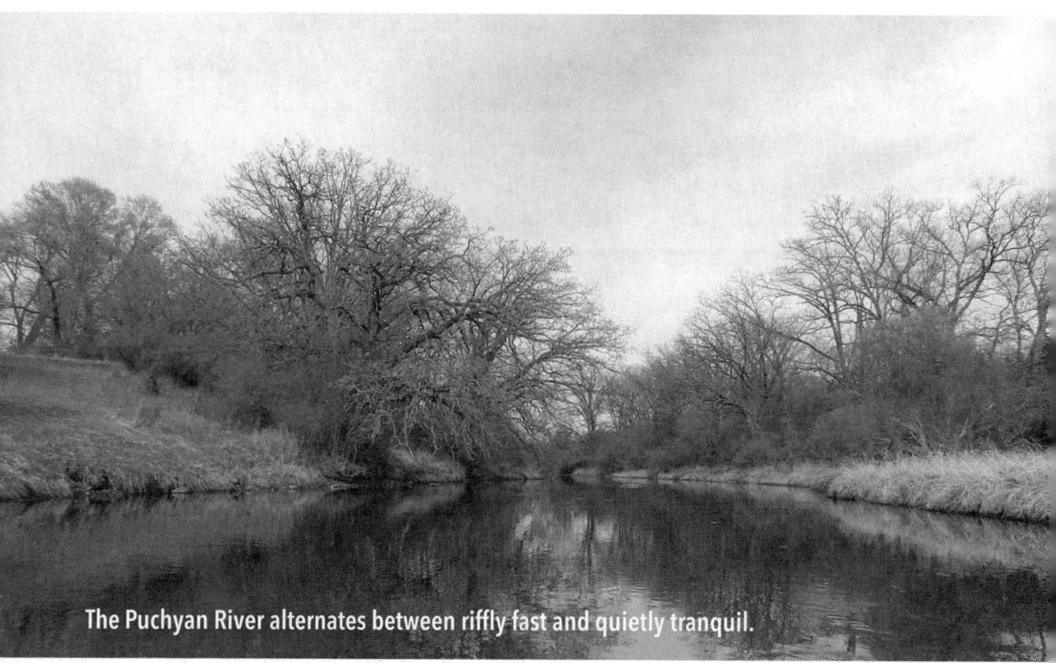
The Puchyan River alternates between riffly fast and quietly tranquil.

The small park here is called Friday Club, so named because a women's club met here in the early 1900s, on Fridays, and assumed custodial responsibility of the park. The river follows the path of a millrace, not its natural meandering course that today lies off to the right. Back in 1850, the millrace was dug to power a four-story gristmill a mile downstream. Today, you'll simply see a few houses on the left as you paddle through the straight, still water. It's a quaint little vignette.

Soon the banks on both sides rise to what feels like a modest gorge, where on your right you'll see the backwaters of where the original stream entered. You'll see and hear the tall spanning bridge of WI 23, but still the scenery is quite lovely due to the tall scale. An island will split the main channel in two.

Below the highway bridge, the river will sprawl and crawl into a millpond; fortunately, it's only 1,000 feet long. The next bridge is at North Lawson Drive. You will want to take out here on the upstream side of the bridge, river left. Why? Because 50 feet below the bridge is a dangerous spillway where the gristmill once stood (today an excavation site). Both sides of the river leading to the spillway are lined with tall concrete walls, so you need to exit and portage beforehand.

(Strictly speaking, one could run the spillway itself, but only true whitewater paddlers would even entertain this notion. Bowling ball–sized boulders lie just below the spillway, making for a bumpy landing after a scraping ride. One then would have to pivot immediately to the right into the middle of the river to attempt a run through a very "bony" boulder garden. It's doable, but you'd really need to know what you're doing to avoid damaging your boat and/or injuring yourself.)

Portage the spillway by following the well-marked makeshift trail on river left through a woodsy corridor. *Where you reenter is up to you.* The river will remain rock-lined and riffly for another couple hundred yards. It's intimate and fun, complete with a picturesque footbridge enhancing its rugged feel; but if the water is too shallow, this will be frustrating to the point of unrunnable. It's wise to scout this before running, as the current is fast, and fallen trees could be problematic. The river will bend to the left briefly and continue straight north again as the current slows down. It will bend to the left at Berlin Road, where there's a fun riffly drop below the bridge.

Below Berlin Road, the Puck will begin to revert to its natural state: a wet prairie meadowlands with a slight rugged feel. With only a few brief exceptions, where the river sweeps along a sloping hill lined with pine trees, you will be out in the sun-basked lowlands until the final 0.5 mile. But what makes *this* section of the Puchyan River so lovely and distinctly different from a monotonous marsh are the many trees just beyond the banks of tall grass and cattails, in conjunction with the soft hills in the background. Clear water and the lush sandy bottom are easy on the eyes as well.

At a bend to the left, you'll pass by what may have been a primitive dam where there are dike-like rows of boulders jutting into the water from both banks. Beyond this is a hermitage of a cabin in a nook of woods. The river will meander to and fro small wooded areas for the next mile. Around a horseshoe bend, you'll hear the sound of rushing water before seeing its cause: a small ledge beneath a low-clearance footbridge. If the water is too high, you must portage around this. If not, it's a fun drop, and beneath it, there's a playful surfing spot, too. The river will lazily loop here and there around small sandbars, where you will almost certainly see sandhill cranes and sandpipers.

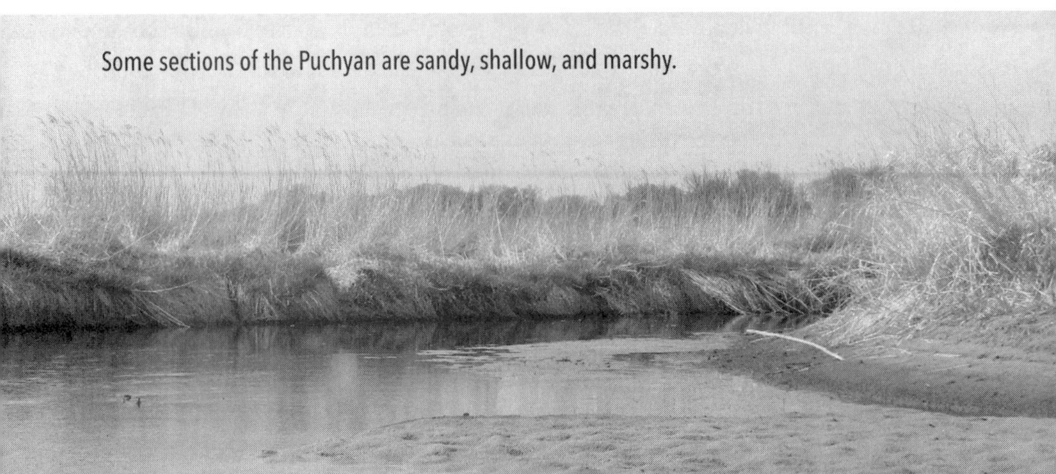

Some sections of the Puchyan are sandy, shallow, and marshy.

The next bridge is at CR A. Just below the bridge is a fallen tree, but there should be an open passage at the far right (**N43° 51.654' W88° 58.591'**); if you have only a small window of time to paddle, you can put in or take out here to break this trip in half. The next few miles are pretty and pleasant as the river saunters this way and that. There will be oxbows galore, but if you follow the current, keeping on the main stream will be a cinch. A long hill will gradually come into view on the right. The landscape remains meadowy and mostly undeveloped; soon thick stands of old gnarled oak trees appear.

You will paddle closer to a pleasant wooded area as the river heads north and then, essentially for the first time, east. Snake Creek will enter on the left, but it's hardly distinguishable from the many oxbows and sloughs upstream. As you round the woods clockwise, the left bank will rise with a backwards lean. Boulders emerge as the current quickens. *This last 0.5 mile will be not be runnable if the water is low.*

Both banks now are roughly 30 feet high. Fun riffles lead up to and lie below the bridge at CR J. Take out on the downstream side on river right.

•THE•FUDGE•

ADDITIONAL TRIPS I don't recommend the last segment of the Puchyan River, from CR J to its confluence at the Fox River between Princeton and Berlin. It's just a flat, slow, monotonous marsh with a handful of frustrating logjams to portage.

Alternatively, some paddlers tool around **Spring Creek,** off of CR A at Sunset Park, south of downtown Green Lake. There are protected wetlands and nature preserves in a large bay surrounded by a couple hills. Development on the shore is limited; most of the bay is pristine and protected. The creek eventually makes its way to nearby Ripon to the east, but it's much too small and shallow to paddle after a point.

CAMPING **Hattie Sherwood Campground** on Green Lake (451 S. Lawson Drive; 920-294-3344)

FOOD FOR THOUGHT Green Lake is a cute town with a number of shops and restaurants to consider if you're hungry or thirsty.

13 Rock River: HARNISCHFEGER PARK TO KANOW PARK

•THE•FACTS•

Put-in/take-out Harnischfeger Park on Crawfish Road/Kanow Park off Rock River Road

Distance/time 10.3 mi/Allow for 4 hrs

Gradient/water level Less than 1 fpm/See USGS gage 05425500, but there should always be enough water.

Water type Quietwater

Canoe or kayak Either

Skill level Beginner

Time of year to paddle Anytime

Landscape Floodplains surrounded by an agricultural valley

OVERVIEW This section of the Rock River is perfect for beginners and offers a pleasant, tranquil trip through a mostly undeveloped landscape of floodplain forests and an occasional quaint farm. There are outstanding facilities at the put-in and take-out, as well as spectacular wildlife opportunities all along the way: songbirds including orioles and goldfinches, sandhill cranes, great blue herons, a yellow-crowned night heron, turtles, hawks, frisky fish, muskrats, wood ducks, woodpeckers, deer, grouse, and cormorants.

SHUTTLE **6.7 miles.** From the take-out, turn right onto Rock River Road and then bear right onto River Valley Road. (*Note:* Rock River is a particularly pretty and rusticated road, but 1 mile of it is unpaved gravel.) Turn right onto Gopher Hill Road and follow up the hill. Turn right onto CR CW, then take your first left after the bridge onto North River Road. Bear left onto Highview Road at the Evergreen Road intersection. Turn right onto Crawfish Road into Harnischfeger Park.

TAKE-OUT N43° 08.546' W88° 33.931' **PUT-IN** N43° 12.614' W88° 32.561'

•THE•FLAVOR•

PUT IN AT THE CONVENIENT BOAT LAUNCH at Harnischfeger Park, where there are full facilities. Take a moment to peruse the helpful kiosk regarding all things Rock River.

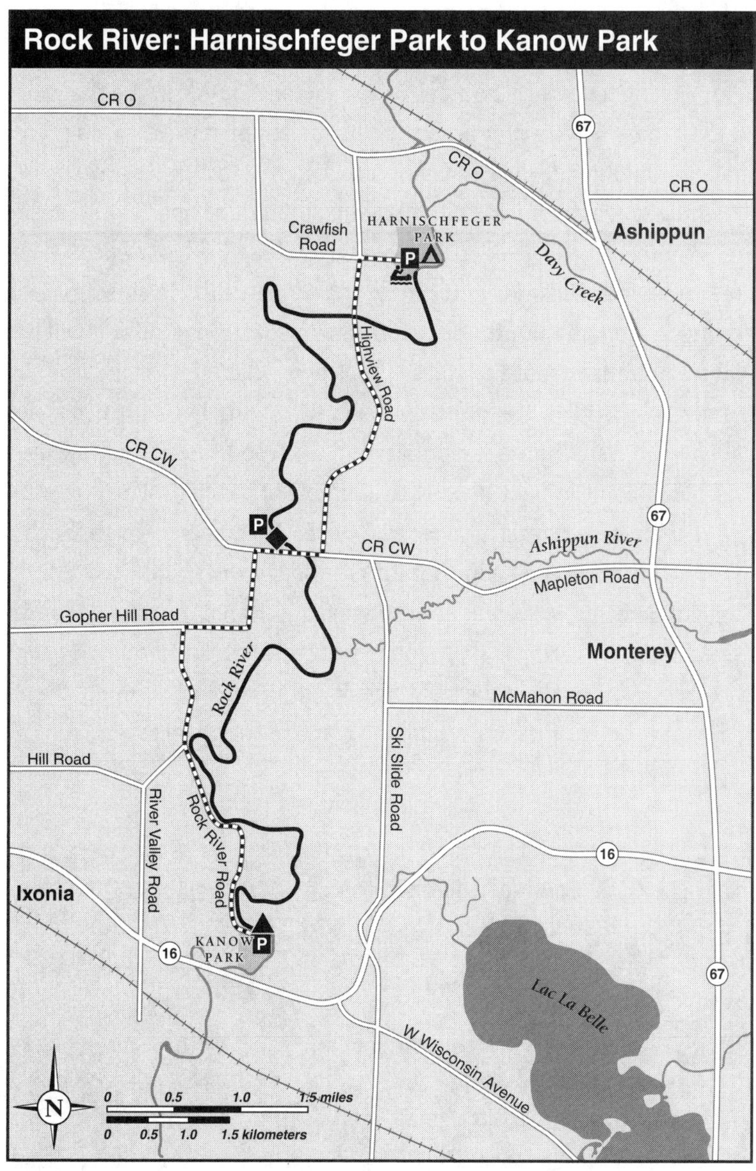

The river here is 100 feet wide and 3–4 feet deep, representative of this entire trip. Unless the river is high, the current will be rather slow. Obstacles should be few to none since this is a well-tended section of the Rock. The left bank will be low, while the right is pleasantly tall and flanked with trees. Soon this will taper and yield to a lush meadow.

All along this trip will be infrequent gentle slopes. In addition, this trip offers innumerable recesses to secretive waters and back-channel sloughs. Some scoff at the Rock River for being too wide, too slow, or too marshy, but I'd argue that, for some, a wide, slow river that takes its time and is unimpeded by obstacles is absolutely perfect. There are moments of terrific wilderness on the Rock—and on this trip particularly.

Half a mile downstream from the put-in, a quaint red barn will appear on the right after a right bend to the east. The Highview Road bridge immediately follows. The next few miles feel wild and wonderfully abandoned. Floodplains line both banks, and the feeling is intimate. But for occasional farm equipment, all you will hear is the melodic babble of birdsong, or the splash of a leaping fish.

The river will bend to the right then sharply to the left as it heads south and east. Four dilapidated shacks are camouflaged in the woods on your left, while there's a skinny strip of land on the right lined with a jumble of concrete slabs sometimes used by folks trying their luck at some of those frisky fish. Clearances through the thin woods on the right provide for teasing glimpses into the soggy wilds to the westward beyond. There's a logjam here, but someone has thoughtfully cleared out an angled passage on the right side. Since the current is slack, maneuvering through it should not pose a problem. Sit back, relax, and soak up the slow serenity; you'll almost certainly see great blue herons in the many trees or patiently stalking lunch in the green grass.

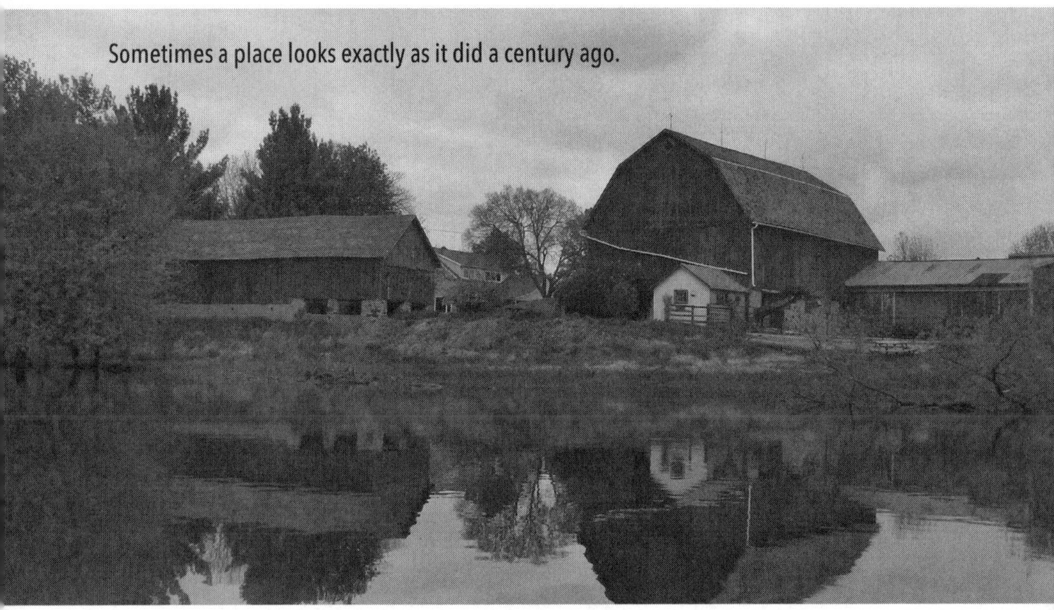
Sometimes a place looks exactly as it did a century ago.

A wayside park on the right marks the basic halfway point of this trip, on CR CW (**N43° 10.864' W88° 33.656'**). There are no facilities here, but it's a good place to stretch your legs or shorten this trip if you're low on time. Below the bridge, the right bank will rise again while the left offers a pastoral panorama. During a graceful bend to the right, you'll see a pretty vignette of a house atop a small hill off to the left. Trees enclose intimately once more. Through the leafy skein, you might discern a church steeple on the right followed by a weeping willow on the left. After a left–right–left buckle of turns, you'll arc past River Valley Road, where you may encounter folks fishing. Just downstream, you'll see a road and a sloping field beyond it. The river then veers off to the east, away from the road. You'll head straight for three houses where the river comes to a T, and it's a little confusing to tell in which direction the current heads. You'll want to turn right, as the slough to the left doesn't really lead to anywhere.

Paddling south now, the stretch here is positively lovely, as tall trees line a nonexistent marshy shore and undeveloped meadows beckon behind them. You'll head back west momentarily and make a sharp turn to the left after a few willows preceding farmhouses. For the last 0.5 mile, the river will run parallel to Rock River Road. You'll see a farm on the right, and then the river will bend to the left, to Kanow (KAY-now) Park. Here, there is no boat ramp, but landing at the designated swath of grass is easy and neat. There are full facilities at this park, too.

•THE•FUDGE•

ADDITIONAL TRIPS At 285 miles, the Rock River is humongous. From Hustisford to Harnischfeger Park are 17 miles of semi-wilderness marsh, while below Kanow Park to Watertown are 14 miles of pretty and rural stretches (including the Oconomowoc River confluence).

The city of Watertown offers a novel urban paddling experience, but there are two dams to portage (both clearly marked). Below Watertown are 13 miles through more semi-wilderness (minus the I-94 bridge). In a rather mundane stretch, the river then passes through the cities of Jefferson and Fort Atkinson but then picks up again to Lake Koshkonong.

The segment below the big lake, all the way to Janesville, is mostly residential, though a number of city parks and two interesting dams add some diversity. The Janesville-to-Beloit trip is quite pleasant and surprisingly natural (minus a few processing plants). Once in Illinois, the Rock flows for another 160 miles to its confluence at the Mississippi River, where the village of Saukenuk, the home of Chief Black Hawk and the Sauk people, once was located.

CAMPING AND RENTALS Harnischfeger Park (W3048 Crawfish Road, Ixonia; 920-474-7178)

FOOD FOR THOUGHT For good local microbrew, head down to Sweet Mullets, on Industrial Road in Oconomowoc (262-456-2843). Or, for an awesome breakfast, check out Burnt Toast (113 S. Main St., Oconomowoc; 262-560-0380).

SHOUT-OUTS Established in 2010, the Rock River Trail is part of our collective past. For everything you ever could want to know about paddling on, pedaling along, hiking near, or driving by the Rock River in Wisconsin and Illinois, check out rockrivertrail.com.

Also worth mentioning: In 1917, WI 16 immediately south of the Kanow Park take-out became the first road anywhere in the nation to be identified by a number. Before then, what few roads there were usually had no names beyond colloquial quirks. As such, one relied on landmarks or just got lost in the countryside. (But why didn't they name it Highway 1?)

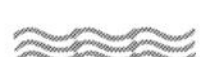

14 Rocky Run Creek and Wisconsin River:
US 51 TO COUNTY ROAD V

•THE•FACTS•

Put-in/take-out US 51/Dekorra Boat Launch (behind Hooker's Resort)

Distance/time 4.4 mi/Allow for 2.5 hrs

Gradient/water level 2.5 fpm/There should always be enough water. At high water, the flooded bottomlands are more accessible.

Water type Quietwater

Canoe or kayak Either, but a kayak works best if exploring the "cave."

Skill level Beginner

Time of year to paddle Anytime

Landscape Hardwoods, marsh, bottomlands, sandbar islands, limestone rock outcrops

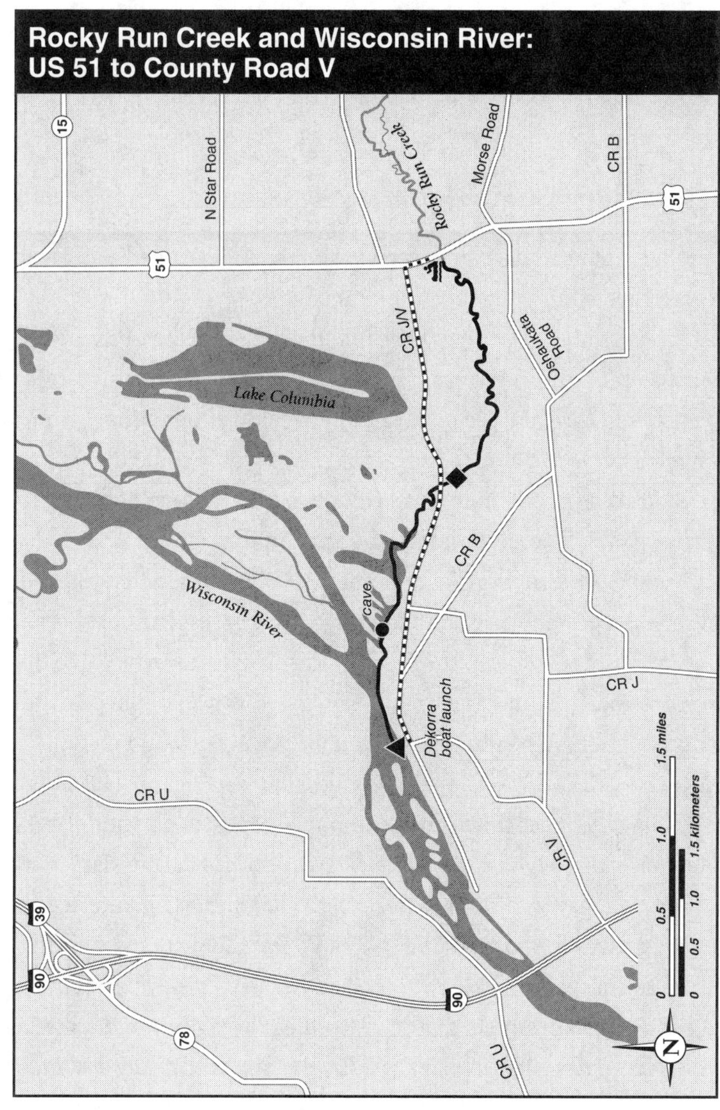

OVERVIEW With this trip, you get two streams for the price of one and three distinct landscapes in under 5 miles, plus a tiny but accessible cave. Expect to see deer, ducks, blue-winged teal, snapping turtles, bald eagles, great blue herons, and even cormorants.

SHUTTLE **3.3 miles.** From the take-out, turn left onto CR V/CR J (the same road goes by both letters) and head east. At US 51, turn right (south). The bridge for the put-in will be just down the road. Look for a trampled footpath leading to the water.

TAKE-OUT N43° 27.548' W89° 28.029' **PUT-IN** N43° 27.346' W89° 24.413'

•THE•FLAVOR•

PUT IN ON THE DOWNSTREAM SIDE of the US 51 bridge, river left. The creek is narrow, only 20 feet wide, but downed trees usually aren't a problem. It's prudent to have a handsaw and a pair of loppers for any low-hanging branches though. The water is attractively clear and sandy. You will not pass a single building from here to the Wisconsin River. Instead, the landscape is simply undeveloped and lovely. In spring, the banks are covered in pungent skunk cabbage.

After a half mile of squiggly meanders, the creek passes a ridge on the left topped with a stand of pine trees. This is an especially beautiful stretch that could be easily mistaken for the Mecan River. The creek will bend away from the woodsy ridge then return to it. At a tight right-hand bend, you'll come upon the remains of a dilapidated footbridge half submerged (that is, unless a flood has washed it out since the last time I paddled here). Portage around it on the right.

Next, you'll pass through a combination of bottomlands and sedge meadow, where solitude is a premium. A railroad bridge more or less divides this short segment in two: Downstream from here, the creek gradually widens from 40 to 80 to 100 feet, while the surrounding landscape becomes marshy. You'll paddle past a deer stand or two, but nothing else. Expect to see a diversity of waterfowl here.

Below the CR V/CR J bridge, the creek narrows again, unless the Wisconsin River is high, in which case it will be pretty much impossible to find the main channel. If the water level allows, you can paddle wherever your heart desires, but for the sake of orientation you may wish to hug close to the left shore, a guaranteed guide to lead you to the attractive rock formations on the Wisconsin just downstream.

(If you do follow your heart for a bit in higher water, you might try your hand at locating one of two channels that leads to the power plant and Lake Columbia; see Appendix B: Honorable Mentions, page 319. The first is basically a ditch on your right at the mouth of Rocky Run Creek; for 1 mile eastward it leads to the public parking. The second, a bit harder to locate, requires that delicate balance of knowing where to paddle and dumb luck, or a GPS. It's roughly 0.7 mile northeast, upstream on the right, from the mouth of Rocky Run Creek and leads to a pretty meadow, then a concrete embankment. Walk up the embankment to the levee, and on the other side is Lake Columbia.)

From the mouth of the Wisconsin, hug the left shore. Immediately the left bank rises and undulates, eventually as high as 50 feet. Soon the indented woods yield limestone outcrops, many with spooky porous borings. At one spot on the left, the rocky facade recedes into a narrow cavity—the "cave" mentioned in "The Facts"—that's easy

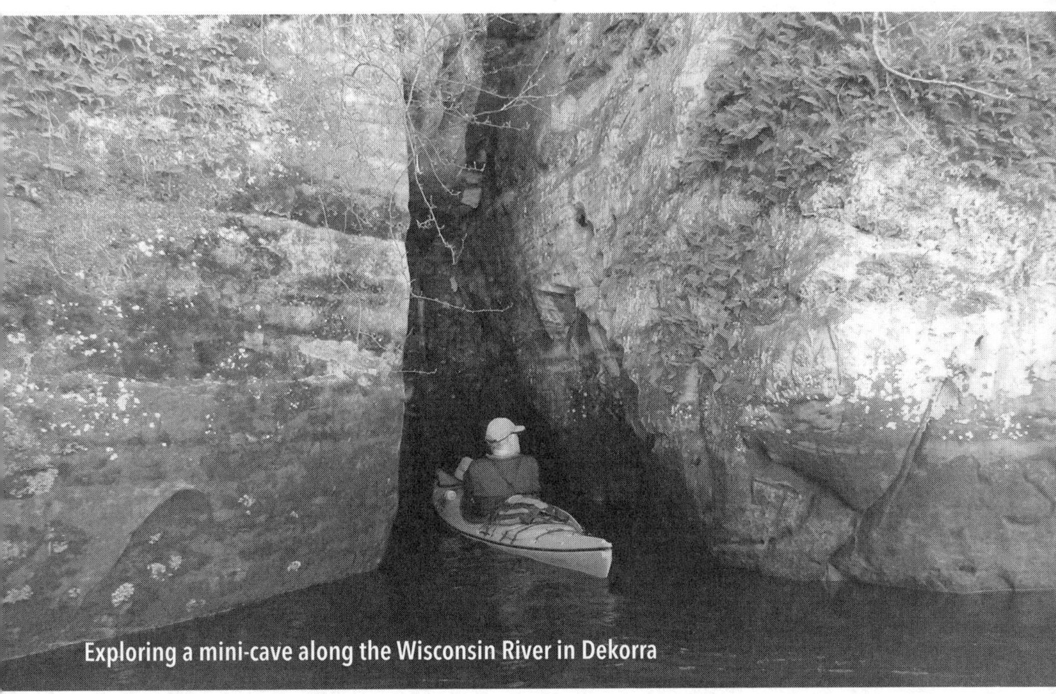
Exploring a mini-cave along the Wisconsin River in Dekorra

to miss if you're not looking for it and is more a cleft in the rock than an actual cave. But can you can paddle inside it and reverse out again. While caving, look for a sapling shooting out from the top of the rock. Inscriptions carved into the rock on the inside wall date to as far back as 1910 (or so the engraving purports).

Back in the open, the rocky left bank continues for a short while but soon fades as the shoreline flattens to signal the town of Dekorra. Here, you have two take-out options, both on the left. The first is not recommended simply because its parking lot is 400 feet away, whereas the second is only 1,000 feet downstream with a parking lot right at the launch (and a pub cheekily named Hooker's Resort).

•THE•FUDGE•

ADDITIONAL TRIPS You can try your luck putting in at Dunning Road, where there is a vast outlay of public land. From here to US 51 are 4 miles of narrow meandering along a rocky bottom with lots of deadfall. The water is shallow thanks to a steep gradient (7 fpm). As such, riffles are constant and there are several small ledges. To paddle this without walking your boat most of the day, you'd have to catch it right after a hard rain.

Farther upstream, the only other access to the creek is at Cuff Road (off WI 22). The creek is narrow enough to jump here, and deadfall is as bad as ever. You're pretty much in the middle of nowhere—the kind of care-forgotten place all the more remarkable for how close it is to both Portage and Madison. It is an enchanting stretch, all of it along the **Rocky Run Oak Savanna,** a state-owned natural area. (If nothing else, go for a hike here. It's 440 acres, hardly visited, and contains a stunning topography combining gentle rolling hills as well as two box canyons through cut sandstone.)

CAMPING **Wunder Er'de Campground,** in Dekorra on the Wisconsin River (N3204 CR V; 608-635-2059)

RENTALS **Rutabaga Paddlesports** (220 W. Broadway, Madison; 608-223-9300)

FOOD FOR THOUGHT What could be more convenient than good food and beer awaiting you at a trip's take-out? **Hooker's Resort** has both (W9370 CR V; 608-635-7867).

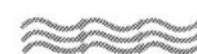

15 Token Creek: PORTAGE ROAD TO CHEROKEE MARSH

•THE•FACTS•

Put-in/take-out Portage Road/boat launch off Wheeler Road. See "The Flavor" for an alternative take-out.

Distance/time 9.7 mi/Allow for 5.5 hrs

Gradient/water level 2 fpm/There is no gage, but there's usually enough water except during dry spells in midsummer.

Water type Quietwater with occasional riffles, flatwater in the marsh

Canoe or kayak Kayak

Skill level Beginner for the first half, then experienced advised for the second half

Time of year to paddle Anytime

Landscape Modest hills, sedge meadows, and a large marsh

OVERVIEW A real gem of a creek too often forgotten or overlooked in the otherwise lake-centric Madison area, this meandering stream trip through public land happens

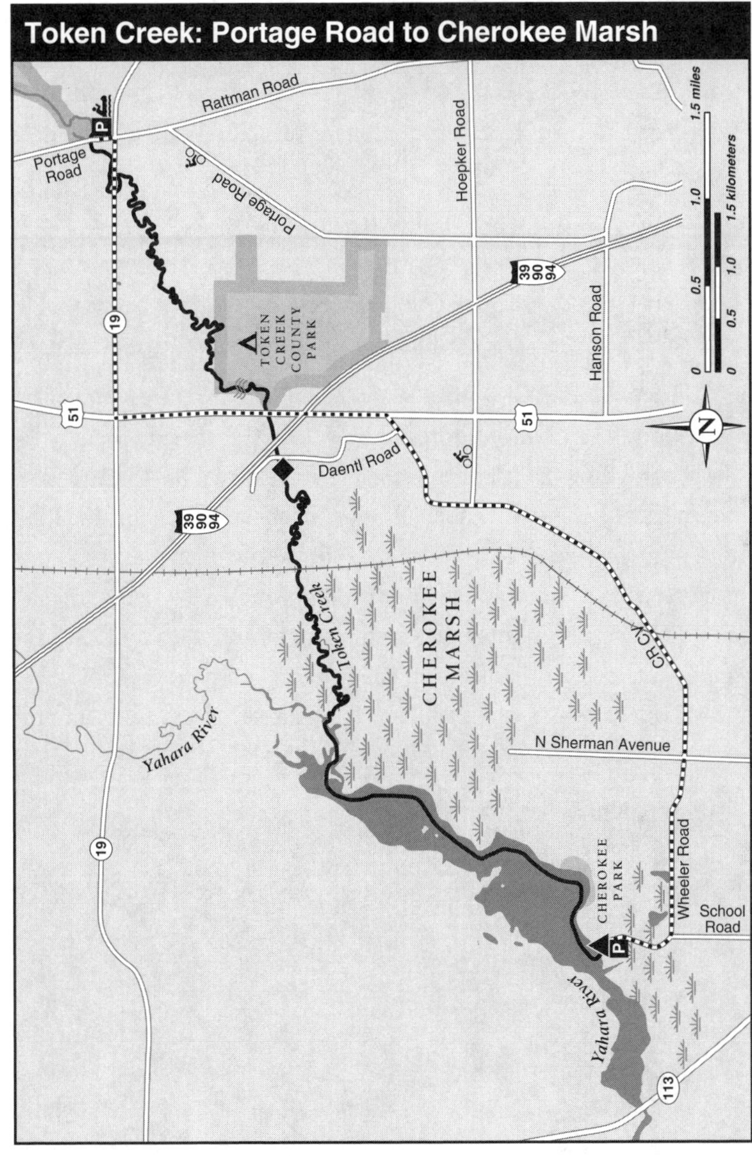

to slip underneath an interstate highway and occasionally has airplanes flying directly overhead. The last third of this trip lies on Cherokee Marsh, a huge wetland area. Expect to see geese, ducks, muskrats, turtles, great blue herons, sandhill cranes, deer, and frogs. During spring and autumn migrations, you might see pelicans, huge flocks of coots, shovelers, and mergansers.

SHUTTLE **7.5 miles.** From the take-out, turn left onto Wheeler Road from the access road, then left onto CR CV. Turn left onto US 51 North, then take the WI 19 exit and turn right to go east on WI 19. Turn left onto Portage Road to the put-in. (If you're bike-shuttling, turn right onto Hoepker Road after CR CV, then left onto Portage Road to the put-in.)

TAKE-OUT N43° 09.224' W89° 22.989' **PUT-IN** N43° 11.798' W89° 17.619'

•THE•FLAVOR•

PUT IN OFF THE SMALL PARKING AREA at Portage Road, on the upstream side of the bridge on river left. The creek is clear and only 15–20 feet wide. Below the bridge, you'll see aptly named Big Hill. The creek runs parallel to WI 19 for 100 yards before passing underneath it, after which it shall begin its characteristic meandering.

A line of pine trees precedes an attractive covered wooden bridge at a private residence. The creek will widen to 30 feet as it flows through a low-lying marsh. Around a few bends, you'll likely encounter a tree to negotiate, but you shouldn't have to portage anywhere on the creek thanks to the dedication and hard work of volunteers at Capitol Water Trails and Mad City Paddlers. There's a low-clearance farm bridge to be

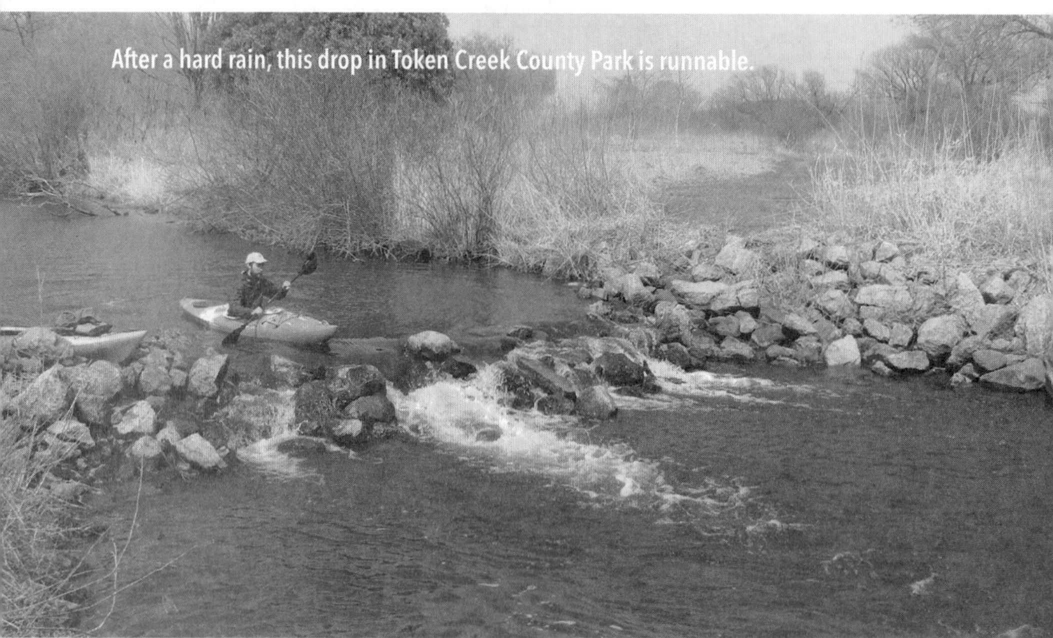

After a hard rain, this drop in Token Creek County Park is runnable.

mindful of that is followed by a sweet run of riffles. Eventually, on your right, you'll see what looks like a feeder stream; it actually connects directly to a random pond. (There's not a whole lot to see, but it's an unusual diversion all the same.)

Chances are good you'll begin to see hikers or at least the occasional section of boardwalk on the left, signaling Token Creek County Park. (Also, you'll definitely hear the din of highway traffic whirring by.) The creek passes through a culvert with a little riffle running through it, below which is a wide pool of sorts, created by a rock dam shortly downstream. Stay to the right shore—the left is a dead end.

You'll see a horizon line at the small dam and, depending on water levels, maybe hear the rush of the rapid. (The drop is only 2 feet, and there's a narrow but not-unsafe slot to line up and run it through, but it's composed entirely of rocks. If there's enough water to run it, I recommend it because it's fun, even if you do scrape a little. Most of the time, though, it will be too shallow to run; portage on the right.)

There will be a few more meanders as the creek approaches the interstate. On the right will be towering signs and billboards. Two tunnels follow in immediate succession: one at US 51 and then one at the interstate. Both are concrete lined, rectangular, safely runnable, and pretty fun, frankly. The interstate right-side tunnel has a downspout, so if it's rained recently there will be a small waterfall effect that's naturally lit from a skylight above. (The tunnel is wide enough to paddle around this without getting showered on.)

Just below the interstate tunnel is a popular, if hard-to-locate, access area off Daentl Road. There's a random parking area up the slope on the right (**N43° 10.891' W89° 19.732'**). At this point, you've paddled 4 miles, and the portion of the trip that's more challenging is about to begin.

The next section, to Cherokee Marsh, has quite a different and wild feel to it (once you're away from the highways and airplanes) but is prone to more obstructions in occasionally swift current. It's for this reason alone that *this second half is more appropriate for experienced paddlers.* It's narrower and it meanders considerably, so you want to be sure you've allowed enough time to paddle it.

For a couple hundred yards, the creek runs straight, lulling you into a false sense of ease. But just after you pass the last house on the right, in a cul-de-sac, the creek will swing to the left and begin a series of frisky switchbacks such that you will face each cardinal direction a couple of times in the next 0.5 mile. A pretty hill faces you on the north. There's a surprisingly reputable current here, which, in conjunction with the narrowness of the creek and an occasional tree to dodge, makes this section a bit difficult, but it's not dangerous.

A low train trestle comes after a brief but welcome straightaway. The environs of the marsh start to take hold after the bridge. There's a delightful feeling of abandon down here, with no buildings or signs of development anywhere. For the most part, the meandering is gentler here than upstream until you reach Cherokee Marsh.

After a couple of sharp switchbacks, the creek widens and you'll see a small island. If there's enough water, take the right channel. If not, paddle clockwise around the island. If in doubt, just follow the path of the current. *Note:* A separate tributary from the south enters at this same junction at the island. Because it's pretty much the same size as Token Creek, it's easy to assume that it's the same stream, but this one will take you *away from* the marsh.

Another couple of zigzags take you into Cherokee Marsh. Turn left to avoid inadvertently paddling upstream the Yahara River, which creates the marsh. You'll pass two sloughs on the left, the second of which is next to a small island. The main stream widens out before you. To the right is the top of the marsh; to the left takes you to the body of the marsh. First, it bottlenecks, then it spreads out widely. The rest of this trip is all flatwater lake paddling. The good news is the marsh is a no-wake zone for motorboats. It's a pretty mosaic of hardwood forests, cattails, tag alder, willows, dogwood, and lots of handsome oaks.

At more than 1,200 acres, Cherokee Marsh is the largest wetland in Dane County. Also, it marks the headwaters of Madison's chain of lakes from here all the way down to Stoughton; the Yahara River is a connecting corridor of wetland complexes. The marsh is part of Madison's parks system and is divided into north and south units. The north is pretty wild and rugged, the left shore in particular (a couple McMansions and an occasional farm are on the right).

Entering the marsh, you'll see a large drumlin far off on the right; it's a hill deposited by receding glaciers. You want to be mindful about paddling the marsh: If you're against the wind, the experience will be frustrating, exhausting, and wet, with whitecaps splashing you; at low water levels, the paddling will be slow going and mucky. I personally recommend staying close to the left shore. Subtle but lovely rolling hills comprising oak savannas lie off to the left. There is a pretty pier here you can dock against to stretch your legs, go for a hike, or have a picnic.

Soon, alas, on the left you'll see a large cluster of houses. Just after these will be a long slough on the left. Turn into the slough if your take-out is off Wheeler Road. A wooden dock extends from a gravel parking area.

•THE•FUDGE•

ADDITIONAL TRIPS If you're wondering what's upstream on Token Creek to paddle, it's not much, and obstructions preclude most of what little there is. Depending on your ambition, you can continue past Cherokee Marsh and into **Lake Mendota,** the largest of Madison's four lakes. Hug the right shore to the mouth of Sixmile Creek (see Appendix A, page 317), turn right upstream, and then turn left at the mouth of Dorn Creek to the bridge.

CAMPING **Token Creek County Park** (6200 US 51; 608-224-3730)

FOOD FOR THOUGHT For a huge menu and a nod to the retro diner, check out **Gus's Diner** in Sun Prairie, just east of the put-in off WI 19 (630 N. Westmount Drive; 608-318-0900). You might also try the **Ale Asylum,** off Packers Avenue on Madison's north side (2002 Pankratz St.; 608-663-3926). Even closer to the take-out is the **Parched Eagle Brewpub,** an excellent new microbrewery on CR M, half a mile from WI 113 (5440 Willow Road; 608-204-9192). And then there's the reliable and slightly cheeky **Nau-Ti-Gal Saloon** at 5360 Westport Road, just downstream from the take-out and essentially accessible by boat (608-246-3130).

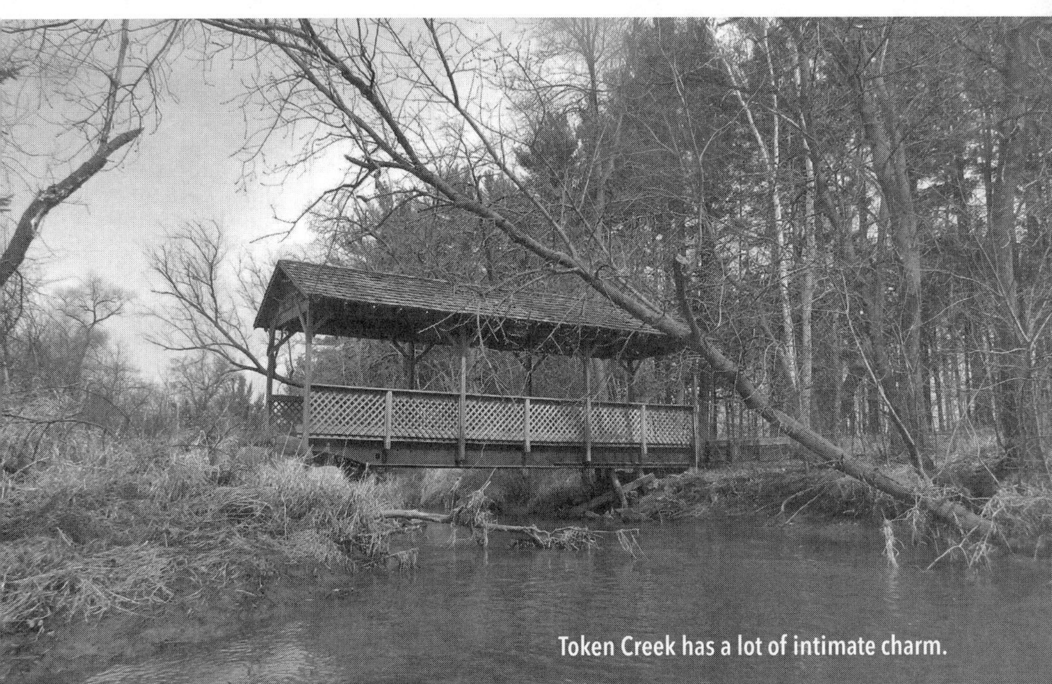

Token Creek has a lot of intimate charm.

16 White River (Green Lake County):
NESHKORO DAM TO WHITE RIVER ROAD

•THE•FACTS•

Put-in/take-out Public park below the dam in Neshkoro/White River Road. See "The Flavor" for two alternative take-outs.

Distance/time 15.7 mi/Allow for 7 hrs

Gradient/water level 2 fpm/There is no gage, but water levels are usually adequate. Call Renewable World Energies at 855-994-9376 for dam-release info. Avoid this trip on windy days.

Water type Quietwater

Canoe or kayak Kayak

Skill level Beginners might want to break this trip up at one of the two intermediate points highlighted, due to its length.

Time of year to paddle Spring or autumn (lots of mosquitoes in summer)

Landscape Tall clay banks with pine trees, prairies, oak savannas, tamarack bogs, a huge wildlife-area marsh, hardwood bottomland swamp

---

OVERVIEW A long, meandering, but exquisitely pristine trip through a huge wildlife area, this stretch of the White River is at its prettiest and most interesting. Expect to see bald eagles, bitterns, crawfish, turtles galore, sandhill cranes, wood ducks, frogs, raccoons, deer, pheasants, groundhogs, plovers, killdeer, beaver, mink, woodpeckers, hooded mergansers, and the ethereal (but endangered) Karner blue butterfly. This is one of those trips where the journey itself is the destination. Two intermediate access points allow for shortening this otherwise-long day trip.

SHUTTLE 11.5 miles. From the take-out, head south on White River Road, one of Wisconsin's premier "Rustic Roads." Turn right onto CR D. Stay straight on County Line Road where CR D bears right, then turn right onto Pond Lily Road. Bear left onto CR DD. Turn right onto WI 73 and follow it into town. Turn right onto Wall Street, then left onto State Street. Turn right into the park, where a dirt road loops around a small pavilion. There is no designated parking, so pull off the loop to allow other vehicles to pass.

TAKE-OUT N43° 55.043' W89° 04.804' **PUT-IN** N43° 57.782' W89° 12.959'

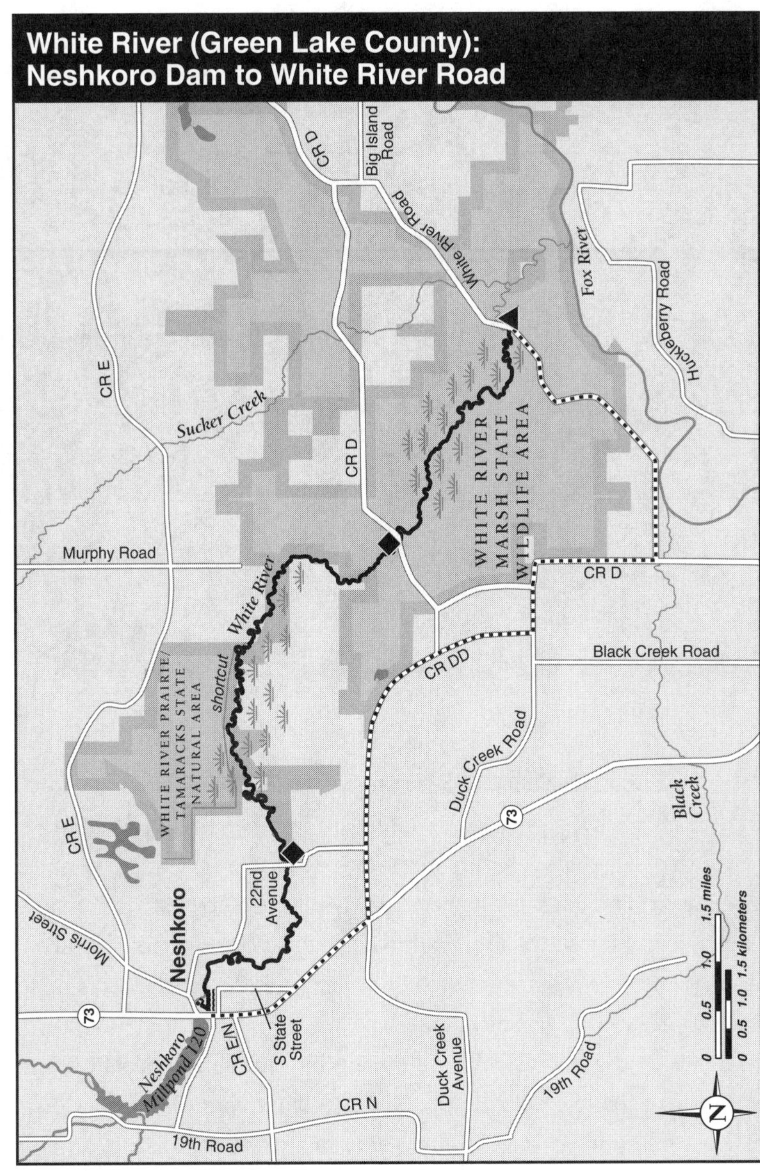

•THE•FLAVOR•

PUT IN ANYWHERE YOU LIKE BELOW THE DAM, as there is no official launch. There's an old red-brick powerhouse that adds an attractive contrast to the blue sky and clear water, along with a natural spring on the south side of the loop road around the park.

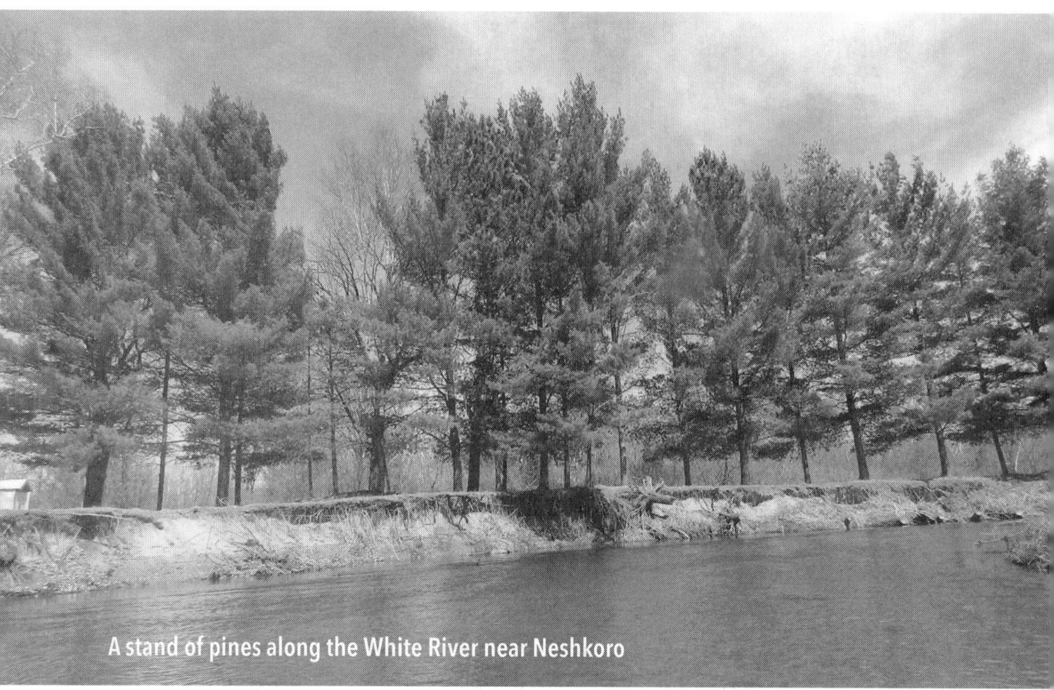

A stand of pines along the White River near Neshkoro

The only riffle on this trip is 25 yards below the dam. Right away, you'll appreciate the color of the water, which will alternate between cream soda and root beer hued. The width of the river here is representative of the rest of this trip: about 50 feet wide. Beige clay and tallgrass banks begin to rise shortly downstream, many punctuated with pine trees. Only for a short mile will you pass by a few houses, all on the left; otherwise, this entire trip bears no signs of development (save the occasional hunting blind, which is prohibited, technically).

Small hills in the background are discernible through breaks in the filigree of trees first on the right, then on the left 1 mile downstream. Beyond a slough on the right, you'll see an antenna tower. Soon a very real sense of isolation and sweet solitude prevails as the river meanders through a lush landscape of scrub brush and oak savanna. As you approach the bridge at WI 22, take note of the fun rope swing on the left, the perfect cure for the common hot of a summer day. Some 75 yards downstream from the bridge is an official access on the right (**N43° 56.967' W89° 11.223'**), a convenient way to shave 3.3 miles off this trip or to take out if you have only the late afternoon to paddle.

The bridge and landing mark the northwestern demarcation of the 12,000-acre White River Marsh Wildlife Area, a place that Aldo Leopold, the father of wildlife ecology, had fought to protect from irresponsible farming. You will be enveloped by public land for the next 12.5 miles, and the feeling of escape is palpable. You can't see it from the river, but in the southwest corner of the marsh lies a small "no entry" parcel dedicated exclusively to the training and releasing of whooping cranes, a critically endangered species. Maybe, just maybe, you'll hear or even see a whooper while on the river!

You'll pass one more house on the left, the very last on this trip. Shortly downstream lie the remnants of a former bridge followed by the inverted root system of some ancient tree, resembling a fortress. A series of squiggly meanders takes you to the periphery of the White River Prairie/Tamaracks State Natural Area, one of the largest tamarack bogs and wet prairies still extant in Wisconsin.

For a fun diversion, and a way to shave off more than half a mile of meanders, turn left into what looks like one of countless oxbows but leads to a millrace canal. In addition to saving time and labor, you'll paddle closer to the haunting tamaracks seeped in sphagnum moss. What's especially nice is that the millrace reenters the river seamlessly. On both sides of the river, you'll see stands of tamaracks in the near distance buffered by marshy sedge.

Soon hardwoods line the banks of the river and the wide-open sky gives way to pleasant tree canopies as the marsh begins to feel more like a swampy bottomlands. Here, you may well encounter the occasional obstacle. Paddlers and tubers alike use the river, so it does benefit from occasional maintenance, but be prepared for ducking underneath low-hanging branches and riding over surface-level logs. In some tight spots, you may need or simply prefer to portage.

The swampy bottomlands continue for another 3 miles, so if this is not your cup of tea, you may wish to take out at the CR D bridge (**N43° 55.999' W89° 07.408'**), newly reconstructed in late 2014. I encourage you to continue on, though. A mile downstream from CR D, the woods give way to a majesty of open marsh, a welcome relief from the woodsy confines of the bog. Why go all the way to Montana when there's plenty of big-sky country right here?

For the last 4 miles, the river runs through the largest southern sedge meadow in all of Wisconsin. A dominion of cattails and shrub-carr islands, the serene simplicity and expanse here is breathtaking. Good luck keeping count of the turtles and sandhill cranes you'll see!

Woods will enclose once more, first on the left, then on the right, with bogs off in oxbows. Savor the moment, as the take-out is located at the next bridge shortly downstream. There's a small parking area on the downstream river-right side.

•THE•FUDGE•

ADDITIONAL TRIPS Continuing past White River Road is not recommended unless you start your trip here and continue onto the Fox River down to Berlin. It's only 2 miles to the confluence of the Fox River, but there are no bridges between Princeton and Berlin, so the shuttle route is 14 miles long.

Upstream of the Neshkoro Dam, the river is too impounded and the banks too developed to recommend paddling. However, there is a make-do access at Czech Lane from which you can paddle upstream against the current; here, the White River resembles its more popular neighbor to the west, the Mecan. There are some cabins and houses, but the environment is otherwise pretty. You may have thought about putting in at the dam on CR YY, but it's not recommended on account of the many obstructions and unpleasant portaging.

CAMPING AND RENTALS **Mecan River Outfitters & Lodge** (W720 WI 23, Princeton; 920-295-3439); **Rendezvous Paddle & Sports** (201 Main St., Montello; 608-297-2444)

FOOD FOR THOUGHT For a delicious vegetarian meal washed down with a local microbrew in a cute setting, stop by **MORE Healthy Foods and Cafe** (15 Main St., Montello; 608-297-8111), located at Marquette County's one and only stoplight. Also darling is **Once in a Blue Moon** (538 W. Water St., Princeton; 608-295-6100). In fact, there is much charm along Water Street in downtown Princeton.

SHOUT-OUT A standing ovation is owed to the tireless efforts of **Operation Migration,** an organization devoted to protecting, rearing, and stabilizing the whooping crane population. Check them out at operationmigration.org.

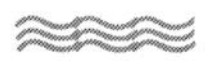

17 Yahara River A: DeForest to Windsor

•THE•FACTS•

Put-in/take-out Veterans Memorial Park in DeForest/Windsor Road in Windsor

Distance/time 5.3 mi/Allow for 2.5 hrs

Gradient/water level Approximately 5 fpm/See USGS gage 05427718. Below 2 feet on the gage, you will scrape quite a bit. This trip is runnable only in spring during the snowmelt or after a mighty hard rainfall. The river can drop 8 inches in 24 hours, so catching it at the right level can be tricky.

Water type Quietwater with several riffles

Canoe or kayak Kayak

Skill level Experienced

Time of year to paddle Anytime there's enough water

Landscape Woods, farms, residential, protected public land corridor

---

OVERVIEW A surprisingly scenic and riffly stretch of clear water surrounded by a protected corridor in an otherwise developed area, this short trip offers moments where it feels like you're in the wild. Expect to see wildlife such as great blue herons, turtles, fish, and deer.

CAR SHUTTLE **2.6 miles.** From the take-out, head east on Windsor Road, then turn left onto Lake Road into town. Veterans Memorial Park will be on your right; the parking lot is south of the river.

BIKE SHUTTLE **4.2 miles.** Follow the Upper Yahara River Trail north from Windsor Road as it parallels the river (for the most part) and wends around subdivisions; then head north on River Road and east on South Street into Western Green Area Park and finally Veterans Memorial Park. It's a pretty and fun opportunity for a bike shuttle.

TAKE-OUT N43° 12.988' W89° 20.973' **PUT-IN** N43° 14.974' W89° 20.614'

•THE•FLAVOR•

PUT IN AT VETERANS MEMORIAL PARK, where there is an information kiosk regarding the Yahara River. The river here is emblematic of this trip: skinny, clear, and rocky, more

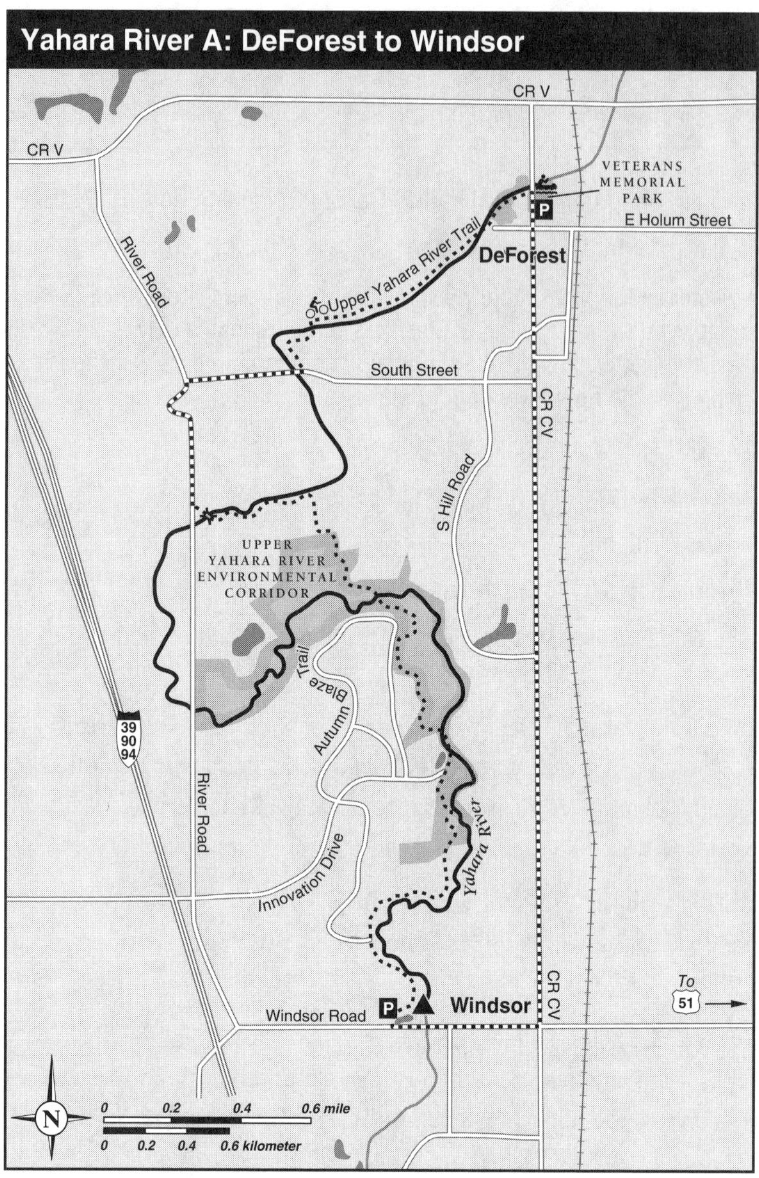

like a creek than a river, and nothing at all resembling the lower Yahara River down in Rock County (see Yahara River B, page 168). For the first mile-and-change, there are almost no meanders, and the current is slow. Don't worry, though; it's not boring. Tiny vignettes of unexpected quaintness sneak up on you: lovely trees, raised banks, open fields, and so on. Consider this beginning a warm-up before the riffles and twists.

Things get interesting at the South Street bridge, where the river narrows considerably and the current picks up. Riffles await underneath the bridge and then again immediately downstream. As the river heads south then west, the backyards of cul-de-sacs will be visible briefly on the right, followed by Sunnybrook Park. You'll pass under one of several attractive pedestrian/bike path bridges as the river begins to meander in earnest.

The riverbanks will gradually rise to 10 feet high, some studded with brief peeks of moss-covered rock outcroppings. Approaching and then following the River Road bridge (the first one; the Yahara passes beneath the road twice), riffles will flourish, modest boulders dot the streambed, and leafy woods will enclose—it's "DeForest," after all! This is a particularly pretty section. You'll probably hear the din of the interstate, but you won't see the highway at any time.

After passing under River Road the second time, a sense of real isolation ensues. There's a temporary break from all the subdivisions; only sparse farmland surrounds you. Here, you're heading east and away from the interstate. Both times I've paddled this trip, I have spotted owls in this stretch.

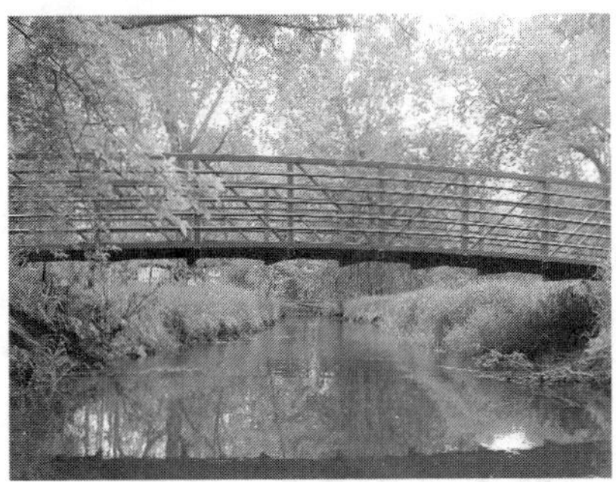

Quaint pedestrian bridge over the river

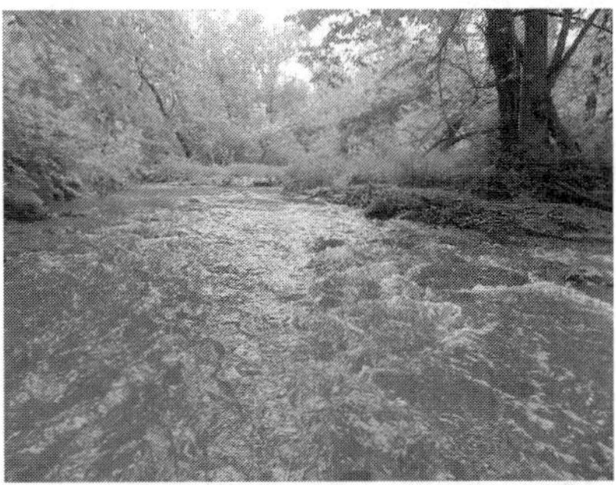

Fast riffles on the upper Yahara

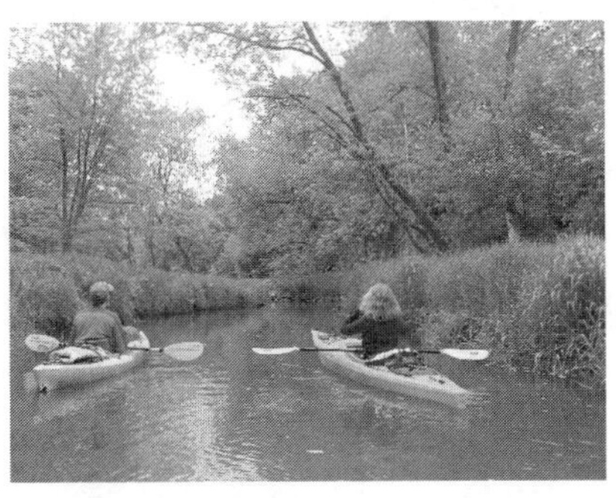

Intimate and naturally secluded

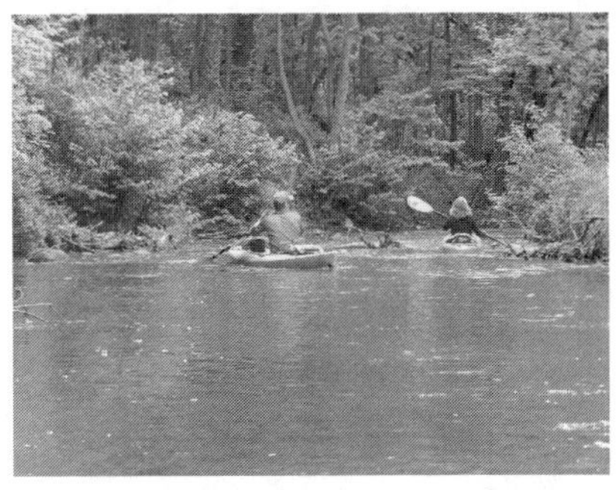

Expect to maneuver around obstructions.

Soon you'll see a very attractive sandstone rock outcrop about 30 feet wide and 10 feet high on your right. A tall ridge lies behind it, and the Upper Yahara River Trail follows its sinuous nature. To be sure, the scenic river inspired the trail, but it took admirable organization and landscape architecture to create the trail in so respectful a manner in the first place. There will very likely be some downed trees to contend with, some of which might well require portaging around or over. Volunteers do an outstanding job of maintaining the upper Yahara, but its tree cover and narrowness make it prone to obstructions.

Swift riffles and shallow water continue as the river heads mostly southward and the surroundings revert to development and subdivisions. Two more steepish banks prevail, and there's even one last small hill on the left before the landscape opens up to grass. You may see the trail on your right once more, now signaling the end of the trip. Take out at Windsor Road on the right, upstream of the bridge. From there, it's a short walk to the parking area.

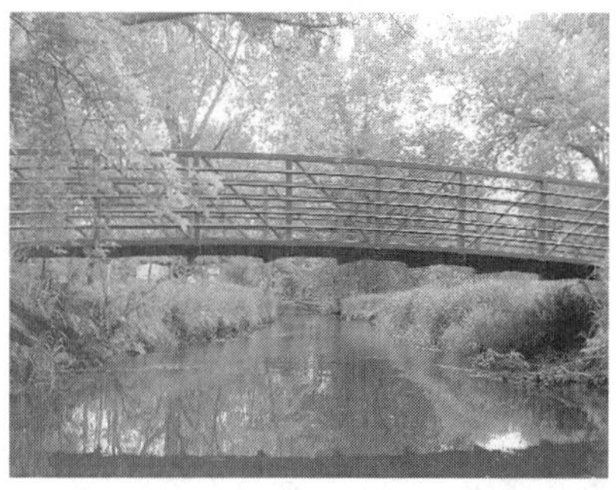

A bit of quietwater before more riffles

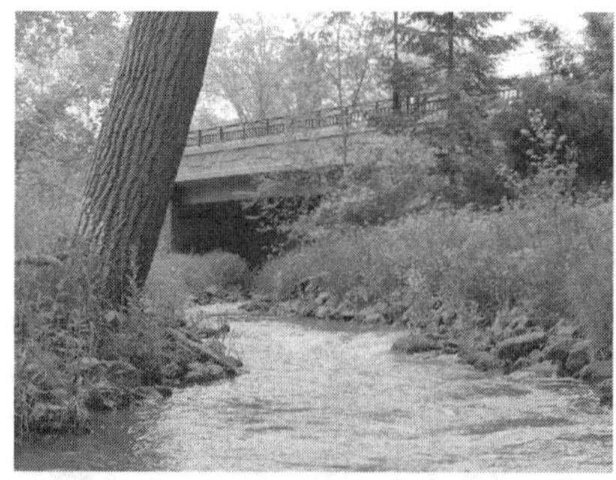

Little ledge below South Street

•THE•FUDGE•

ADDITIONAL TRIPS You can add 1.5 miles to this trip by putting in upstream at Yahara Road, but it's undeveloped and there's only roadside parking. The river environs are a mix of agricultural and industrial, and deadfall can be problematic.

Continuing past Windsor Road is not recommended because there's a golf course immediately on the other side. Saying nothing of the rather undesirable potential for being struck by golf balls *or* steely gazes from disapproving golfers who'd just as soon not see kayakers paddling through their game, there are lots of low-clearance bridges throughout the course, some of which require you to portage around.

The Yahara flows beneath the interstate, then WI 19, and then into Cherokee Marsh, but this section is a horror show of logjams and fallen trees.

CAMPING Token Creek County Park (6200 US 51; 608-224-3730)

RENTALS Rutabaga Paddlesports (220 W. Broadway, Madison; 608-223-9300)

FOOD FOR THOUGHT Why not end your trip with a slice of pie—or *lefse*? The Norske Nook Restaurant & Bakery (608-842-3378), at the intersection of Main and Holum Streets in DeForest, specializes in pie, as well as traditional Norwegian meals.

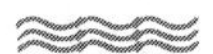

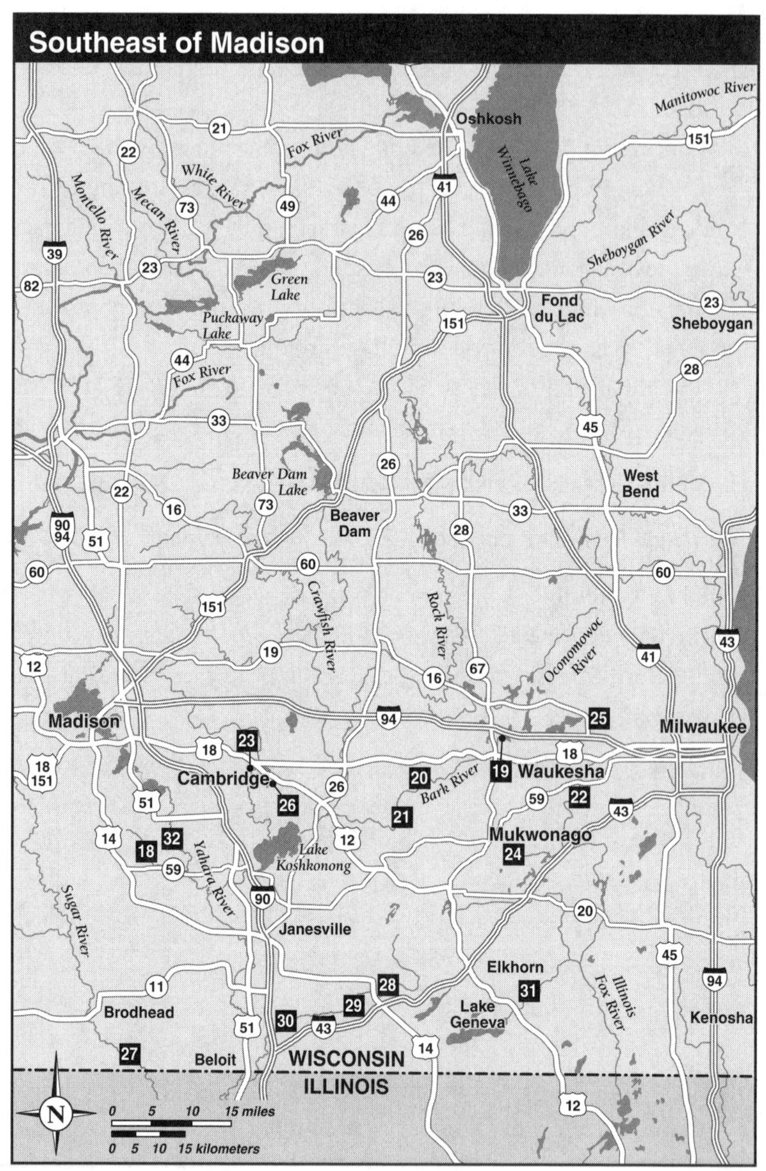
Southeast of Madison
Oshkosh
Lake Winnebago
Manitowoc River
Fox River
White River
Mecan River
Montello River
Sheboygan River
Green Lake
Puckaway Lake
Fox River
Fond du Lac
Sheboygan
Beaver Dam Lake
Beaver Dam
West Bend
Crawfish River
Rock River
Oconomowoc River
Madison
Milwaukee
Cambridge
Waukesha
Bark River
Mukwonago
Lake Koshkonong
Yahara River
Sugar River
Janesville
Elkhorn
Illinois Fox River
Brodhead
Lake Geneva
Kenosha
Beloit
WISCONSIN
ILLINOIS
0 5 10 15 miles
0 5 10 15 kilometers

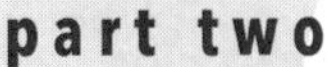

part two

SOUTHEAST OF MADISON

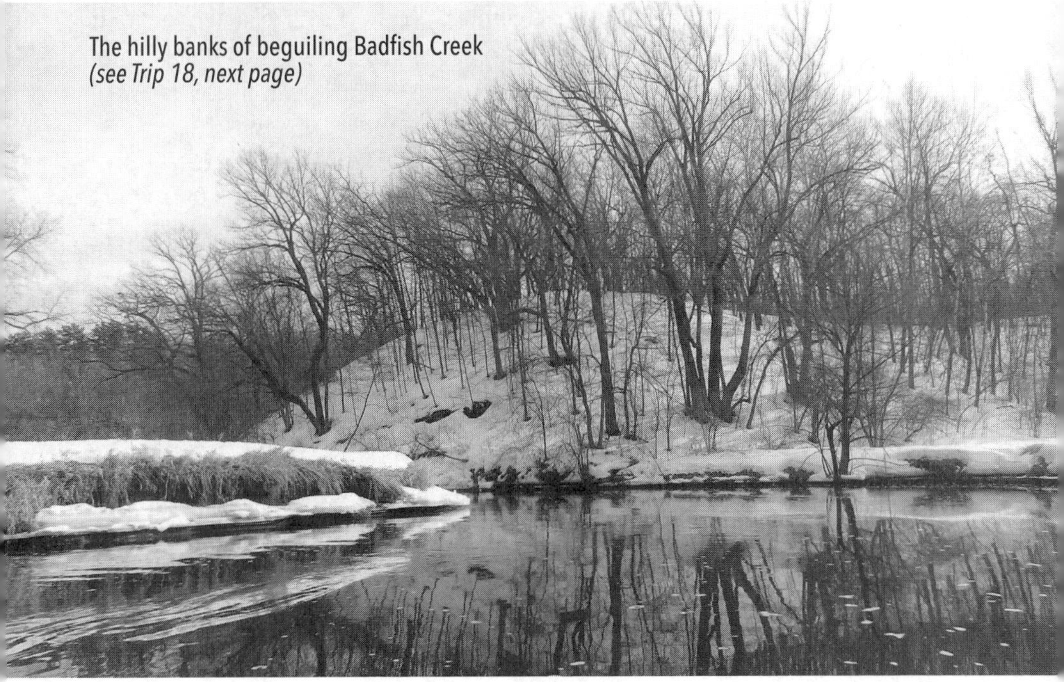

The hilly banks of beguiling Badfish Creek
(see Trip 18, next page)

18 Badfish Creek: OLD STAGE ROAD TO CASEY ROAD

•THE•FACTS•

Put-in/take-out Old Stage Road/Casey Road

Distance/time 6.8 mi/Allow for 3 hrs

Gradient/water level Approximately 5 fpm/See USGS gage 05430150. Best at 130+ cfs but can be paddled as low as 60 cfs.

Water type Riffles and light rapids

Canoe or kayak Kayak preferable, but a canoe will work

Skill level Experienced

Time of year to paddle Anytime

Landscape Hardwood forests with small hills, pastures, and prairie remnants

---

OVERVIEW One of the best secrets in south central Wisconsin, Badfish Creek has everything you can want in a stream: clear water, swift current, riffles and light rapids, pretty scenery, sandbars, some small hills, a sense of remoteness, and lots of twists and turns. Not for beginners, the Badfish requires solid boat control and river-reading skills. Expect to see deer, muskrats, ducks, geese, turkeys, hawks, great blue herons, fish, and bald eagles.

SHUTTLE 5 miles. From the take-out, drive south on Casey Road, then turn right on WI 59. Turn right on WI 138 in Cooksville. Turn left on Old Stage Road to the put-in. There is parking along the road at the Casey Road bridge. At the put-in, there is a small parking area.

TAKE-OUT N42° 50.012' W89° 11.477' **PUT-IN** N42° 51.180' W89° 15.400'

•THE•FLAVOR•

THERE ARE MANY ASPECTS THAT MAKE BADFISH CREEK WONDERFUL, chief among them its swift current, clear water, meandering nature, and surrounding environment. Throw in some small boulders, sandbars, great wildlife, and gentle hills juxtaposed with open meadows, and it's all within a half-hour drive from downtown Madison. This trip is a perfect length for many paddlers—the current doesn't require strenuous

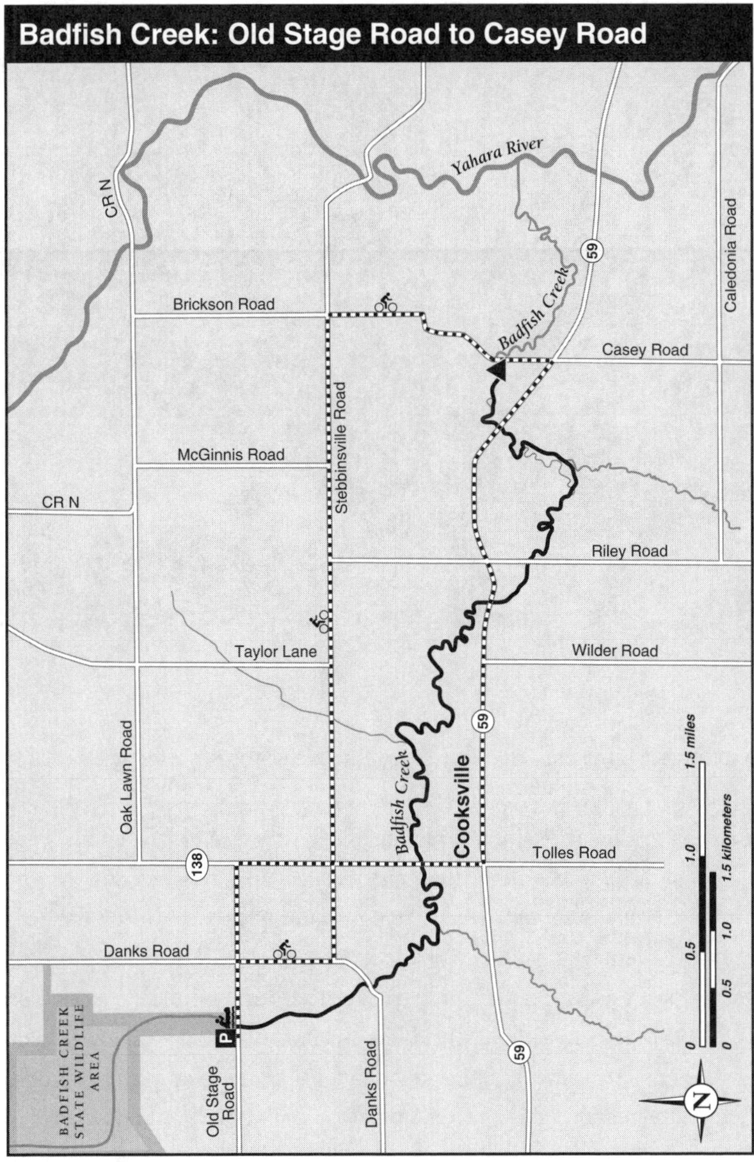

effort, and you can take your time soaking in the scene, even picnicking at one of the many small islands.

The creek is a great place to practice reading a river, as there are many shallow spots, typically in the more open sections where the stream widens. That said, it should be noted that Badfish Creek daily receives Madison's treated wastewater. While that

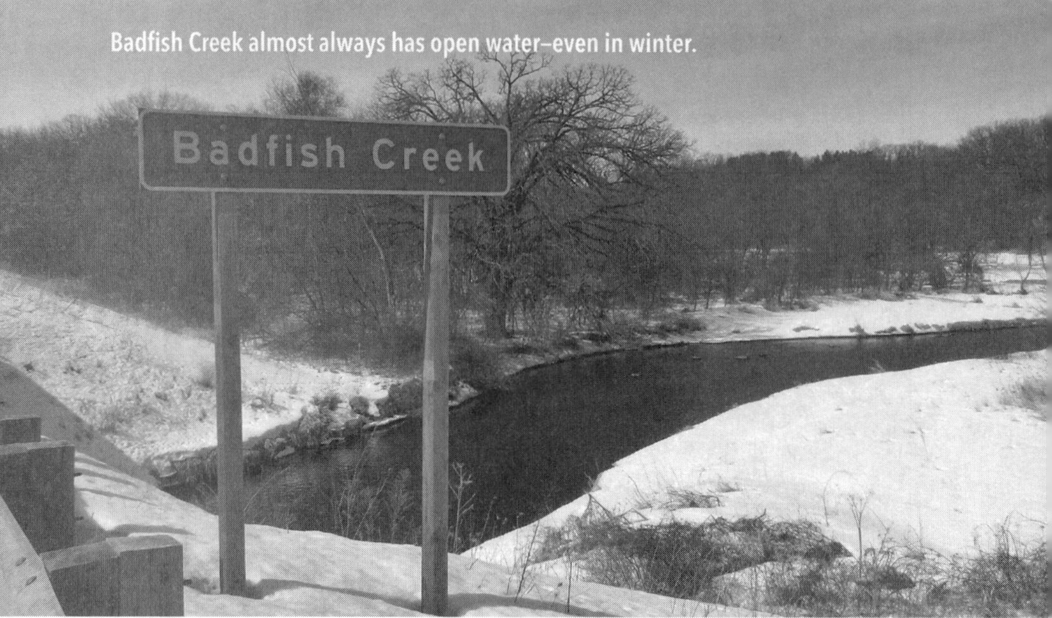

Badfish Creek almost always has open water—even in winter.

fact may sound disagreeable in theory, in reality the water is perfectly clean and clear. (I grew up near the Passaic River in New Jersey, so I know polluted waterways!) There is a chemical aroma in the air—a by-product of the effluent being treated by UV light, not chlorine—but it is no worse than the pungent scent of a nearby farm. Moreover, the benefit of this is there is almost always enough water to paddle the Badfish.

Put in off the parking area for Badfish Creek Wildlife Area at Old Stage Road. There's a short schlep along a path to the water that can be a little muddy (also watch for ticks). For the first mile, trees provide a shady canopy and narrow banks enclose the creek. The current is swift, the water clear. The creek is atypically straight in this section, which makes for a good warm-up before the many twists downstream.

There are a few houses in this stretch, but they are the exception to the rule. There used to be a rustic truss bridge at Leedle Mill Road, which enhanced the romantic nostalgia of this trip, but it was replaced in 2011 by a mundane modern bridge. A small rapid lies downstream of the bridge, one of the best on this trip. Boat control is important here as the river makes a sharp bend to the left below the bridge. A mix of trees and open meadow follows, at which point the Badfish will begin to meander considerably.

At this point, the Badfish is nonstop fun. A few houses can be seen again approaching the WI 138 bridge. Another delightful and easy rapid lies below the bridge. After this bridge, development is sparse to nonexistent. The landscape gets hillier and more remote. The Badfish passes under three more bridges: twice at WI 59 and under Riley Road in between. There is another fun light rapid after the first WI 59 bridge. The woods are thicker and the banks steeper approaching and following Riley Road. This is an especially pretty area with a rugged feel. By the second WI 59 bridge, the landscape is more open. Here and there, you will pass clusters of old oak trees and even a stand of pines atop a small hill. The peppy Badfish sweeps past a tall, attractively eroded bank of sand on the right.

You'll see the name "Viney" on the proverbial broadside of a barn off to your left. When you see the fifth bridge come into view, make your way over to the left bank. This is Casey Road, which means that this trip is over. (If in doubt, look for neon-green tape on the bridge itself, someone's landmark.) Take out on the upstream side of the bridge on the left where there is a small cleft in the bank to safely wedge your boat into. Look for two ropes on the bank to help pull yourself out of the boat.

•THE•FUDGE•

ADDITIONAL TRIPS Putting in farther upstream is not without its charms, but I don't recommend it. There are more than 10 miles of accessible creek upstream of Old Stage Road, including a designated wildlife area, but deadfall is quite problematic below Old Stone Road, and the creek is predominantly channelized (it's just one straightaway after another).

Downstream from Casey Road, there are 2 more miles until the confluence at the Yahara River. There is some deadfall to contend with in this section, but it should be quite manageable. The first available access here is the bridge at WI 59 on the upstream river-left side of the Yahara. Parking is much more limited here, however, and vehicles drive fast on the road.

If you're feeling ambitious, you can paddle the final miles of the Yahara until its confluence at the Rock River for a three-for-one paddling trifecta (see Yahara River B, page 168). While the current is swift, this makes for a long trip at 16.5 miles. It's great fun, though, and how often do you get to be on three rivers in one day?

CAMPING **Lake Kegonsa State Park** (2405 Door Creek Road, Stoughton; 608-873-9695)

RENTALS **Rutabaga Paddlesports** (220 W. Broadway, Madison; 608-223-9300); **Stoughton Canoe Rental** (2598 CR B, Stoughton; 920-728-0420)

FOOD FOR THOUGHT **Wendigo** (608-205-2775) and the **Viking Brew Pub** (608-719-5041) both offer good beer and food. **Fosdal Home Bakery** (608-873-3073) will fix your *lefse* and *krumkake* cravings, while **Laz Bistro & Bar** (608-492-0781) offers great entrées in a fun setting. Stoughton claims to be the home of the coffee break, and the **Koffee Kup** (608-873-6717) is a charming throwback in time. All of these establishments are on Main Street.

SHOUT-OUT Spend a little time in downtown **Stoughton,** a real gem of a place with a Main Street that feels exactly as Main Street should. There are lots of great shops and eateries and a great deal of Norwegian pride.

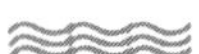

19 Bark River A:

NEMAHBIN LAKE TO ATKINS-OLSON MEMORIAL PARK

•THE•FACTS•

Put-in/take-out Sugar Island Road public boat launch/Atkins-Olson Memorial Park

Distance/time 9 mi/Allow for 5 hrs

Gradient/water level 1.5 fpm/Look for 90 cfs minimum at USGS gage 05426250 to avoid scraping. Above 150 cfs, you will likely need to portage around some of the farm bridges between Crooked Lake and WI 67.

Water type Flatwater and quietwater

Canoe or kayak Either

Skill level Beginner

Time of year to paddle Anytime

Landscape Glacial lakes, sedge meadow marsh, bogs, fens, hardwood forests, residential

---

OVERVIEW This is a truly adventurous trip, where the crystal-clear Bark River connects to glacial lakes and then meanders quietly through sedge meadows, bogs, and fens, on into downtown Dousman, and finally through a pretty hardwood area of little development. There are some obstructions, including a low-head dam, five low-clearance bridges, and downed trees toward the take-out, but all of these are

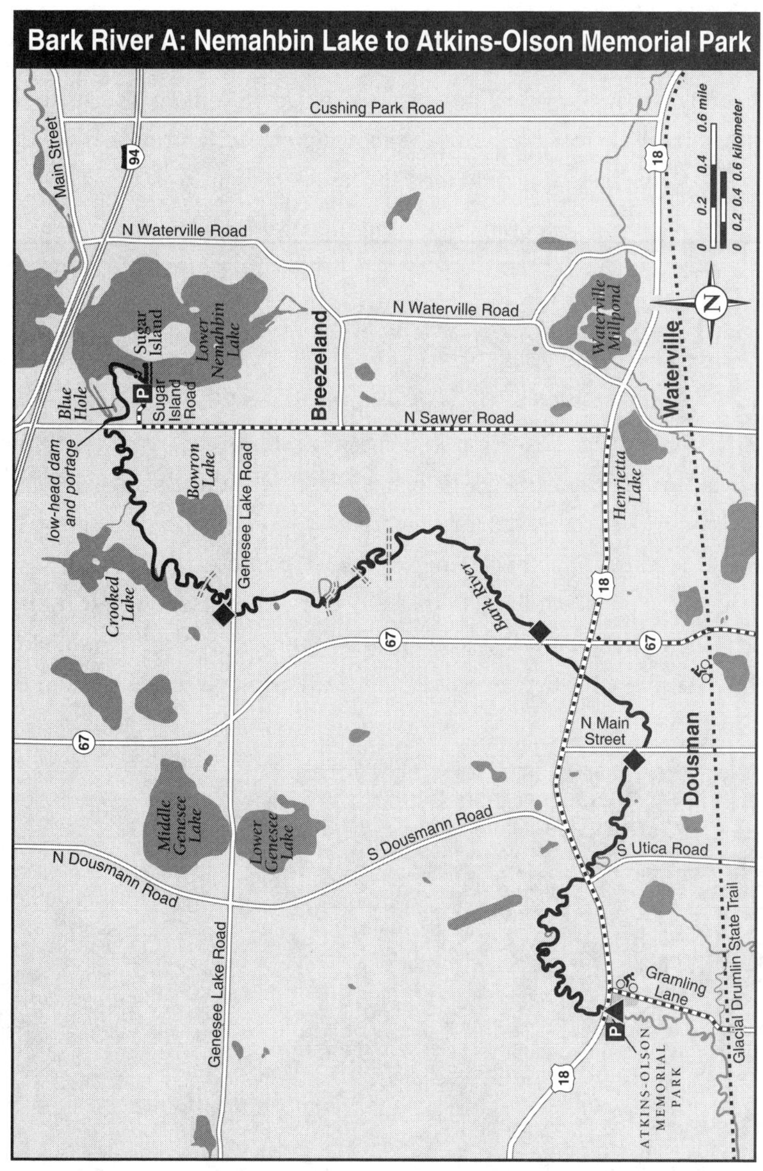

easily negotiated and worth the effort. Expect to see great blue and green herons, turkey vultures, sandhill cranes, duck varieties, owls, kingfishers, woodpeckers, frogs, muskrats, mussels, damselflies, and even freshwater sponge.

CAR SHUTTLE **5.3 miles.** From the take-out, head east on US 18 (a.k.a. Sunset Drive). After WI 67, turn left on CR P, then right on Sugar Island Road. Put in at the lake.

BIKE SHUTTLE 6.6 miles. Head east on US 18, then take your first right on Gramling Lane. Cross Scuppernong Creek, then turn left on the Glacial Drumlin State Trail. Follow the trail east across WI 67, then parallel to US 18. Where it turns to the right (south), you'll want to cross back into the shoulder of US 18 for only 100 yards, then left onto CR P to the put-in, as described above.

TAKE-OUT N43° 01.174' W88° 28.353' **PUT-IN** N43° 03.220' W88° 26.313'

•THE•FLAVOR•

PUT IN AT THE BOAT LAUNCH at the end of Sugar Island Road. The lake here is called Lower Nemahbin (the upper portion is on the other side of the I-94 bridge). The water clarity is excellent. Across from the launch is a large island with a dozen cabins on it but no roads or bridges to it. I don't recommend spending too much time on the lake, as it's large and rather popular with the powerboat, pontoon, and Jet Ski crowd.

You'll paddle northward less than 1,200 feet until you see a cleft in the shoreline, which is where the Bark River resumes its course. Here, the 70-mile-long Bark is roughly at its midpoint between Bark Lake, in Washington County, and the Rock

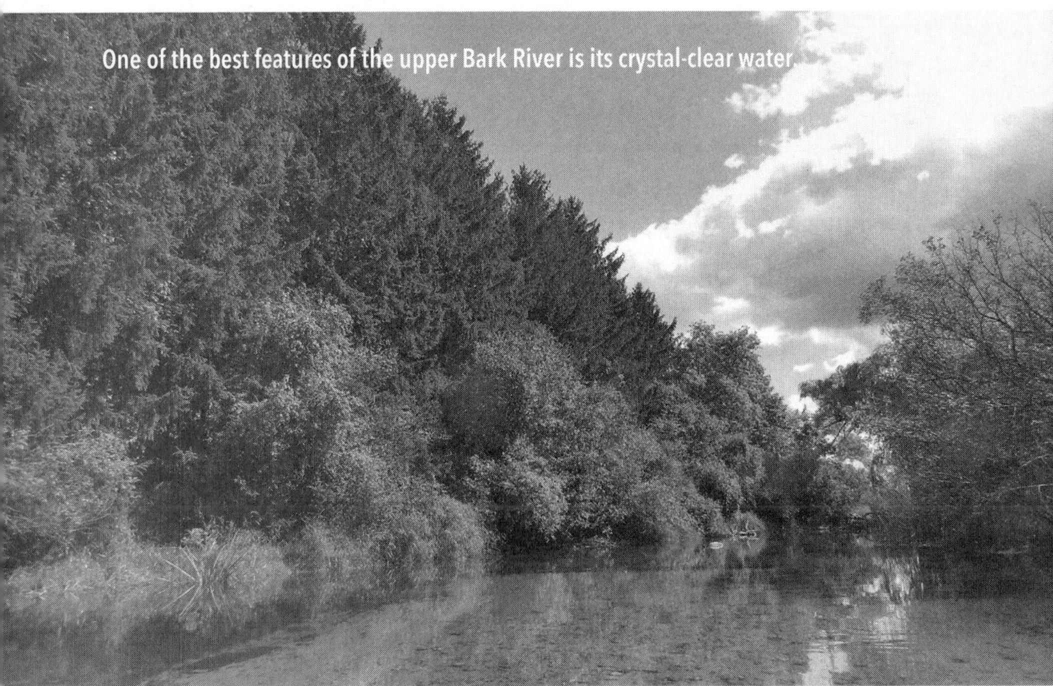

One of the best features of the upper Bark River is its crystal-clear water.

River, in Fort Atkinson. Only 20 feet wide for a while, the river is lined by cattails and aquatic plants in the absence of banks. You'll see an open channel on the right; it leads to a hidden pond called Blue Hole, whose color is cast by marl, a bog limestone found in shallow glacial lakes.

There's an abrupt right-hand turn where cute cottages line the dry land followed by the humbled remains of a long-forgotten canoe. There's a small low-head dam at the CR P bridge that monitors the lake level. Due to the low-clearance bridge immediately below the dam, it's unsafe to try to run this and best instead to portage around it on the right. It's a fun swimming hole, though.

Next, the Bark meanders through one of the prettiest stretches on this trip: a large cattail marsh all the way to Crooked Lake. About midway, you'll see a side channel on the right that takes you to the northern side of the lake, where it's undeveloped. This diversion is pretty and worth poking around for a look-see; or, you can simply continue on the main channel. Either way, once it reaches the lake, the main channel makes a tight horseshoe bend to the left and exits the lake as quickly as it came. This novelty of lake–river–lake–river paddling is quite splendid and truly lends itself to a sense of an adventure. Most of the time, you'd have no idea you were in suburbanized Waukesha County.

Below Crooked Lake, the streambed changes from silt and sand to softball-sized rocks. The current picks up a little (but not much), and the river is shallower. It's mostly on account of the next few miles that you don't want to paddle this trip below 90 cfs, unless you enjoy scraping and bottoming out. That said, in between Crooked Lake and WI 67 are five low-clearance farm bridges. In high(er) water, at least a couple of these will dictate portage. (One of these has an actual garbage can on the upstream side and a basketball net downstream.) Shortly after the first of these is Genesee Lake Road, where there's a convenient access on the upstream side of the bridge on the right. But for the farm bridges punctuating the river (and suggesting nearby farms), there's wonderfully nothing in the way of development out here.

Just before the next farm bridge will be the first of two large and lovely islands with attractive tamaracks. After this, the river will alternate between meanders and straightaways. In some sections, long stands of glorious pine line the left bank. Together with the crystal-clear water, it's easy to forget you're near Milwaukee, not Upper Michigan. (Alas, you'll also see a ditch with psychedelic algae that leads to a sewage-treatment plant.) You'll begin to see star grass shimmering in the current below you, a sometimes hypnotizing effect. The next two bridges are very low. The first is a required portage, while the second, at WI 67, is a probable one. There's a make-do access at WI 67 on the upstream side of the low bridge, on the left.

Town does encroach upon the ear for a little bit, mostly the sounds of traffic. After the first of several US 18/Sunset Drive bridges, you'll see a truly handsome set of Masonic Lodge buildings (though at the time of this writing these were slated to be razed) and a narrow, shallow channel that leads to a natural spring. These in turn are followed by a delightful arching footbridge. A mixture of backyards and thin woods encloses the river in the section leading to Main Street.

After Main Street and the municipal garage, you'll cross US 18 twice more; the second crossing signals the take-out. In this section, the Bark is very pretty and remote. The wildlife in particular is outstanding—seeing green herons and owls is a good bet—but the water loses its clarity as the landscape becomes boggy. This section also is prone to downfall. Much of it has been cleaned up and is now passable, but conditions change all the time. As such, I encourage you always to have a trusty handsaw with you and help saw off whatever obstructions you care to take on. Together, we can ensure that this bottom section is safe and fun. Understandably, though, you may wish simply to avoid this and take out at Main Street on the downstream side of the bridge, river left. The take-out just after the second US 18 bridge is at the small but convenient Atkins-Olson Memorial Park, on the right.

•THE•FUDGE•

ADDITIONAL TRIPS Continuing below the take-out is not recommended because the river becomes channelized and monotonously agricultural. Also, before you even arrive at Rome, you must paddle through a humongous pond, then reconcile the dam that created it.

Much more sanguine are the varied sections of the river upstream of the interstate. From its headwaters at Bark Lake to this trip's put-in, the Bark River flows for some 25 miles past a mixed palette of marsh, drumlins, rock quarries, public parks, one swamp, a couple of huge lakes, a few dams (one with a historic mill in Delafield), a charming urban downtown, and a lot of backyards. There is an exciting light whitewater stretch for 1 mile through Hartland, from Bark Park to Nixon Park. (The only section definitely not worth your time is from Willow Creek Road to County Line Road—a hell of impenetrable alders.) Catching the river with enough water will be tricky, though.

CAMPING **Kettle Moraine State Forest-Lapham Peak Unit** (W329 N846 CR C, Delafield; 262-646-3025)

RENTALS Sherpers (225 E. Wisconsin Ave., Oconomowoc; 262-567-6847).

FOOD FOR THOUGHT For some great authentic Mexican dishes, check out Sunny Side Up, at 159 WI 67 in Dousman (262-965-5745). It looks like a tacky family restaurant from the outside—OK, from the inside too—and the name connotes a basic breakfast menu, but you can order dishes like *lomo de res en chile de arbol, pollo o carne asada a la tampiqueña,* and even Mexican fried ice cream.

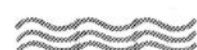

20 Bark River B: ROME DAM TO HEBRON

•THE•FACTS•

Put-in/take-out Rome Dam off County Road F/Hebron Campground. See "The Flavor" for three alternative access points.

Distance/time 10.6 mi/Allow for 5 hrs

Gradient/water level 4.5 fpm/See USGS gage 05426250. You'll need a minimum of 80 cfs to avoid scraping. Ideal levels are between 120 and 180 cfs.

Water type Quietwater, countless riffles, two Class I rapids, one Class I–II ledge

Canoe or kayak Either

Skill level Experienced

Time of year to paddle Anytime, but duckweed flourishes in high summer heat.

Landscape Hardwood forest, marshy bottomlands, glacial valley with drumlins

---

OVERVIEW Wend your way through picturesque hardwood forests, drumlins, and wetlands on clear water created by an ancient glacier in a predominantly undisturbed area. With outstanding wildlife opportunities and a handful of riffles and rapids, this is a superior stretch of the Bark River's 70 miles. Expect to see sandhill cranes, great blue and green herons, hawks, osprey, turkeys, turkey vultures, turtles, frogs, fish, mussels, mink, and deer.

SHUTTLE 6.7 miles. (*Note:* Before deciding on your shuttle route, you may want to read through "The Flavor," where I've mentioned alternative access points, in case you want to make this trip shorter.) From the campground take-out, turn right onto

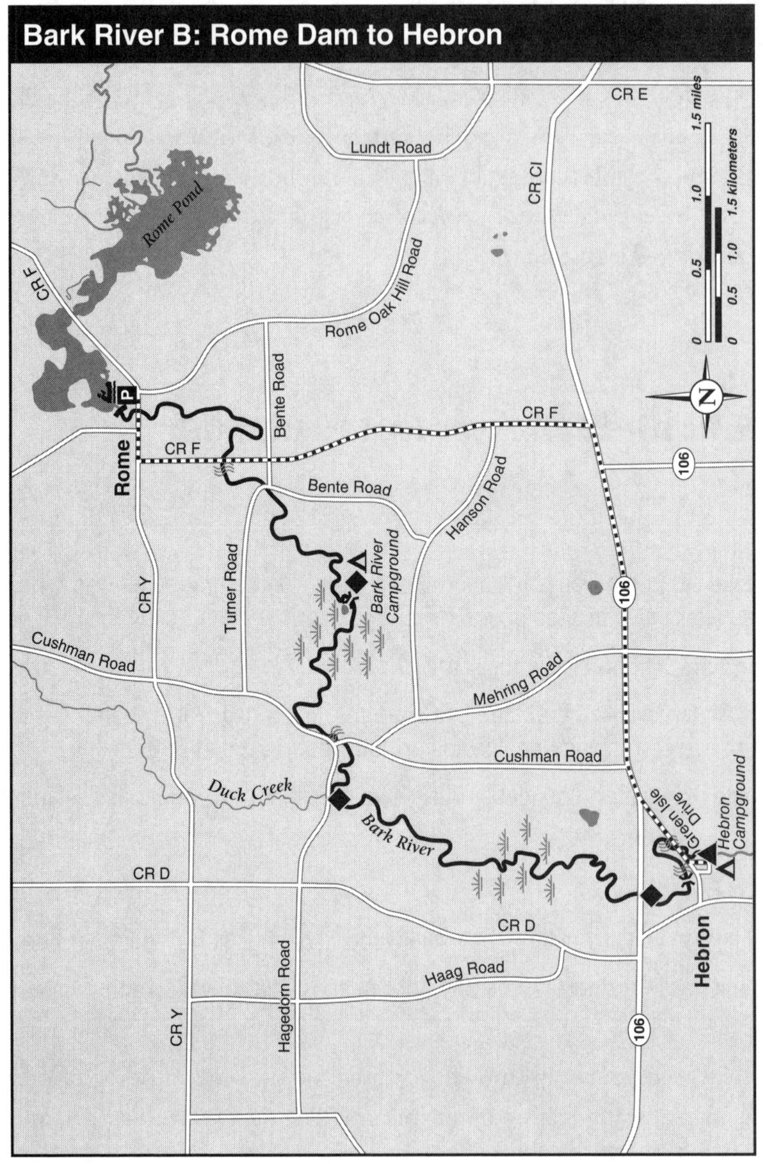

Green Isle Drive. When crossing the bridge, look left to visually scout the Class I–II ledge for obstructions or hazards. Turn right onto WI 106. Turn left onto CR F just after WI 106 turns south. Travel north on CR F to the stop sign in Rome; turn right onto Main Street (also CR F). After crossing the river, turn left onto the dirt road next to the old mill. A public parking area is up ahead.

TAKE-OUT N42° 55.455' W88° 41.201'

PUT-IN N42° 58.902' W88° 37.676'

•THE•FLAVOR•

FROM THE PARKING AREA, you'll walk 500 feet to the dam. There is no designated boat launch, but it's easy to access the river here; just don't get too close to the dam. As you approach the attractive old mill on the left, you'll see an outflow from the former millrace. Delightful riffles or light rapids (depending on water levels) await underneath the Main Street bridge. On your right, you'll see an alternate access point to the river at the parking lot of Pickets Country Store (a great place for supplies, by the way). Take a moment to turn around, facing upstream, to appreciate the sweeping view of a luxurious weeping willow, the first of many on this trip, and the old Rome Feed Mill behind it.

For the first mile, you'll pass a large campground on the right with two canal-like inlets and a cattail-marsh environment. You'll pass a gentle hill on the left at the top of which is a small cemetery; many of the gravestone surnames are of prominent families who settled the area, after whom several area roads are also named. Delightful riffles flourish underneath the Palmyra Road and Turner Road bridges. At Turner Road, there is a makeshift access to the water on both banks (**N42° 58.031' W88° 38.270'**). Putting in here cuts off 2 miles from Rome.

A straightaway leads to an iconic brick farmhouse nestled at the base of a prominent drumlin that diverts the river to the right. Unless the duckweed is high, which does happen in the heat of summer, the water clarity on the Bark is outstanding. Consisting mostly of sand and gravel and large boulders (called *erratics*) here and there, the Bark is a great example of a glacial stream. A couple of zigzags left and right take you past another campground, where there's access on the right before a pedestrian bridge (**N42° 57.556' W88° 39.156'**). Putting in here cuts off more than 3.5 miles of paddling from Rome.

For only 100 yards, you will pass sites on your left, after which the river will bend to the right, and you will quickly feel transported to a blissfully abandoned landscape. The river will split in two around a giant island in a mixed setting of marsh and hardwoods that feels wild and looks wonderful. Both channels are pleasant and allow passage, but I recommend going right, which is usually deeper. The right channel will then also split, and this time I recommend choosing the left channel, which will take you closer to an attractive wooded drumlin, the river following a flowy, cursive letter *S* from top to bottom. Really, though, any route you choose should be fine.

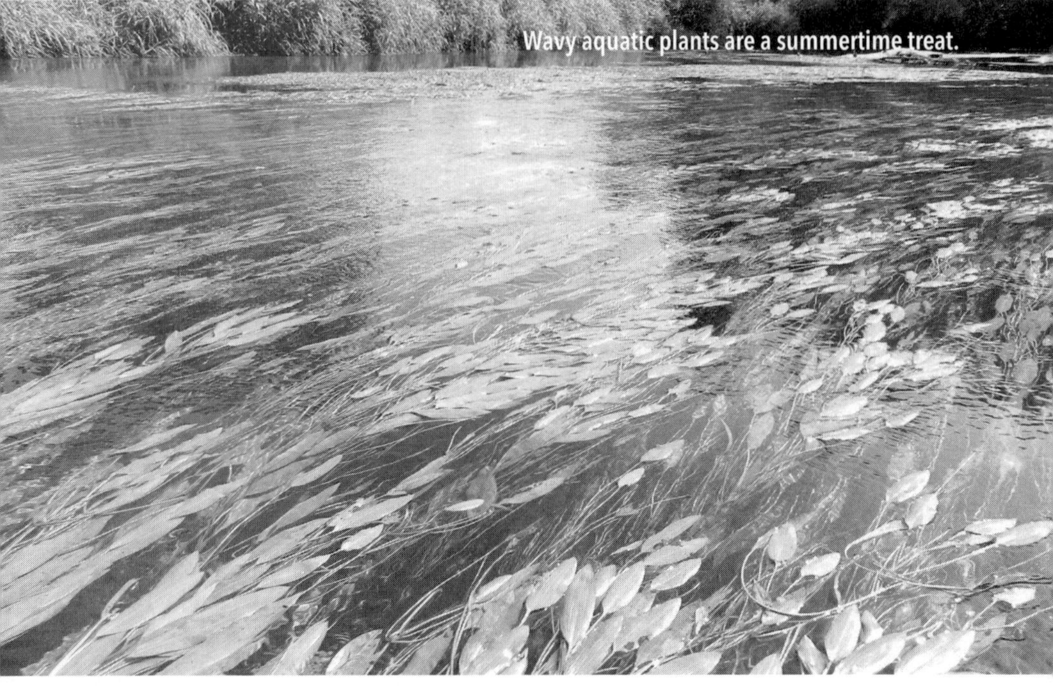
Wavy aquatic plants are a summertime treat.

As you slalom south then north through two modest drumlins, you will enter what used to be a prominent pond that was a popular resort back in its day. The river will make an abrupt left-hand bend near Cushman Road and course through a modest valley where the banks constrict and the river bottom becomes rocky and shallow, tumbling toward the bridge. Here is the site of a mill that had created the dam upstream, once a stagecoach stop between Madison and Milwaukee with a premier dance hall. Today there is a pleasant Class I rapid where the dam used to be. Riffles will whisk you westward below the bridge as the river meanders past the mouth of Duck Creek on the right.

The water here is crystal clear and the river bottom sandy for a short while. By midsummer, many plants will wave in the current. The`width will vary between 30 and 50 feet. Tree-lined banks lend a sense of privacy on the water. It's mostly farm fields anyway, so the sense of isolation is delightfully real. You'll pass a large triangular island after a short straightaway, followed by an attractive farm bridge. Woods will enclose both banks in another straightaway.

You'll find innumerable log stumps in the river on this trip, none too difficult to dodge. However, you may well encounter one ugly clog of downed trees to portage during this stretch. Once things open up again, an agricultural ditch will be on your right, followed by a couple of meanders leading to another straightaway. The left bank will rise to 6 feet, a mix of sand and soil.

Soon you'll begin seeing oxbows everywhere in a classic bottomlands floodplain; just follow the direction of the current and you'll be fine. The environs here feel completely different than upstream. Gone are the drumlins and cattail marshes, replaced by a swamp of thick woods through which the river slowly meanders. The diversity is intriguing, and a lush canopy of leafy green trees provides welcome shade in the summer heat. There's even a heron rookery off to the left; look for the cluster of large nests in the treetops.

On the downstream side of the WI 106 bridge on the left is another alternative access point (**N42° 55.852' W88° 41.466'**). If you wish to skip running or portaging around the Class I–II ledge in Hebron, you might want to take out here instead of downstream at the next campground.

The gradient will gradually increase in the next mile, the river bottom rocky and shallow. After an abrupt left turn, riffles will pick up in earnest, leading you to an attractive red bridge. Fun standing waves form here when the river is high. It's this section of the trip that earns it the 80-plus-cfs requirement. It's not dangerous, but you do have to navigate some boulders and tree limbs in swift current.

The river then makes an unusual mushroom-shaped curve before heading due south to a fun Class I–II drop of 2 feet where a dam was removed (another fortuitous casualty of the 2008 flooding). It's wise to scout this on the right shore before running it or from the road during the shuttle. You can portage around it on the right, but it

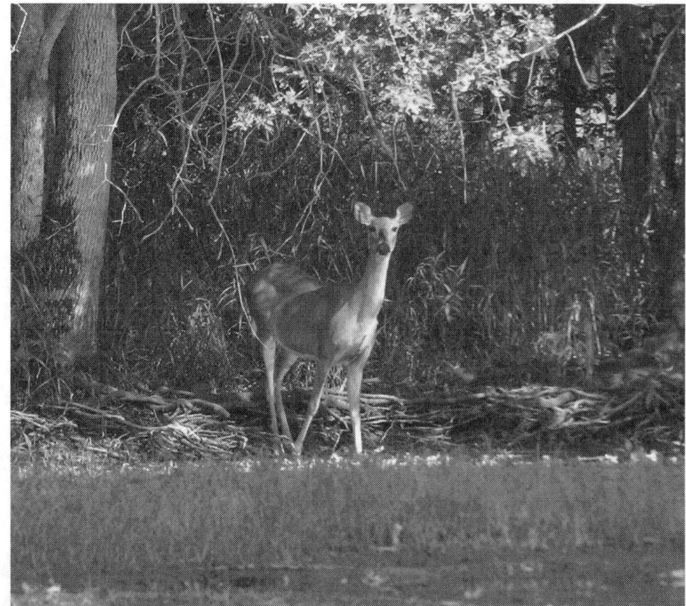

The wildlife sightings along the Bark River are excellent.

will be tricky. Small boulders lie on the right and left below the drop, so it's best to run the drop just to the left of center. Be careful of the potential backroller at the bottom of the drop when the river is high (above 200 cfs).

The river remains shallow below the next bridge, and the water turns muddy. Alas, this turbidity shall be found for the remainder of the Bark River to its confluence with the Rock River in Fort Atkinson. After a couple of easy curves, you'll see the cute Hebron Campground on the right. Again, there is no designated launch, so take out on the right where it's least obtrusive but still comfortable.

•THE•FUDGE•

ADDITIONAL TRIPS One can paddle downstream an additional mile to Koch Road and take out on the upstream side of the bridge on river left, but it's steep and rocky. Upstream of Rome, there is a huge pond created by a dam. Beginning in Sullivan via CR E, the Bark is quite wild and marshy before becoming full-on lake paddling.

CAMPING **Bark River Campground & Resort** (W2340 Hanson Road, Slabtown; 262-593-2421); **Hebron Campground,** at the take-out (N2316 Museum Road, Fort Atkinson; 262-593-8765); or **Rome Riverside Campground** (N3780 W. Water St., Sullivan; 262-593-8663)

RENTALS **2 Rivers Bicycle & Outdoor** (33 W. Sherman Ave., Fort Atkinson; 920-563-2222)

SHOUT-OUTS For a delightful and admirably researched book about the Bark River from both a paddling and historical perspective, check out ***The Bark River Chronicles: Stories from a Wisconsin Watershed,*** by Milton J. Bates.

Special thanks to **Hebron Campground** for generously allowing noncampers to use their grounds to take out for this paddling trip without charging a fee. Please consider patronage, whether camping, dining, or purchasing supplies. It is, of course, still courteous to let someone know that you are there to paddle and will be leaving a vehicle. Ask for Joanne or Ralph. (*Full disclosure:* Joanne trained me as a letter carrier at the USPS for a very short-lived stint during a particularly frigid January.)

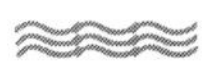

21 Bark River C: KOCH ROAD TO BURNT VILLAGE PARK

•THE•FACTS•

Put-in/take-out Koch Road/County Road N

Distance/time 10.2 mi/Allow for 5 hrs

Gradient/water level 1 fpm/See USGS gage 05426250. Levels are reliable year-round, but I don't recommend paddling this when the river is too high, as it will be virtually impossible to follow the main channel in the Prince's Point floodplain forest.

Water type Flatwater

Canoe or kayak Kayak preferred until CR D, due to the many meanders and obstacles to maneuver

Skill level Experienced

Time of year to paddle Anytime, though especially lovely in spring. Expect duckweed in late summer. This is a good trip to paddle after rain to wash downstream some of the natural muck.

Landscape Hardwoods, marshy bottomlands, meadows, and savannas

---

OVERVIEW The most primitive section anywhere on the Bark River, here you will paddle through the heart of a spectacular wildlife preserve and see virtually no development whatsoever until the final mile of this slow yet truly tranquil trip. What you will likely see, however, are songbirds, sandhill cranes, great blue herons, great egrets, hawks, wood ducks, woodpeckers, painted and softshell turtles, frogs, fish, clams, kingfishers, swans, and deer.

SHUTTLE 5.6 miles. From the take-out, turn right onto CR N, cross the river, then turn right onto Lower Hebron Road. Most of the shuttle is on this road, which is particularly pretty and rural. After a right-hand bend, turn left onto Hoffman Road. Turn right onto CR D, then take your first left onto Koch Road. Park along the road.

TAKE-OUT N42° 54.901' W88° 46.760' **PUT-IN** N42° 54.778' W88° 41.176'

•THE•FLAVOR•

PUT IN AT THE UPSTREAM SIDE of the Koch Road bridge on river left. It is not a designated landing, and the slope is steep; but the vegetation is light and the launch

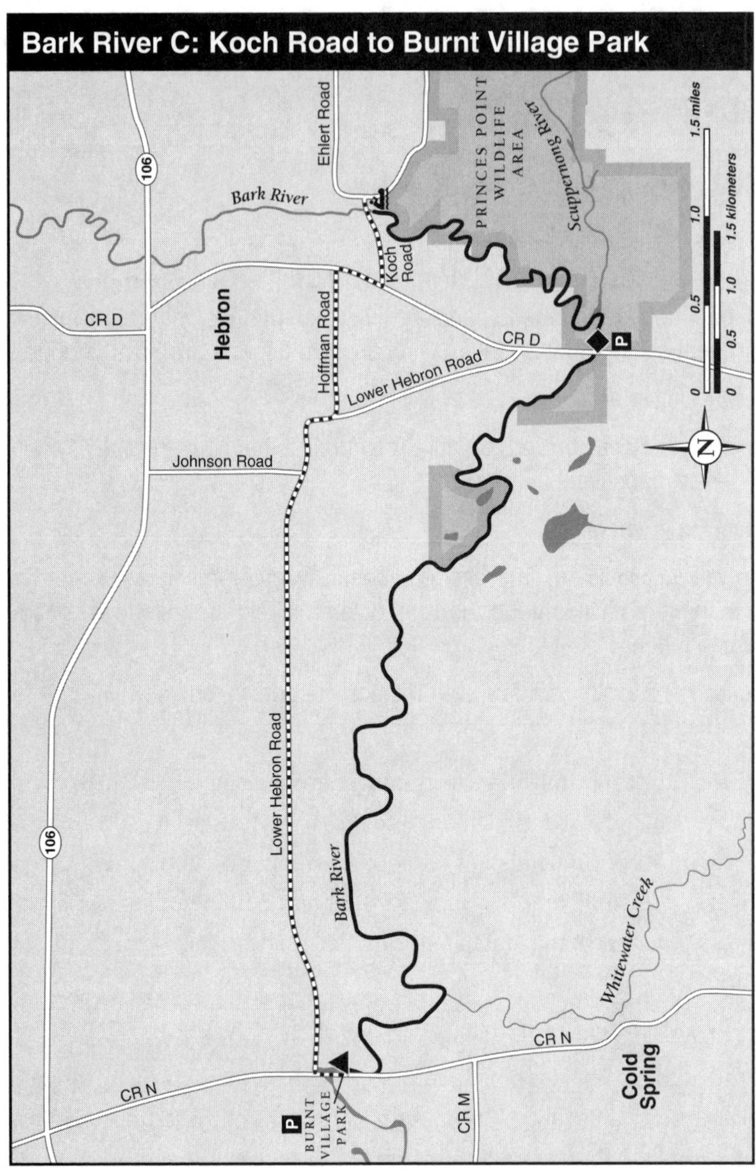

is from rocks, not mud. If there is any doubt of the suitability, put in at Hebron Campground 1 mile upstream instead (see previous trip). Here, the Bark is still narrow, at 40 feet wide, but deeper than upstream. The river will flow due south for 100 yards before swinging to the right past a quaint red barn, one of very few buildings you'll see on this trip, and then making a sharp left bend. A straightaway follows; embrace it, for downstream there are constant meanders and maneuvering around downed trees.

Soon woods enclose. You are now entering the gorgeous and utterly secluded Prince's Point Wildlife Area, a bottomland hardwood forest and open-water marsh 2,000 acres large. A series of long-abandoned drainage ditches like clefts in the landscape will be seen on the right. Some are interesting to explore, particularly in hopes of spotting wildlife, but none leads to anywhere in particular.

For the next 1.5 miles, the river will switchback, but the landscape is striking; you'll be glad to take the time. Rows of random wildflowers add colorful contrasts to the brown water and green leaves. Where it is marsh, the landscape is low but lush; the woods are haunting. Considerable work has been done to keep the river clear of formidable obstructions while retaining its natural and wild feel.

There will be at least one fallen tree that will require portaging over or around it. To be sure, downed trees are numerous until CR D. Getting over, under, and through these should not be difficult, but the maneuvering will be constant for the first 3 miles. Don't worry: The views of a preserved setting and the outstanding flora and fauna don't make this section feel like work. Clumps of cottonwoods line the right bank, swampy and exotic. Attractive views of rising uplands to your right will balance out the bottomlands.

At a certain point, the river will run parallel to a large ditch (this time on the left), separated only by a 70-foot-wide isthmus. It lies only 0.25 mile downstream from two consecutive ditches on the right. It's worth getting out of your boat (if it

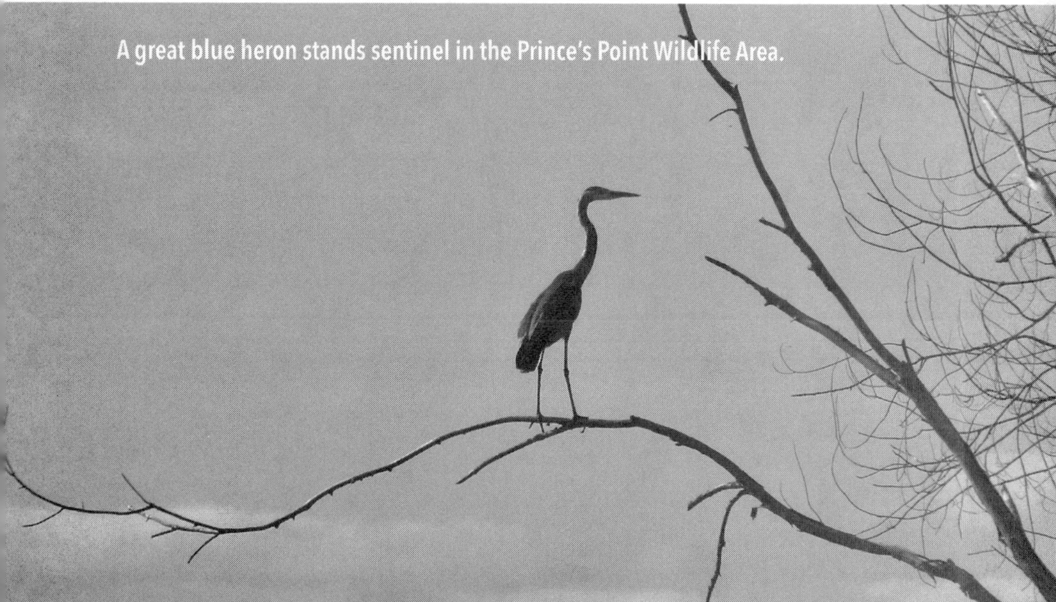
A great blue heron stands sentinel in the Prince's Point Wildlife Area.

isn't too muddy or the vegetation too overgrown and potentially tick-ridden) and onto terra firma for a look around. In early spring, most of the bottomlands will be flooded, allowing you to paddle pretty much wherever you wish.

That said, without banks it's easy to become disoriented and not know where the main stream is. Added to that confusion is the confluence of the Scuppernong River coming in from the east only 1,000 feet upstream from the CR D bridge. If you have the time and inclination, paddling upstream the "Scup" is a beautiful diversion. Otherwise, keep to the right past a lovely meadowy marsh off to your left. After the confluence, you'll enter a short corridor of hardwood bottomlands thick and deep heading toward CR D. If you wish to shorten this trip, there is a dedicated boat landing 200 feet upstream of the bridge, on the left at a convenient gravel apron (**N42° 53.653' W88° 42.068'**).

Below the bridge, the river bulges to 70 feet wide and the need to maneuver obstructions will abate. Alas, the current will slow down considerably. Lush tree canopy prevails for the next mile before the landscape opens up unto lovely marsh and meadows. After it does, the vast vacancy takes your breath away, so different in feel than the previous 4 miles. Egrets and herons should be numerous.

Be sure to wear sunscreen here, as there won't be much relief for quite a while. By contrast, on an overcast or even lightly drizzling day, this stretch can become positively melancholy. Here and there, you'll see the peripheries of rising uplands, mostly to your right, off to the north. After a series of gentle meanders, you'll relax on a pleasant straightaway along which a knoll of conifers is mirrored in the still water against a spectacular sky.

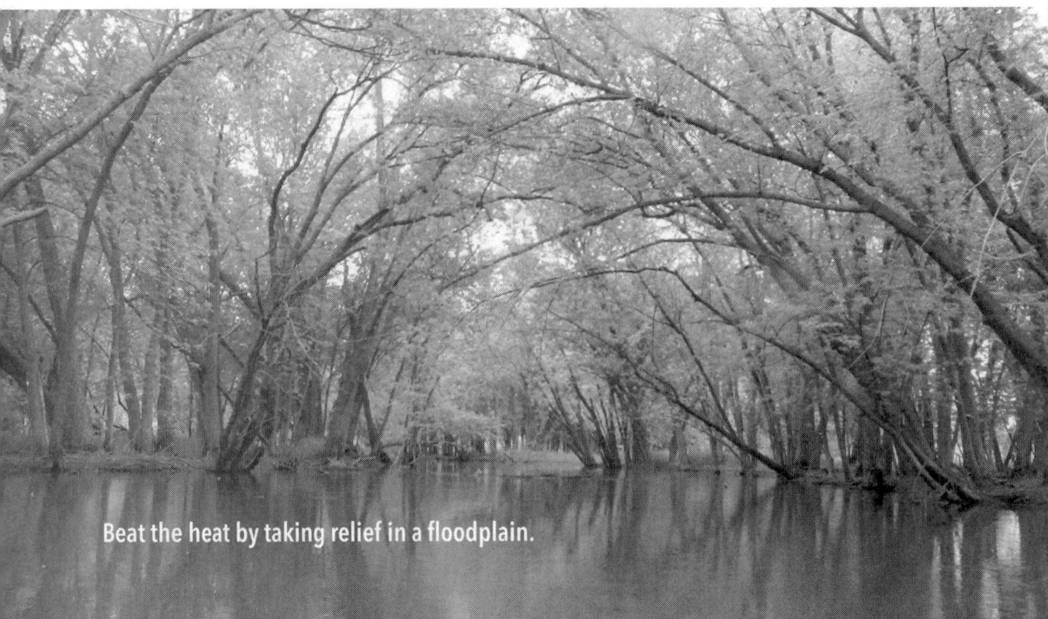
Beat the heat by taking relief in a floodplain.

Soon the river will narrow modestly, and the banks rise to 10 feet. You'll come upon a long line of seemingly random riprap on the right near a private residence before the final mile that feels lush and wild. At the bottom of an S-curve toward the right, you'll pass the mouth of Whitewater Creek on your left and an attractive truss bridge. (Incidentally, this creek can be paddled, but it's monotonous and nondescript.)

A straightaway, bend to the left, another straightaway, and bend to the right are all that remain until the take-out. After the right-hand bend, you'll hear passing cars along CR N, which will run parallel to the river. Modest riprap will line the base of the left bank signaling the property of Burnt Village Park. Take out at the boat landing on the left, upstream of the bridge.

•THE•FUDGE•

ADDITIONAL TRIPS Downstream from Burnt Village Park are the Bark River's last 6 miles before it meets the Rock River in Fort Atkinson. It's pretty and pleasant in its own right, but it's more developed and louder than this trip, and it offers nothing that you don't already experience in between Prince's Point and Burnt Village. Conversely, for an all-in-one trip, combine parts of this and the previous sections of the Bark by putting in at Bark River Campground and taking out at Prince's Point (an 11-mile trip).

CAMPING **Hebron Campground** (N2316 Museum Road, Fort Atkinson; 262-593-8765)

RENTALS **2 Rivers Bicycle & Outdoor** (33 W. Sherman Ave., Fort Atkinson; 920-563-2222)

SHOUT-OUTS The Bark River received its name from the peeled bark used for shingle-clad dwellings by the Ho-Chunk (Winnebago) Indians, who revered the river.

Burnt Village Park is the site of a military encampment where US Army Gen. Henry Atkinson stayed with his men while pursuing Chief Black Hawk during the Black Hawk War in 1832. Before the troops arrived, the site had been an Indian village, but it was burned down during an intra-tribal conflict and abandoned.

22 Illinois Fox River: COUNTY ROAD H TO COUNTY ROAD ES

•THE•FACTS•

Put-in/take-out County Road H/County Road ES. See "The Flavor" for an alternative access point.

Distance/time 11.4 mi/Allow for 5.5 hrs

Gradient/water level 1 fpm/minimum 100 cfs at USGS gage 05543830

Water type Quietwater

Canoe or kayak Either

Skill level Beginner

Time of year to paddle Anytime, though especially lovely in spring and autumn

Landscape Wetlands, cattail marsh, fens, glaciated hills

OVERVIEW This trip along an especially pretty section of the Illinois Fox or "Little Fox" River that meanders through the heart of the Vernon Wildlife Area is sure to reward you with tranquility and exquisite wildlife. Expect to see great blue herons, blue-winged teals, red-tailed hawks, great horned owls, bald eagles, sandhill cranes, pelicans (in season), minks, muskrats, beavers, turkeys, turkey vultures, turtles, otters, frogs, pheasants, swans, hooded mergansers, wood ducks, coots, even coyotes.

SHUTTLE **8 miles.** From the take-out, head east on CR ES, then turn left onto CR XX. Turn left onto CR I at the intersection. Turn right onto CR H. You'll come to the bridge in half a mile.

TAKE-OUT N42° 52.556' W88° 18.370' **PUT-IN** N42° 57.828' W88° 16.691'

•THE•FLAVOR•

PUT IN ON THE DOWNSTREAM SIDE of the CR H bridge on river right. (Alternatively, you can put in at Fox River Park, part of the Waukesha County parks system, but it costs $4 a day to leave your vehicle there, and it's not much of a boat launch besides.)

The river here is about 70 feet wide, which, with the exception of some narrow bends, will remain to be the case for most of this trip, though it will swell to a range

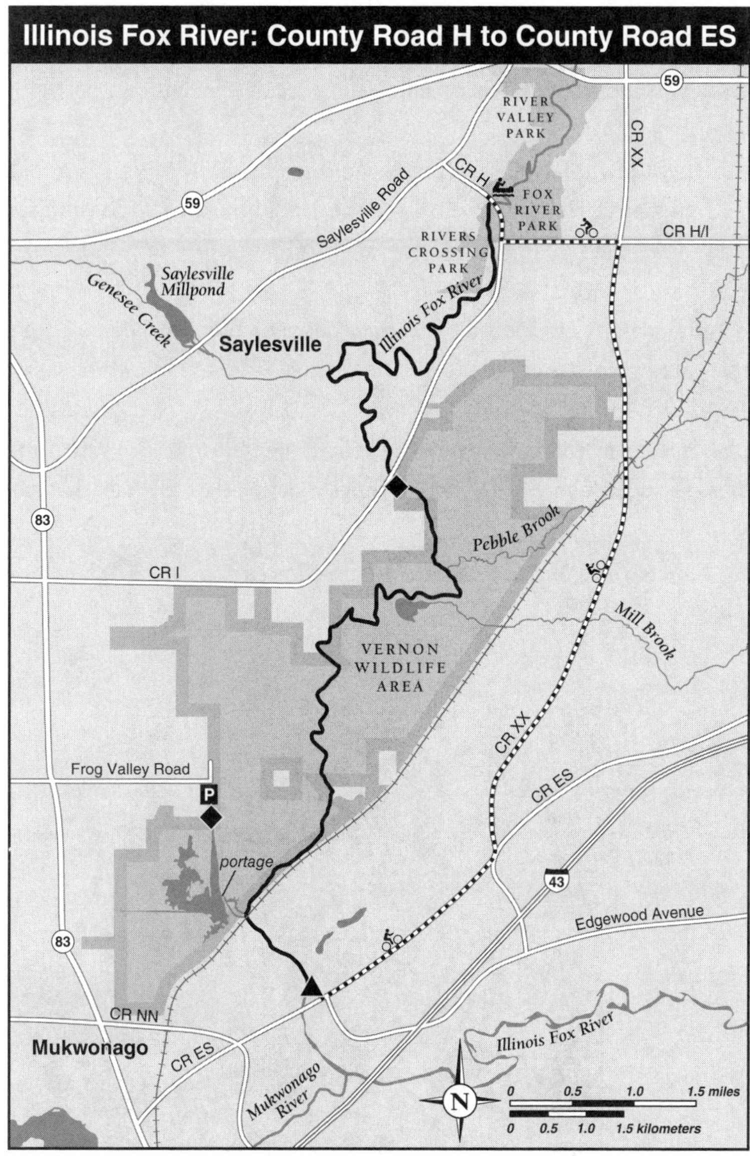

of 80–100 feet toward the take-out. Despite its width, the Illinois Fox is not a terribly deep river; so you don't want to paddle it if it's shallow, as you will scrape quite a lot. The clarity of the water is only so-so, but the bottom itself is predominantly sandy and attractive. While there is a small subdivision off to the right, you'll see it only briefly. Besides, the right bank rises to 10 feet high.

Just downstream from the put-in, a pleasant pedestrian bridge spans the river. It is followed by an appreciably undeveloped modest wetlands complex between the river and some humdrum subdivisions. On the left, however, are two soft-blue barns, both easy on the eye.

For the next few miles, CR I will run close to the river, so you'll probably hear some cars driving past. Here, too, you'll see the same housing subdivision for a brief moment, but after the river bends to the left, you'll escape the trappings of settlement as you enter the woods.

If mountains first have foothills that precede them, then consider the next 2 miles as the gentle gateway into the splendor of the Vernon Wildlife Area. The river will begin to meander in earnest, but the turns are easy to anticipate, so even canoes can handle these deftly. Tree cover will begin to increase incrementally, which in turn makes the trip feel more secluded, even if the surroundings remain relatively flat. That said, off in

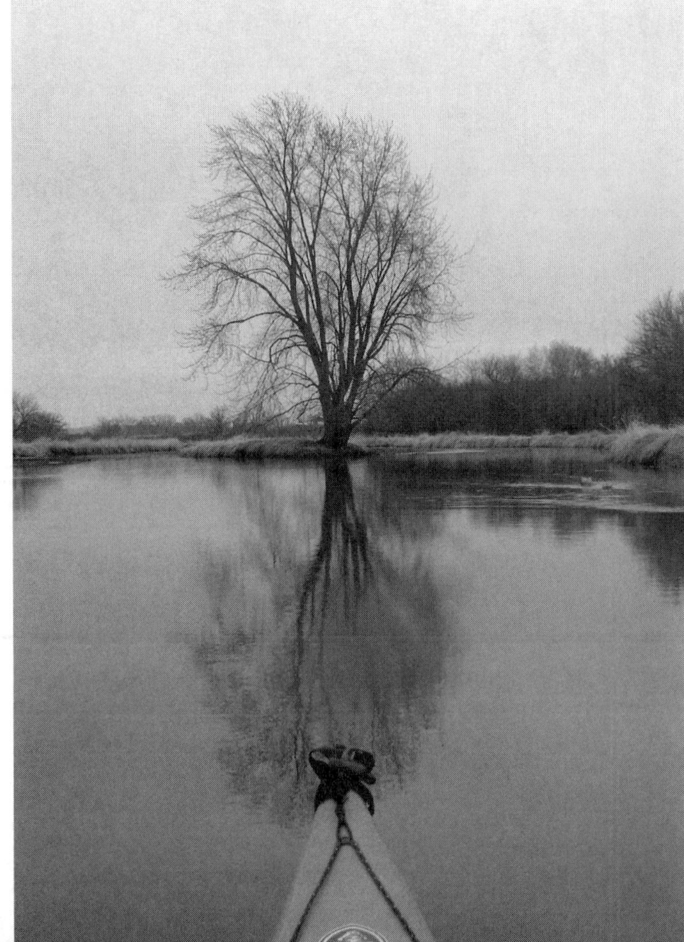

Stillness and solitude abound in the pretty Vernon Wildlife Area.

the distance you will begin to see some peek-a-boo glimpses of raised glacial moraines through occasional clearings, foreshadowing what's to come downstream.

In the meantime, simply relax and soak up the solitude. On a sunny day, going with the slow flow, a trip like this offers that rare passport back in time to simpler paces and sparser places. The environs are lush, and the wildlife is spectacularly diverse. You'll come upon beaver dams and certainly the tooth-gnawed whittling of tapered trunks, as well as bald eagle nests at the apex of abandoned trees. Beneath you, fish will swim and muskrats will dive once discovered. You may even see a mink or otter running on the banks or floating on its back.

More creased meanders take you to a raised left bank and some small islands. Soon you'll see on the right two buildings, one red and the other white. Just downstream is the only road bridge on this trip, at CR I, which offers a relatively easy alternative access point on the downstream side, river right (**N42° 56.024' W88° 17.580'**).

After the bridge, you'll enter into the heart of the marsh. The refuge is a 4,600-acre wetlands area with woods and a calcareous fen, a rare substrate of nonacidic peat in a wetlands complex reported to exist in only 10 states in the country. At a sharp left-hand turn, the left bank will be lined with riprap, allowing for easy access. If you get out of your boat here to stretch your legs or heed nature's call, you'll be atop a unique isthmus between the river and Pebble Brook.

As you continue downstream, the glimpses of glacial moraines increase. The contrast of cattails in the foreground and soft hills in the background is especially pleasant. By now, chances are pretty good that you'll have heard a train off in the distance. But it isn't until the last couple of miles that you'll see the accomplice to this bygone soundtrack: On the left, you'll see train tracks leading to a railroad bridge spanning the river. These trains haul freight, so if you can catch one, long as a man-made millipede, crossing over the river in its color-variegated carapace, the view is impressive, and your timing excellent.

As the river bends to the right to go underneath the railroad bridge, you'll see another marshy flowage on the right, this one marking the evocatively named Frog Alley. You'll have to portage over another isthmus and then paddle up to its northernmost reach, but it's an idyllic diversion if you have the time and inclination.

After the railroad bridge, there's only a little more than half a mile to the take-out on the upstream side of the bridge, river left. You'll probably hear traffic on CR ES, signaling the necessities of being back in a car yourself momentarily, but the view of a wooded hill on the left bank keeps you anchored to the memories of this special trip while looking forward to the next time you'll be here, perhaps in a different season, to appreciate this special place in a different shape.

•THE•FUDGE•

ADDITIONAL TRIPS Upstream of the put-in from downtown Waukesha is clogged with development and subdivisions and not worth your time. Downstream from the take-out, it's less than a mile before the confluence of the Mukwonago River, where the Illinois Fox takes a sharp swing to the east toward Big Bend, a pleasant enough 8-mile trip.

CAMPING **Mukwonago County Park** (S100 W31900 CR LO, Mukwonago; 262-363-7658)

FOOD FOR THOUGHT (AND RENTALS) For a comforting meal in a classic Wisconsin bar on the lake, check out **Eagle Springs Pub** (W345 S10463 CR E, Mukwonago; 262-594-2337), just west of the put-in. They also rent paddling equipment.

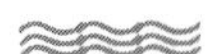

23 Koshkonong Creek: CAMBRIDGE TO HOOPEN ROAD

•THE•FACTS•

Put-in/take-out Water Street behind CamRock Cafe & Sport *or* dock off Water Street/ Hoopen Road. See "The Flavor" for an alternative take-out.

Distance/time 5.6 mi/Allow for 3 hrs

Gradient/water level 3 fpm/There is no gage, but water levels are usually reliable. Call CamRock Cafe & Sport (608-423-2111).

Water type Quietwater with some riffles

Canoe or kayak Either

Skill level Experienced

Time of year to paddle Anytime

Landscape Tree-canopied forest, rolling hills, bottomlands

OVERVIEW This trip on a cute creek half an hour outside of Madison runs through and along public land and offers options for trip lengths and a reputable current with intermittent riffles. The trip alternates between tree-canopied intimacy, wide-open

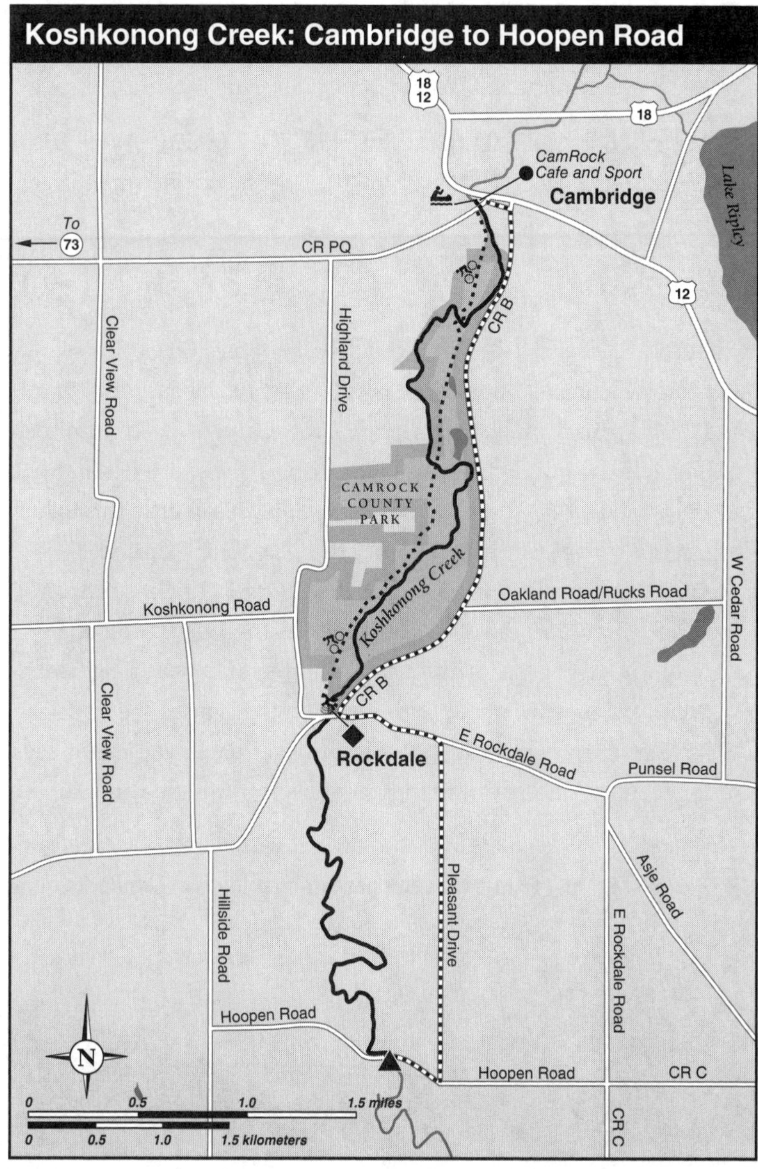

rolling hills shaped by glacial retreats, and some steep banks. Expect to see turtles, great blue herons, muskrats, songbirds, frogs, and maybe even a beaver and a bald eagle.

SHUTTLE 4.7 miles. From the take-out, head east on Hoopen Road, then turn left on Pleasant Drive. At the stop sign, turn left onto East Rockdale Road. In Rockdale, turn right onto CR B/Water Street. *If bike-shuttling, cross the intersection here and take the* *footbridge over the creek to the other side, then head north on the trail to Cambridge.* Take CR B into Cambridge. After South Street, on the right, turn left onto Spring Water Alley, then left onto Water Street.

TAKE-OUT N42° 57.077' W89° 01.620' **PUT-INS** N43° 00.212' W89° 01.192' (CamRock Cafe & Sport), N43° 00.179' W89° 01.156' (dock off Water Street)

•THE•FLAVOR•

WITH ITS HEADWATERS NEAR SUN PRAIRIE, Koshkonong Creek flows for some 40 miles before emptying into its namesake lake by Fort Atkinson. From Cambridge to Rockdale the "Kosh" runs through public land: the beautiful 440-acre CamRock County Park. It's a short bur tranquil 3-mile jaunt. This trip can be shortened in Rockdale for a pleasant 3-mile paddle that combines a fun 2.5-mile bike shuttle through CamRock County Park; this is a great way to experience the bike-shuttle option.

Put in at Water Street on river right behind CamRock Cafe & Sport or at the dock on river left. There may be a few obstacles in the first 0.5 mile; any that you encounter should be negotiated cautiously. Volunteers do admirably clear out this section, but what you encounter always depends on the time of the last cleanup.

CR B parallels the creek on the left. On the right bank, you might see an occasional hiker or bicycler. The surroundings here begin through a tree canopy in the

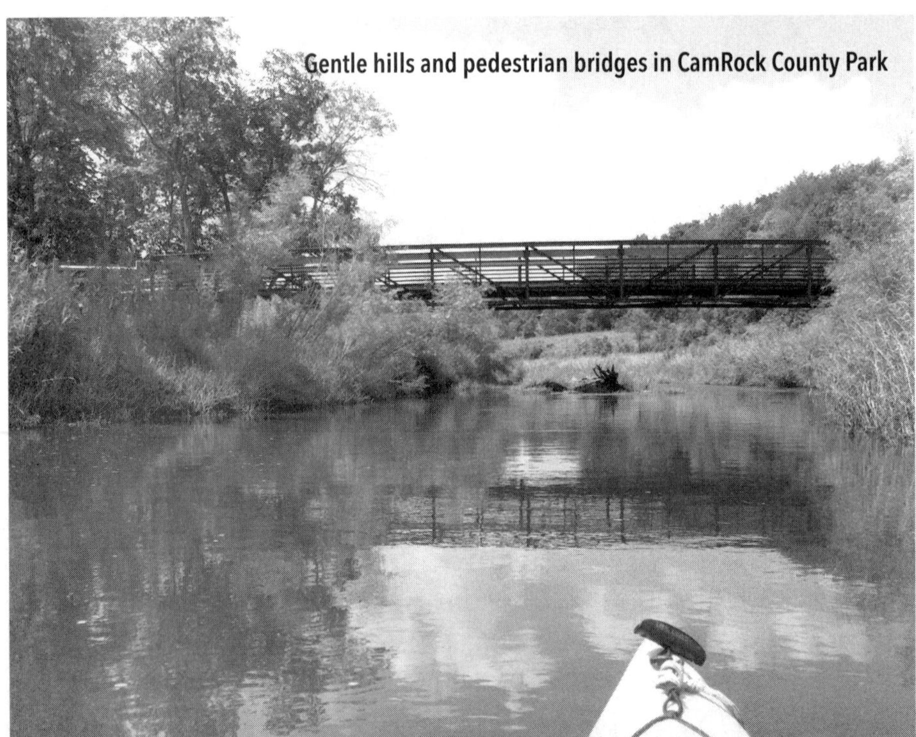

Gentle hills and pedestrian bridges in CamRock County Park

Photo: Barry Kalpinski/MilesPaddled.com

northern portion of CamRock County Park, making for a pleasant respite on a hot summer day. Shortly after you pass under the first footbridge, the trees will begin to thin out and the landscape widen. This is probably the prettiest portion of this trip, as the rolling terrain and hills left by the retreat of the last glacier open up before you.

Just downstream of the second footbridge, a few large islands in this section offer different channels through which you could paddle. As the creek swings to the east, you'll see the largest hill in the park to the west, where there is a pavilion and picnic area at the top.

Approaching the third and final footbridge, you will begin to see houses off to the right. A fun series of riffles and a very small drop below the CR B bridge in Rockdale await you. It's not whitewater, but it's a lot of fun just the same. Or you can take out just upstream of the riffles, on the left, at the grassy slope that leads to a small parking area on Water Street (**N42 58.375' W89° 01.931'**).

Downstream of Rockdale, the creek has an entirely different feel, with more leafy greens and bottomlands but still with a good current. In Rockdale, you'll pass a half-dozen houses on the left bank. After this, there's no development but an occasional farm until the take-out. At times, the isolation feels wild and remote. After some pleasant meandering comes a long straightaway south toward Hoopen Road. The creek turns sharply left. The take-out is on the downstream side of the bridge on the right. *Note:* On the upstream side is private property—*do not take out there.*

•THE•FUDGE•

ADDITIONAL TRIPS Farther downstream of Hoopen Road presents more obstacles and poor access options. There are 9 miles of creek between Hoopen Road and Rockdale Road that you can paddle, but it's hardly different than what you've experienced here. Below Rockdale Road to Lake Koshkonong is a nightmare of logjams and swamp. If you try to put in at Britzkie Road, the creek is channelized and access is difficult.

CAMPING **Sandhill Station State Campground** (N5584 Mud Lake Road, Lake Mills; 920-648-8774)

RENTALS **CamRock Cafe & Sport** (217 W. Main St., Cambridge; 608-423-2111)

FOOD FOR THOUGHT For thoughtfully prepared sandwiches and salads or a good bottle of local beer, stop by **CamRock Cafe & Sport**, or for good ol' bar food, stop by the **Rockdale Bar and Grill** (222 Water St., Rockdale; 608-423-3323).

24 Mukwonago River: COUNTY ROAD LO TO COUNTY ROAD I

•THE•FACTS•

Put-in/take-out Parking area off County Road LO/County Road I

Distance/time 4.7 mi/Allow for 2.5 hrs

Gradient/water level 3.5 fpm/minimum of 70 cfs at USGS gage 05544200 to avoid scraping

Water type Quietwater with riffles and two small Class I ledges

Canoe or kayak Kayak

Skill level Experienced

Time of year to paddle Anytime there's enough water

Landscape Rolling hills, kettle ponds, tallgrass prairie, wild-rice beds, oak savanna, cattail marsh

---

OVERVIEW A beautiful clear stream surround by Kettle Moraine topography that is virtually undeveloped, the Mukwonago is just a delight and worth the drive. Expect to encounter muskrats, ducks, geese, great blue herons, sandhill cranes, red fox, fish, mussels, and maybe even a mink.

SHUTTLE 2.9 miles. From the take-out, head north on CR I for 900 feet, then turn left onto CR LO. Turn left into a small parking area 1.2 miles after Beulah Road. The river is 400 feet south of the parking area.

TAKE-OUT N42° 51.622' W88° 21.923' **PUT-IN** N42° 51.332' W88° 25.088'

•THE•FLAVOR•

DESIGNATED ONE OF WISCONSIN'S "Last Great Places" by the state chapter of The Nature Conservancy, the Mukwonago River watershed is a living laboratory of healthy wetlands set in the topography of the Kettle Moraine State Forest. As such, the river is home to a wide diversity of cool critters, like mink, salamanders, tree frogs, and the longear sunfish. Even that veritable curmudgeon of the piscine family, the longnose gar, can be found trolling these waters. Indeed, more than 50 varieties of fish and 15 different

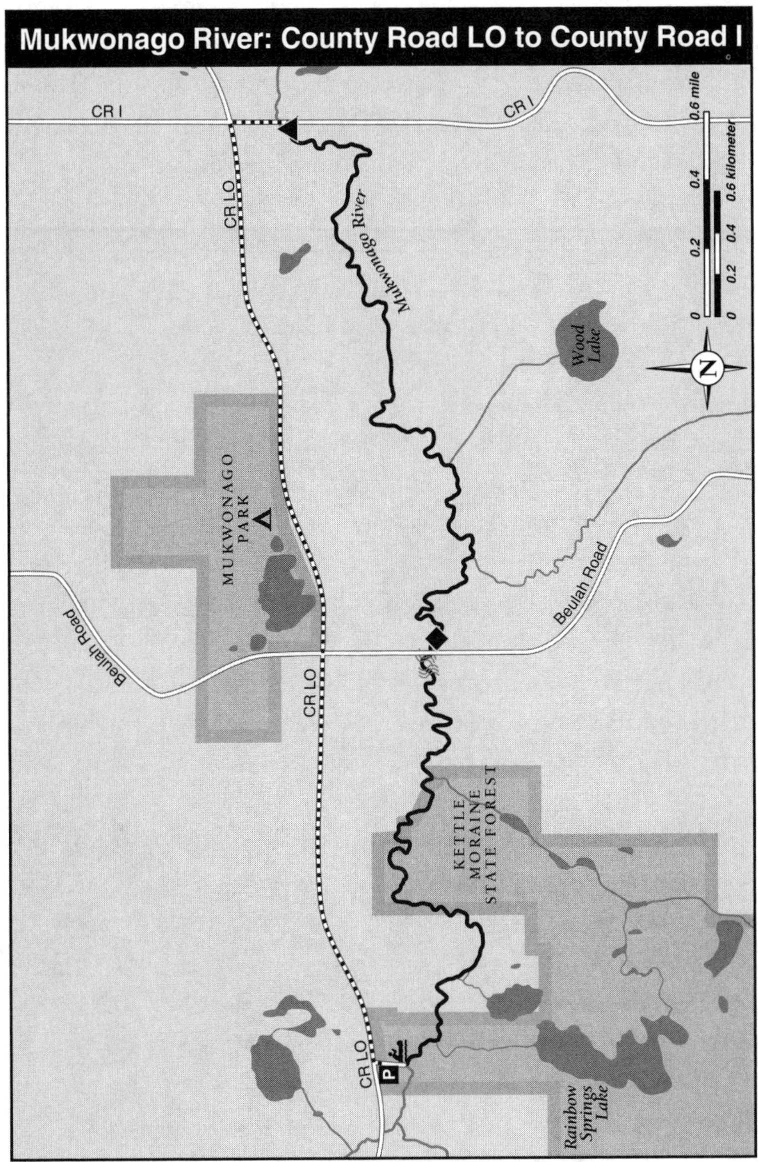

species of freshwater mussels have been found in this rather tiny stream, a remarkable testament to its health and wellness. Altogether, the watershed is a mosaic of wetlands, pine plantations, oak savannas, streams, and kettle lakes, much of it publicly protected.

Put in on the downstream side of the bridge culvert, river left. Since this is a short trip, you may try your luck paddling upstream, but it's a little more than a mile, very shallow, sluggish against the steady current, and prone to deadfall. It's much more practical to begin below the culvert. The river—it's really more like a creek—is only 20 feet or so wide, and there are obstacles to dodge, duck under, and slide over. But these vestiges preserve the wild beauty of the place; there's no airbrushed makeover here.

That said, the good folks at Friends of the Mukwonago River do an outstanding job of keeping an open channel to prevent the need to portage. The river meanders with a cursive grace, not the seeming indecisiveness of some streams that switchback in oxbow sloughs. Gentle hills slope near the banks in the near background, many comprising gnarled oaks in a sun-washed savanna. The water is crystal clear, the bottom alternating between sand, silt, and rocks. The Mukwonago is adorned and adoring.

About a mile in, you'll begin seeing golf balls on the bottom of the river—a lot of golf balls. Before the land was enveloped as a parcel in the state forest, it had been a golf course and resort, the operation of which came to an abrupt end after a fire in 2003. The state acquired the property five years later to keep it protected from development and promoted for recreation. Today, a cluster of white golf balls on a bank looks like so many duck eggs for want of a nest. A kid could do well collecting the balls and selling them back to unsuspecting golfers. Talk about water hazard.

Soon you'll see a green lamppost on the left, indicating private land; the right bank remains predominantly part of the forest. The river then makes a few sharp chevron-shaped turns before coming upon a low-clearance wooden footbridge. The

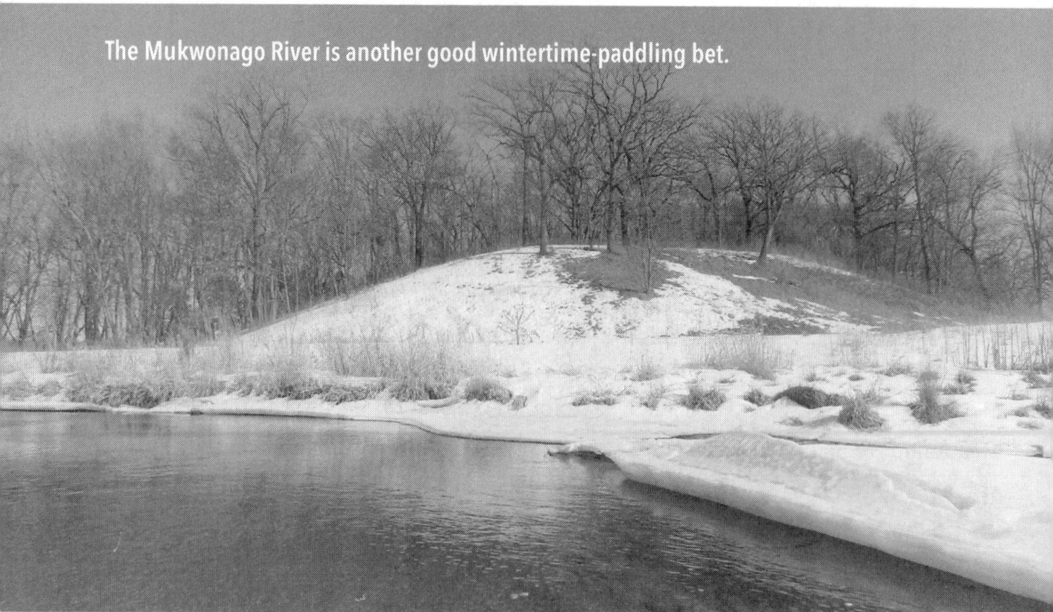
The Mukwonago River is another good wintertime-paddling bet.

right-hand side is slightly higher than the left. A quick left turn follows, with a short straightaway leading to a house (and another green lamppost).

Here, the river bends to the right and leads to a nice Class I ledge. Be careful, though: There's a low-clearance bough from a toppled tree just above the small drop. This is followed by another fun little chute underneath the Beulah Road bridge. There's a convenient access point on the right downstream of the bridge. For the next hundred yards, the gradient increases, making this area rather shallow. A few meanders lead to a straightaway beneath a towering set of power lines. The river begins to widen some as the landscape changes before your eyes from hardwood forest to wild rice beds and cattail marsh; small hills still slope in the background, though.

A feeder stream will appear on your right, which will add to the river's width even more, alas, but not necessarily to its depth. The Mukwonago is too splendid to paddle in low water; you'll be forfeiting the experience due to frustration from getting stuck. After passing a hill on the right, you'll be facing north and see a pretty ridge off in the near distance; it's part of Mukwonago Park, a Waukesha County park with a lake, a dog park, and even camping. For a great little weekend getaway, I wholly recommend paddling this trip one day and Lulu Lake the next (see "Additional Trips" for more info).

If the water is high, you'll delight in floating over rice beds, sometimes not knowing where the main channel is. Think of this like walking through a field of sunflowers or wheat. Just follow the current, and it will lead you to where you need to go. Some of the stalks rise as high as 10 feet in late summer, maintaining a truly isolated feel to this final section. Alas, a wide straightaway leads you directly to a small hill with a couple houses on it. Together with yet another set of power lines and maybe the sound of a car driving down the road, you know the take-out is near.

The river bends to the left and away from the houses, shows off one more pretty savanna, then turns to the right, where you'll see on the right-hand side a clearing in the cattails from the water to the road. Take out here, not at the bridge 200 feet downstream. There's a shoulder on the road to leave at least two vehicles.

•THE•FUDGE•

Additional Trips Put in at the public boat launch off Wambold Road (behind Eagle Springs Pub), paddle southwest across Eagle Spring Lake to the inlet, then head up the feeder stream to **Lulu Lake,** a protected state natural area featuring a clear-water, 40-foot-deep kettle lake left behind by a receding glacier.

Exotic wildflower species such as dragon's mouth orchids and kitten tails, along with a bog-and-tamarack forest, and rolling hills, are additional benefits of this trip. While it's mostly lake paddling, this is a fun exploration, since the lake is entirely protected and otherwise inaccessible. As the crow flies, Lulu Lake is 1.5 miles from the boat launch (plus that distance paddling back), and the lake itself is a little more than 1 mile to paddle around.

You could also put in below the dam in Mukwonago, paddle through the pretty **Mukwonago River State Natural Area,** and then paddle into the Illinois Fox River to **Big Bend** for a 9-mile trip. You will be able to see and hear I-43, though, during about a third of this trip.

CAMPING **Mukwonago County Park** (S100 W31900 CR LO, Mukwonago; 262-363-7658)

FOOD FOR THOUGHT (AND RENTALS) For a comforting meal in a classic Wisconsin bar on the lake, check out **Eagle Springs Pub** (W345 S10463 CR E, Mukwonago; 262-594-2337), just west of the put-in. They also rent paddling equipment.

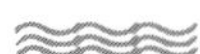

25 Pewaukee River and Illinois Fox River:
PEWAUKEE TO WAUKESHA

•THE•FACTS•

Put-in/take-out County Road M in Pewaukee/Grebe Park in Waukesha

Distance/time 8.3 mi/Allow for 3.5 hrs

Gradient/water level 10 fpm in parts, 1–3 fpm in others/Look for a minimum of 40 cfs at USGS gage 05426067 (Bark River in Delafield) for the Pewaukee River portion and a minimum of 50 cfs at USGS gage 05543830 for the Fox River portion.

Water type Quietwater, riffles, Class I rapids, and flatwater

Canoe or kayak Kayak preferable, but canoe is feasible

Skill level Experienced

Time of year to paddle Anytime the water is high enough (but not too high)

Landscape Marsh wetlands, industrial park corridor, light residential, secluded woods, and urban downtown

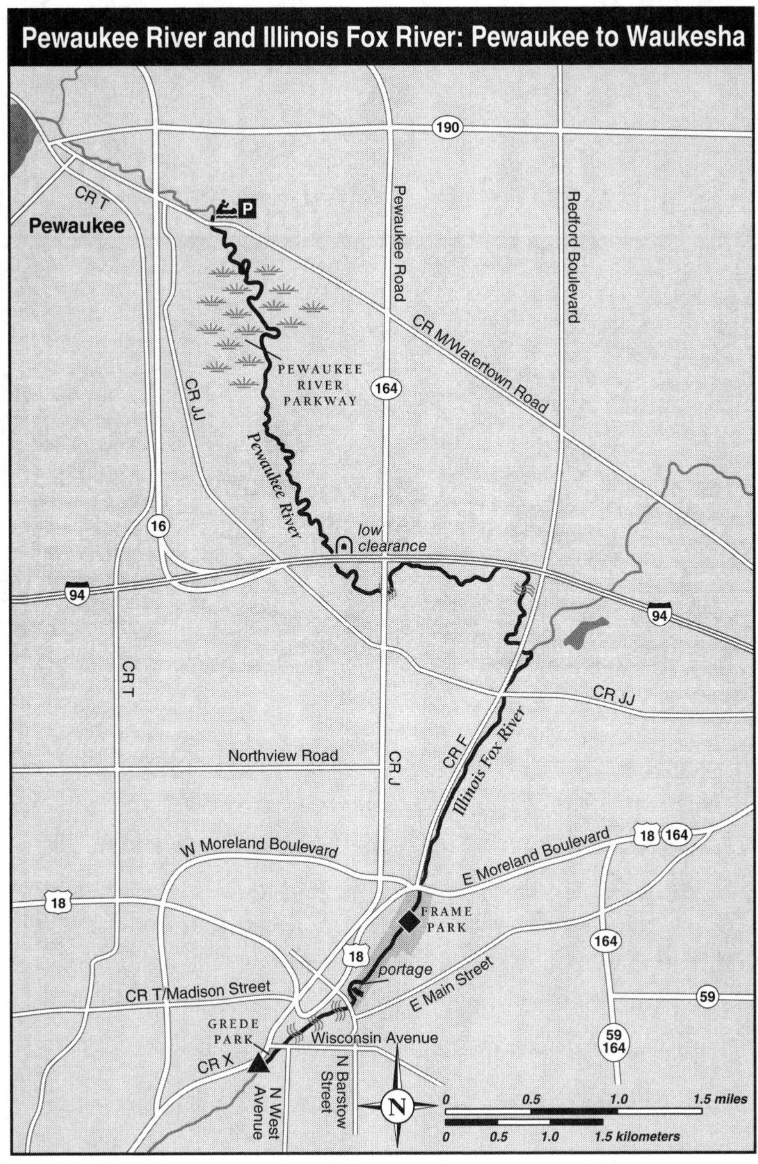

OVERVIEW Here is a truly varied trip that begins in a tranquil wetlands, heads underneath an interstate highway, rushes down a fun set of rapids, and merges with a different river into downtown Waukesha before more Class I rapids. Along the way, you'll see turtles, frogs, hawks, great blue herons, deer, and songbirds.

SHUTTLE 5.9 miles. From the take-out, drive south on Riverwalk Drive, then turn right on North Prairie Avenue and right again onto West St. Paul Avenue. Turn left

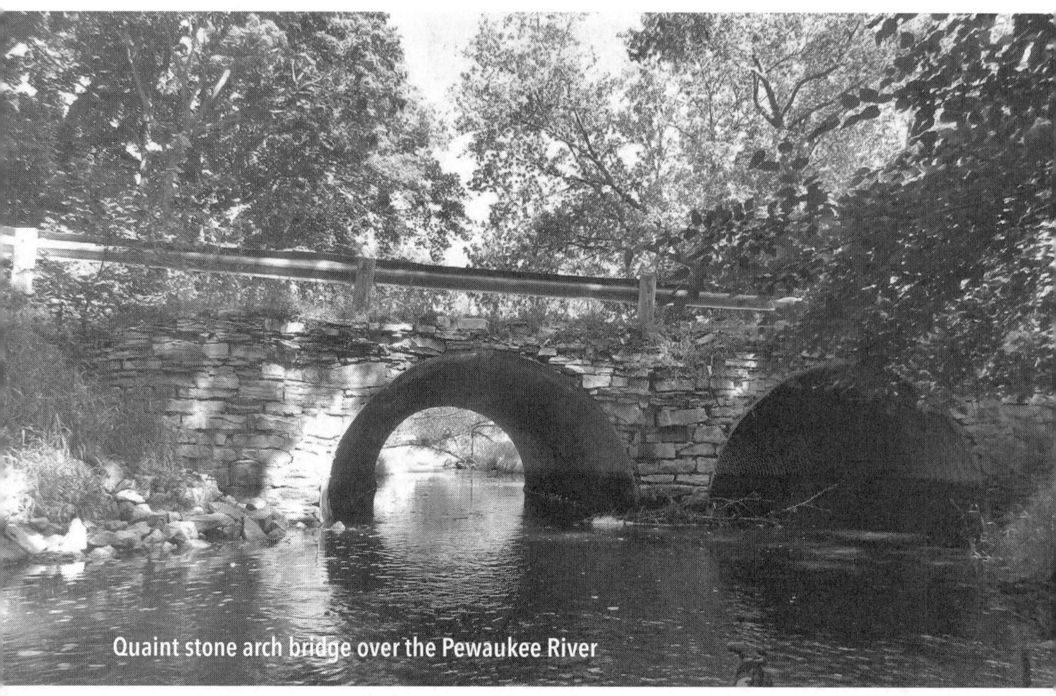

Quaint stone arch bridge over the Pewaukee River

on West Moreland Avenue at the US 18 intersection, then take your first right on Pewaukee Road. Turn left on CR JJ/Bluemound Road; follow it to its intersection with CR M/Wisconsin Avenue, and turn right. Cross the bridge and turn left into a small parking area for the put-in.

Note: To determine visually whether there is adequate water, scout at the Pewaukee Road bridge during this shuttle. If it's shallow there, it will be shallow elsewhere. From this bridge to the Fox River confluence, the river drops 10 fpm, which will mean a lot of unhappy scraping and walking your boat if the water is low.

TAKE-OUT N43° 00.505' W88° 14.365' **PUT-IN** N43° 04.573' W88° 14.675'

•THE•FLAVOR•

THE PUT-IN IS NONDESCRIPT. It is located immediately north of the CR M bridge (also East Wisconsin Avenue). Turn into the unpaved lot and park near the river out of the way. Launch 15 yards upstream of the bridge from a small gravel bar. Below the bridge, there will be a few houses on the right, after which you won't see any until several miles more downstream.

Soon you will be surrounded by the Pewaukee River Parkway, a pretty, marshy public area that is rather large and fairly undeveloped. There will be mostly long stretches of straightaways for the first mile or so, and the current is slack. The water is delightfully clear, and the width of the river is only 20 feet wide here. (Both the Pewaukee and Illinois Fox Rivers feel and look more like creeks than rivers.) There will be some downed trees to negotiate, but volunteers do a great job of clearing out nuisances. In fact, there is a race annually held in May that begins at the put-in and concludes at Frame Park in Waukesha.

You'll see a large office building improbably appear on the left, which in turn signals the beginning of two things: the end of the parkway, as civilization again encroaches, and the beginning of many meanders. A second large office building will appear, again on the left, followed by a brief woods leading up to the interstate bridge. The bridge is more of a concrete-lined tunnel with a very low clearance. The downstream side actually is shorter than the upstream side, so you need to be careful lining up and confident that you will have adequate clearance, lest you get stuck. It will be up to your own comfort level whether to bend down forward in your boat or lie back. This safety concern being what it is, there is a small thrill in passing beneath an interstate highway (one you've been on probably dozens of times as a driver).

Pass through the attractive culvert bridge at Busse Road and get ready for the first of two sets of fun Class I rapids on this trip. Here, riffles usher you around the Steinhafel's Furniture Superstore before becoming splashy rapids, as the river heads south again. (The second set of rapids lies below the dam in downtown Waukesha.) Thrilling rapids next to a parking lot and interstate highway make for a strange but engaging juxtaposition.

The river races through more woods and a surprisingly natural setting (considering its proximity to highways and superstores). Before reaching the Illinois Fox River, you'll pass under three more bridges in quick succession: the entrance to Steinhafel's, CR F, and a small railroad bridge. Minor rapids will be found at each. Be careful at the railroad bridge, as it is low, the current can be a little pushy, and there are some random pieces of concrete to maneuver around. Before you catch your breath, you've reached the confluence at the Fox River—turn right.

Immediately downstream lie the remnants of old bridge pilings, now statuary and picturesque in their random abandonment. The Illinois Fox is considerably wider than the Pewaukee but only a little bit deeper. A long straightaway connects the Pewaukee confluence and dam in downtown Waukesha. Water clarity remains impressively clear given the environment. This segment of the river is industrial bizarre. For one, the Bluemound Road/CR JJ bridge towers above you, yet the banks are totally undeveloped, even neglected.

Just past the huge bridge, large quarries operate on each side of the river. Neither can be seen from the river (and only barely from the road), but you can hear them and they are gigantic, with quite awesome rock outcrops; alas, both are strictly private property. Approaching the US 18 bridge, the "Little Fox" has tripled in width to 200 feet, and the current has ground to a halt, due to the dam downstream.

Below the bridge (adorned with fox statues, incidentally), beautiful Frame Park will line the left shore for the next 0.25 mile. There are multiple docks on each side of the river, as well as an official boat launch on the left bank. You might even see a pink-flamingo paddleboat.

The outline of downtown buildings comes into focus as you make your way through the lake-like impoundment. The dam itself, really a decorative spillway, will first be signaled by spritzing water fountains in the river, then the horizon line. A CANOE PORTAGE sign on the right indicates more or less where to take out; reenter below the dam. (Along the portage trail is a cool iron map embedded in the sidewalk of the whole city of Waukesha.) A cove-like concrete amphitheater, downstream on river right, provides the best access for reentry.

Get ready, because there's only a little more than half a mile left in this trip—and it's all down a series of super-fun Class I rapids. The first rapid lies below Barstow Street, the first bridge below the dam, immediately followed by a pedestrian bridge with more riffly fun. You'll see statues of three bears on the right preceding an ornate pedestrian bridge, below which is a long Class I rapid. You'll pass under a bridge that feels more like a parking ramp. After this, the river looks slightly less urban as trees begin lining the banks.

Attractive rock rubble on the left leads you past a modern apartment building and pedestrian bridges, with one more pleasant riffle before the Wisconsin Avenue bridge. As the current slackens, you'll see the take-out on the right shortly before, you guessed it, another pedestrian bridge. Eight miles is not that long of a journey, but you've come a long way since the slow wetlands in Pewaukee.

•THE•FUDGE•

ADDITIONAL TRIPS You can add 1.3 more miles upstream by putting in below the dam at Pewaukee Lake, but it's mostly residential and industrial. Alternatively, you can take out at West Sunset Drive and add 2.4 miles downstream, but it too is mostly a mix of residential and industrial environs.

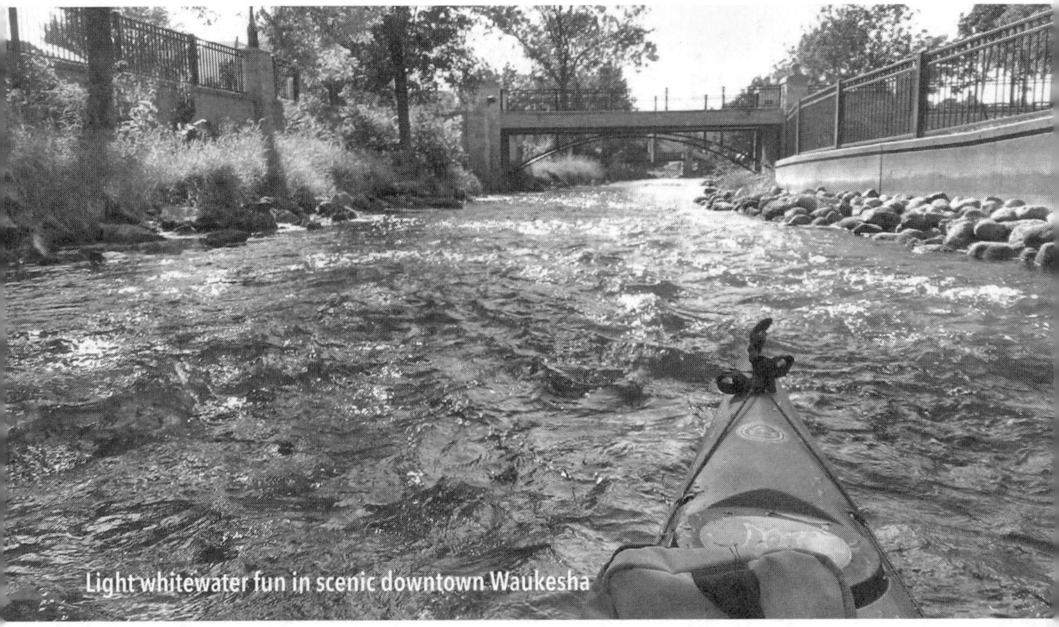

Light whitewater fun in scenic downtown Waukesha

CAMPING **Kettle Moraine State Forest–Lapham Peak Unit** (W329 N846 CR C, Delafield; 262-646-3025); **Menomonee Park** (W220 N7884 Town Line Road, Menomonee Falls; 262-255-1310); and **Muskego Park** (S83 W20370 Janesville Road, Muskego; 262-679-0310)

RENTALS **Smokey's Bait Shop (129 Park Ave., Pewaukee; 262-691-0360)** and **High Roller Fun Rentals** (Frame Park, 1128 Baxter St., Waukesha; 262-524-4008)

FOOD FOR THOUGHT For great pizza, check out **Doc's Dry Dock,** right on the lake in Pewaukee (N38 W27091 Parkside Road; 262-691-9947). For lip-smackin' barbecue, head over to **Pat's Rib Place** (151 E. Sunset Drive, Waukesha; 262-544-4099). Get your java on at **Cafe de Arts** (830 W. St. Paul Ave., Waukesha; 262-446-1856). Or, for a swanky brunch, poke in at **Taylor's People's Park** (337 W. Main St., Waukesha; 262-522-6868).

SHOUT-OUTS For information about the **Frame Park Canoe Race,** call Pewaukee Kiwanis (262-695-8745).

Waukesha is the birthplace of the legendary **Les Paul,** without whose ingenious inventions and guitar contributions rock 'n' roll as we know it would not be the same.

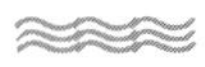

26 Red Cedar Lake State Natural Area:
CAMBRIDGE IN JEFFERSON COUNTY

•THE•FACTS•

Put-in/take-out Public boat landing off Brosig Lane

Distance/time 4.2 mi round-trip/Allow for 2–3 hrs

Gradient/water level N/A

Water type Flatwater

Canoe or kayak Either

Skill level Beginner

Time of year to paddle Best in spring, prettiest in autumn, very weedy in summer

Landscape Cattail marsh surrounded by a gentle topography of pines, hemlocks, and oaks, not to mention innumerable submerged and emergent aquatic plants, such as pickerelweed, water milfoil, water shield, lily pads, and the carnivorous bladderwort

---

OVERVIEW A beautiful lake enclosed within a state natural area for canoes and kayaks only, with outstanding wildlife opportunities and cool aquatic plants, this trips offers encounters with frogs, turtles, black terns, turkey vultures, great blue and green herons, sandhill cranes, bitterns, blackbirds, owls, and lots of cute coots.

SHUTTLE N/A **PUT-IN/TAKE-OUT** N42° 59.024' W88° 58.447'

•THE•FLAVOR•

PUT IN AT THE CONCRETE LANDING. What follows is a long corridor 1,000 feet long with turtle-lined logs on the left and tamaracks off to the right. A small swell of open water is followed by an even narrower path through cattails, on the other side of which is the lake proper. It's a unique and very cool way to begin a paddling trip. It feels like a gateway entrance to a hidden place, which as a protected state natural area, Red Cedar Lake essentially is.

While I sometimes scoff at paddling lakes simply because what you see is what you get, and thus there's little to no sense of a journey, here it's different. With a little imagination, the shoreline of Red Cedar Lake resembles Lakes Michigan and Huron (only significantly smaller), thanks to a peninsula that bisects it. Each half has its own

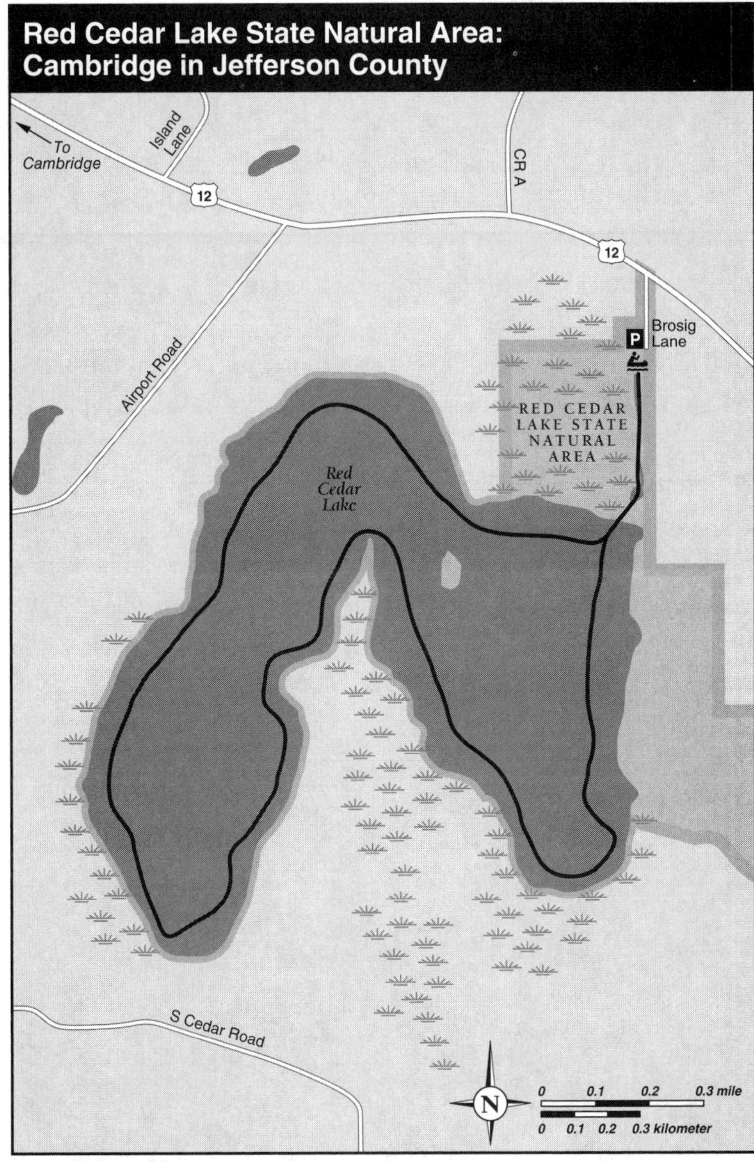

feel. This tour runs clockwise from the paddler's perspective, meaning it starts north and heads south, hugging the eastern shore.

Cattails line the eastern shore on your left. As is true for all of the lakeshore, how close you can or wish to line the limn of the land will be dictated by the watershield plants and lily pads. You will notice these immediately upon entering the lake. The water is clear despite a mucky, dark bottom. On a bright day, the color of the underwater stalks is positively vivid—bright reds and greens struck against a stark black background. And they just hover there, seemingly motionless, as though in dark outer space. Also, the lake itself is rather shallow (90% of it is less than 3 feet deep, and it's only 6 feet at its deepest). Paddling south, you'll see an attractive knoll rise from the eastern shore, followed by a line of various Bob Ross trees in several shades of happy green. The only houses near the lake are on the eastern shore, all but one tactfully camouflaged by foliage. The southern edge of the eastern "lobe" of the lake is an impenetrable cattail marsh with more tamaracks farther back where you will likely hear if not also see lots of sandhill cranes.

As you turn north to paddle along the eastern shore of the peninsula, you'll see a red barn off in the distance ahead. A mix of hardwoods develops on the left. Soon you'll see a break in the cattails where a beckoning woodsy shore comes right up to the water's edge. You may explore this if you wish, but there are no trails. Cattails resume, this time in a beguiling labyrinth you can paddle through or around (the former is more fun). In a short distance straight ahead, you'll see a 1-acre-large island that you can circumnavigate now or wait until later (alas, there's no accessible shoreline).

A receding edge of cattails marks the tip of the peninsula, along with a dilapidated wooden crate. Turn left here to paddle back south. Around the peninsular tip,

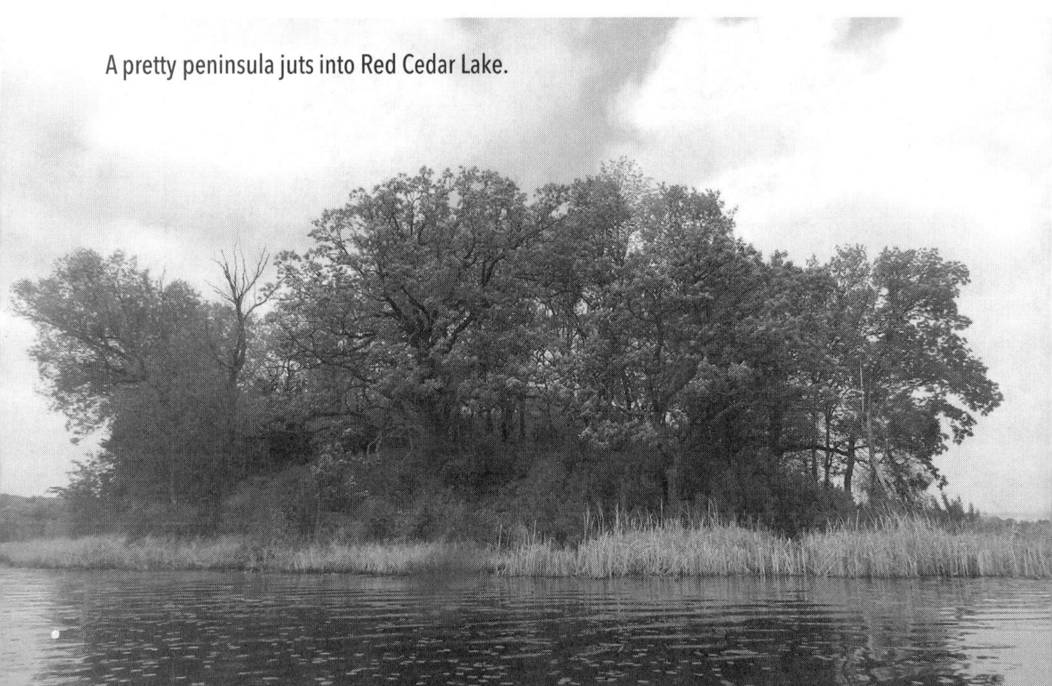

A pretty peninsula juts into Red Cedar Lake.

the shoreline is shallow and unusually gravelly. At first, the left shore (the western shore of the peninsula) is just a thin strip of mixed trees along a bank that is about 15 feet high. But a bulge of land will jut out beyond this, creating a pleasant North Woods feel (as long as you ignore the sprawling cropland in the southwest quadrant of the lake). There are a few spots here along the shore where paddlers of times past have gotten out and walked along the peninsula. In this section, there are no NO TRESPASSING signs; however, farther south on the left, you will see a few signs announcing private property.

A huge complex of cattails dominates the southern section of the western lobe, so it's best just to turn around and paddle north. The left shore here is a continuation of cattails with a large sloping hill marked by wide fields of crops, a patchwork of green and beige conspicuously distinct from the rest of the land surrounding the lake, which is otherwise undeveloped or at least integrated. As you make your way up to the northernmost section of the lake, you'll have begun to see strange tubular objects, organic and usually long, bobbing atop the surface. While they look like a cross between spinal columns and tentacles, they're actually lily pad roots—just thick as squid. They're a little grotesque but in a cool sci-fi way, as if a spawn of misbegotten mutant centipedes started taking over the lake, complete with suction cup–like nodules and spindly legs. Moving eastward, the view on the left (the north shore) is lovely: a tree-lined slope of land with a savanna-like system of grasses and shrubs. The edge of this juts out into the lake, making an attractive mound. The acre-sized island is on your right, while cattails make a standing ovation on your left. Follow the cattails to the opening to take you back into the corridor to the boat launch.

•THE•FUDGE•

CAMPING **Sandhill Station State Campground** (N5584 Mud Lake Road, Lake Mills; 920-648-8774)

FOOD FOR THOUGHT (AND RENTALS) For thoughtfully prepared sandwiches and salads or a good bottle of local beer, stop by **CamRock Cafe & Sport** (217 W. Main St., Cambridge; 608-423-2111), where you can also rent gear.

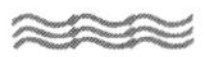

27 Sugar River C:
AVON BOTTOMS TO YALE BRIDGE ROAD IN ILLINOIS

•THE•FACTS•

Put-in/take-out South Nelson Road, Avon Bottoms Wildlife Area/Yale Bridge Road, Colored Sands Forest Preserve

Distance/time 7.8 mi/Allow 3 hrs

Gradient/water level 2 fpm/reliable throughout the season, though 340 cfs at USGS gage 05436500 is excellent

Water type Flatwater and quietwater

Canoe or kayak Either

Skill level Beginner

Time of year to paddle Anytime, though spring and autumn are particularly nice

Landscape Hardwood forests, bottomlands, sand bluffs

OVERVIEW Slow-paced and pretty but still wild-feeling, this remote trip along the Sugar River begins in the hardwood floodplains of far southern Wisconsin and ends along tall, sandy bluffs in northern Illinois, the two points linked by quiet and solitude. Expect to see great blue herons, yellow-crowned night herons, turkey vultures, hawks, frogs, songbirds (especially warblers), snakes, wood ducks, muskrats, and redheaded woodpeckers.

SHUTTLE **6.1 miles.** From the take-out, head west on Yale Bridge Road, then turn right onto Wheeler Road. Follow Wheeler as it doglegs north and west and eventually turns into State Line Road, which is contiguous with the Illinois–Wisconsin border. Make a right into Wisconsin on South Nelson Road, then take another right into the public-access parking area and boat launch, about 1,000 feet south of the bridge.

TAKE-OUT N42° 28.397' W89° 14.946' **PUT-IN** N42° 31.130' W89° 18.338'

•THE•FLAVOR•

PUT IN AT THE BOAT RAMP at the public-access parking area. Here, you're in the southeastern quadrant of the huge Avon Bottoms Wildlife Area, nearly 3,000 acres

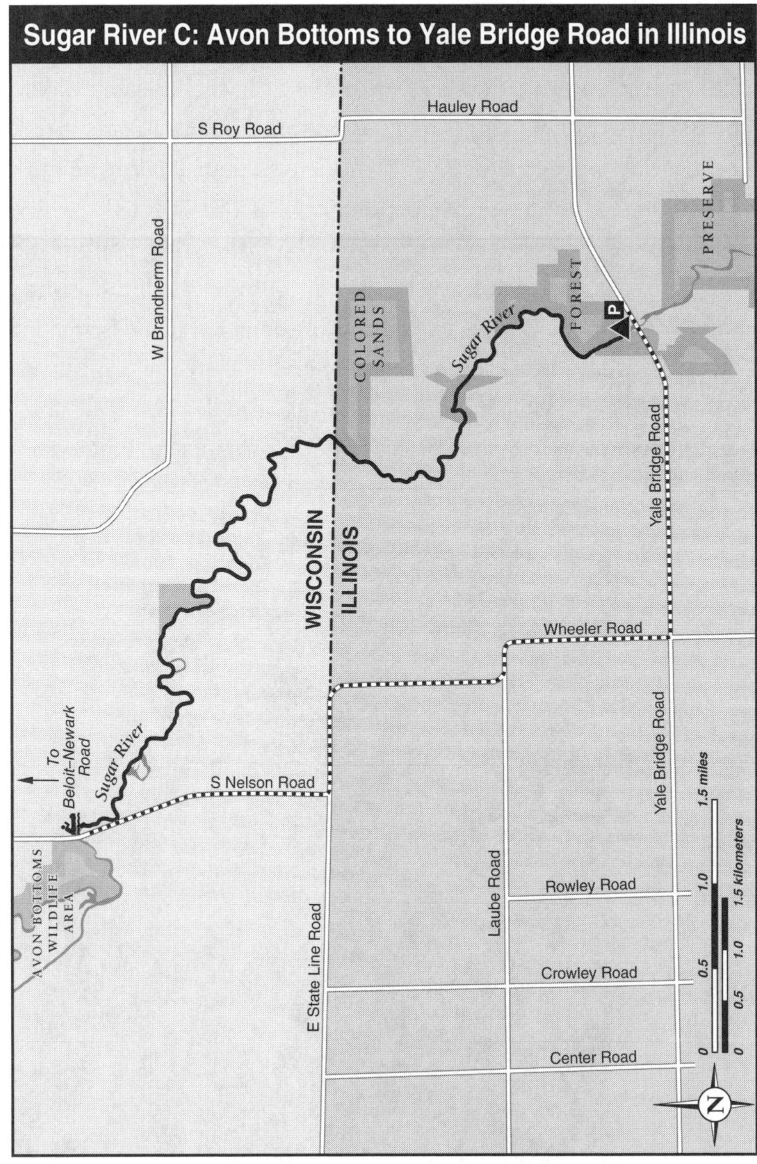

large. The river will range from 70 to 100 feet wide along this trip, and the depth ranges from a few inches to a few feet. The river bottom is consistently sandy, though the banks remain mostly muddy in the beginning, gradually becoming sandier as you head into Illinois. The landscape is scenic, if simplistic: a canopy of trees along both banks and receding beyond to mysterious sloughs and swampy ponds. (This will change some by the time you enter the forest preserves in Illinois, where the landscape is hillier.)

It's the sense of isolation, the slow pace of the river, the excellent wildlife opportunities, and the novelty of crossing state lines that are the salient features of this trip. There will be some obstacles in the stream to maneuver around, but none too difficult. Volunteers have done a commendable job keeping this part of the Sugar River open and accessible—a considerable undertaking given the surrounding bottomlands of silver maples, swamp oaks, sycamores, ash, basswood, cottonwoods, hickory, and willows.

A number of quaint and attractive islands break up the main stream into inviting side channels. It's easy to track the current to know where the main channel is, in spite of the many oxbows. While it's sometimes fun to paddle a floodplain area in high water, since it offers unique access to places not otherwise able to be paddled, I don't

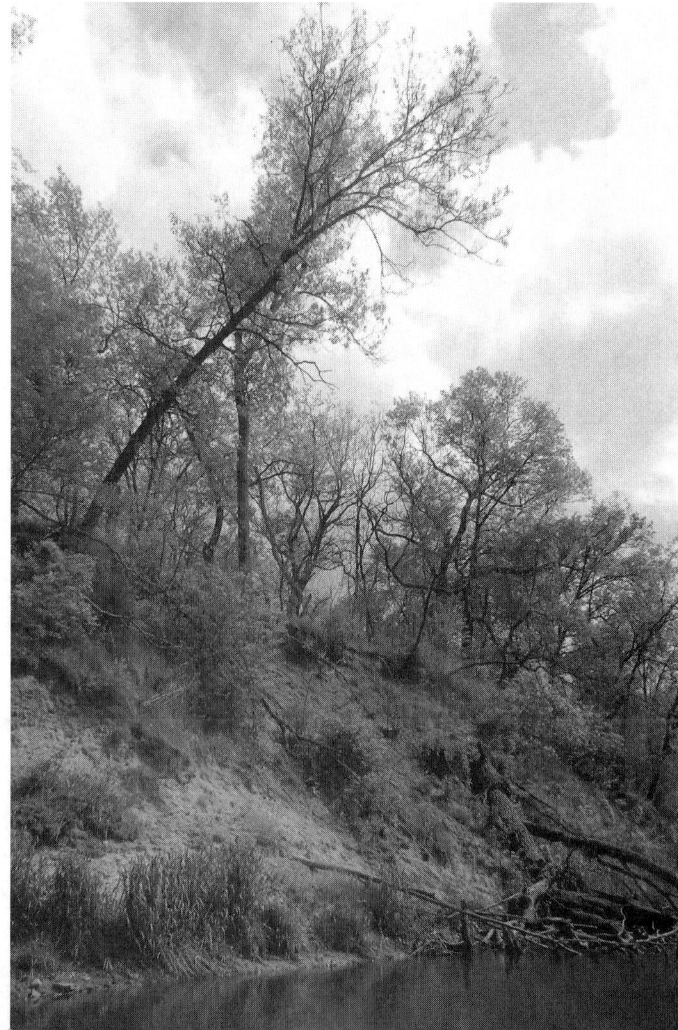

Tall, sandy banks in Colored Sands Forest Preserve, just across the Illinois border

recommend doing that here, because it will quickly become disorienting as to where the main channel is, due to the meandering nature of the river. You do *not* want to get lost down here; it's quite primitive and downright spooky at dusk. Some even claim there's a "swamp monster" in the Avon Bottoms: a "bear–wolf" hybrid or a Yeti-like beast covered in mud and weeds, depending on whom you ask. Rumors abound, too, of the Bottoms having been a depository for the slain enemies of Chicago mobsters in the 1920s and 1930s.

After a mile or so, the river will bend south toward the perimeter of the wildlife area in close proximity to the adjoining croplands beyond. But then a tight left-hand turn takes you north and back into the bottomlands. After more meanders, you'll come upon a large island; take the left channel (the two will converge 0.5 mile downstream). As you head farther east and south, the banks will become sandier and less muddy. While there is no WELCOME TO ILLINOIS! sign along the river, there is an official ILLINOIS NATURE PRESERVE sign more or less at the porous border.

As soon you do cross the state line, the land along the entire left bank is an alder forest more than 500 acres large. With the exception of two small noncontiguous parcels of land that are private, all of the Sugar River along the left bank in the Illinois section of this trip travels through two public nature preserves. Another nice feature is the general straightening out of the river once you're in Illinois. In one pretty stretch, the river gently sweeps along an eroded sandy bank bordering a farm on the right, while a long sandbar lines the left bank at the inside bend. You'll sneak back into the thicketed forest after that and pass a colorful shack called "Hillbilly Haven," complete with a plastic pig and two domestic-beer cans adorning its shingle.

The final mile of this trip is the prettiest. On the left, you'll pass a sign indicating that you're now within the Colored Sands Forest Preserve, more than 300 acres large. After meanders and a left turn, you'll come upon a 20-foot-tall sandbank directly before you. A second one, now 50 feet tall, follows just downstream and lines the river for several hundred feet. As it tapers in height, the right bank begins to open up upon an undeveloped savanna. Trees line both banks again in one last woodsy corridor that leads up to the bridge at Yale Bridge Road. Take out on the left, upstream of the bridge, at the designated boat launch, where there are bathrooms and water.

•THE•FUDGE•

ADDITIONAL TRIPS You can add another 4.2 miles to this trip by putting in upstream at the boat launch just below the Beloit–Newark bridge (the official take-out for Trip 43, Sugar River B; see page 219). The landscape is much the same, though deadfall and necessary portaging can be problematic. If you do add this segment, paddle into the right channel at an island about 1.5 miles from the put-in; the left channel is very narrow and is clogged with obstructions.

CAMPING **Sugar River Forest Preserve** (10127 Forest Preserve Road, Durand, Illinois; 815-877-6100) is a few miles downstream from the take-out. Some sites are located along the river itself.

SHOUT-OUTS As you drive to the put-in, you can't help but notice the time-forgotten desolation of the town of **Avon,** seemingly one heartbeat away from being a ghost town. Abandoned cars and broken-down barns enhance the scene as if it were straight out of *The Grapes of Wrath* or a Hollywood horror-movie set. The railroad bypassed Avon, favoring Brodhead, and the rest was history.

One of the largest small-bird-banding stations in the country is located at **Colored Sands Nature Preserve** (10602 Haas Road, Durand, Illinois; 815-877-6100).

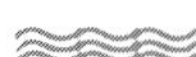

28 Turtle Creek A:
FAIRFIELD AREA IN WALWORTH AND ROCK COUNTIES

•THE•FACTS•

Put-in/take-out School Section Road/South O'Riley Road. See "The Flavor" for three alternative access points.

Distance/time 8.2 mi/Allow for 3–4 hrs

Gradient/water level 3 fpm/Look for at least 130 cfs on USGS gage 05431486.

Water type Quietwater

Canoe or kayak Either

Skill level Beginner

Time of year to paddle Anytime

Landscape A mix of agriculture and woods, with some modest rock outcrops

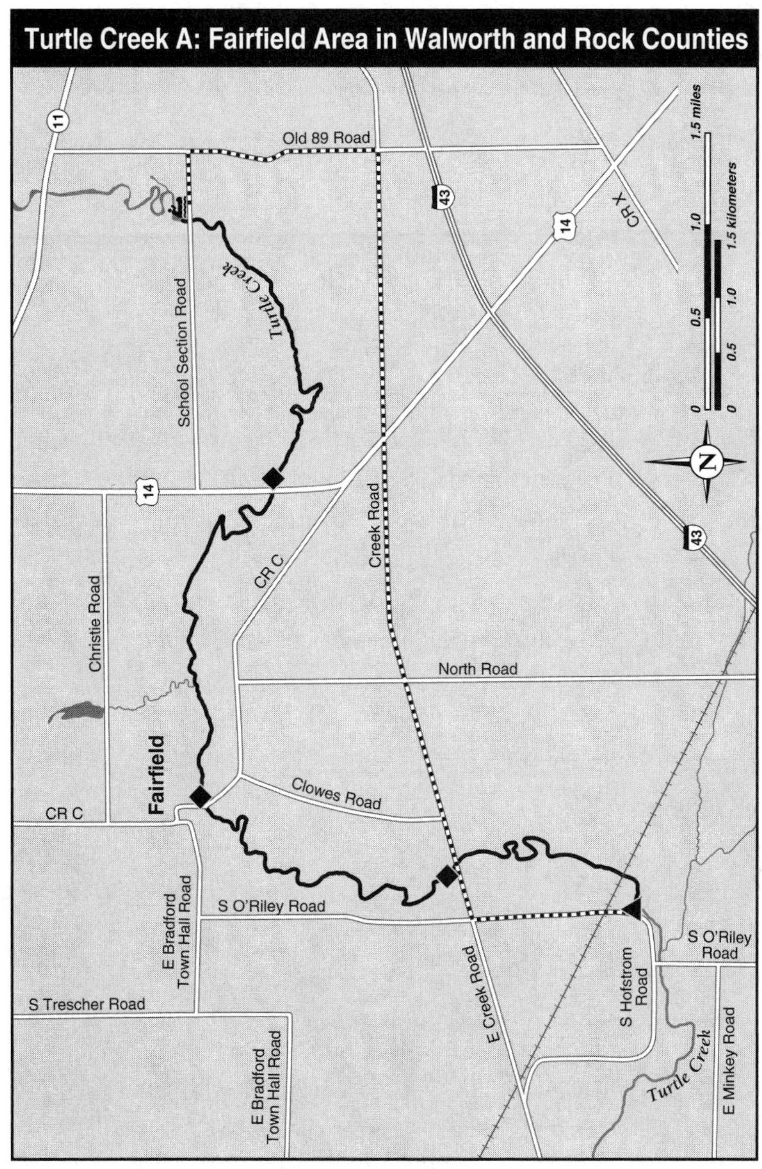

OVERVIEW Combining the best of lush scenery, minimal to nonexistent development, superb wildlife, reliable water levels, and easy current, this first trip on wonderful Turtle Creek has something for all paddlers. You'll see great blue herons, hawks, turkey vultures, songbirds, turtles, deer, dragonflies, and fish.

Though this trip is only 8.5 miles, it has three alternative access points where bridges cross the creek. Uncannily, the bridges neatly dissect this trip in 2-mile sections, which helps you feel oriented and paced. Moreover, one can easily begin or end a trip on Turtle Creek at any of the bridge options in between or even after this trip's take-out, making this stream paddler-friendly and flexible in a way that few others are.

SHUTTLE 6.3 miles. From the take-out, head north on South O'Riley Road. Turn right onto East Creek Road. Stay straight through the US 14 intersection. Turn left onto Old 89 Road, then left again onto School Section Road. Park along the road.

TAKE-OUT N42° 35.842' W88° 47.108' **PUT-IN** N42° 37.915' W88° 42.907'

•THE•FLAVOR•

EVEN THOUGH IT'S CALLED A CREEK, the Turtle has all the look and feel of a river, thanks in large part to its width ranging between 50 and 100 feet. And with only a few meandering exceptions, it flows in broad straight strokes past wavy grass in the water. The bottom will be mostly sandy, and the water is terrifically clear at lower levels. Right away, the landscape is awash in greenery: grassy banks, small hills undulating in the background, even a mix of conifer trees along with the predictable deciduous varieties of southern Wisconsin.

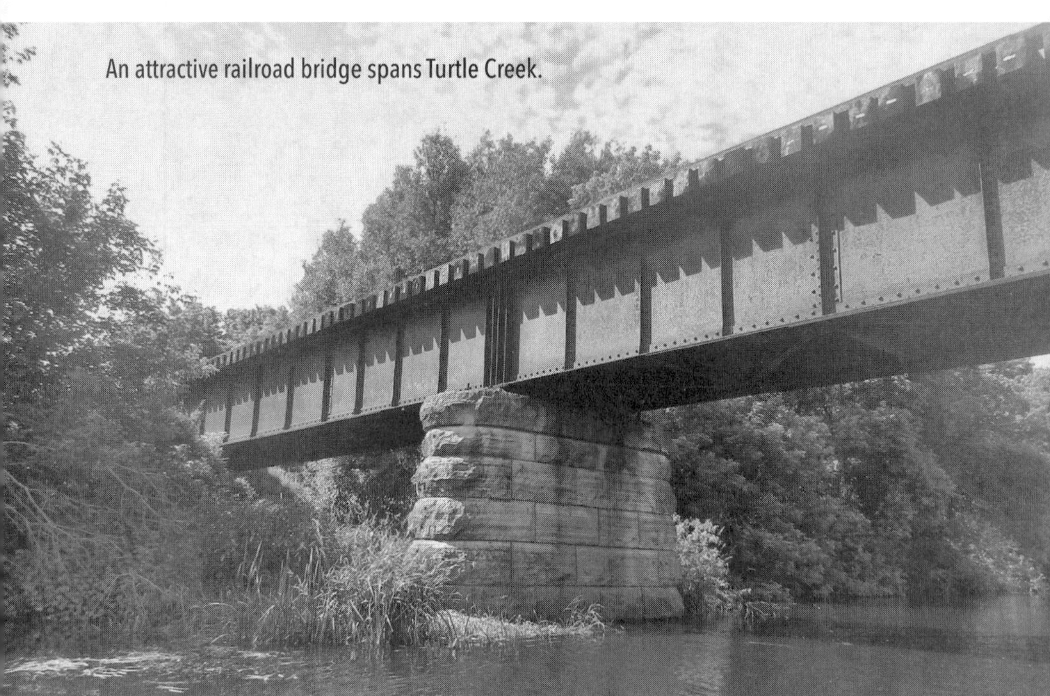

An attractive railroad bridge spans Turtle Creek.

To be fair, Turtle Creek is not an escape from civilization; rather, it's surrounded by roads and large farms. But Turtle Creek and this trip in particular are a case in point for this guidebook's core argument that one can seek and discover natural splendor in our own backyards without a full tank of gas. On this whole trip, you'll see at best two or three buildings, period. Practically all of the thousand-acres-large Turtle Creek Wildlife Area protects both banks of the creek, resulting in a palpable feel of undeveloped naturalness.

Put in on the upstream side of the bridge at School Section Road, on river left. A small path leads to the water, so access is easy. If the creek is high and the current swift, you might want to paddle upstream a few strokes and then turn around in order to line up to pass through one of the culverts at the bridge.

Around a small horseshoe bend, you'll come upon the exoskeletal remains of an attractive iron truss bridge. After a zig and a zag, a long straightaway follows, with a wink of quiet riffles here and there. US 14 (**N42° 37.535' W88° 44.530'**) and then County Road C (**N42° 37.846' W88° 46.484'**) mark the next two bridges. Between the two, a gentle ridge rises off to the right and will continue for a couple miles. Past the three-culverts bridge at CR C, one of the prettiest segments anywhere on the Turtle awaits. The creek will meander gently around a woodsy ridge on the right, a notable punctuation on this otherwise topographically challenged trip. Here, as elsewhere on the Turtle, you'll be treated to a perfect mix of sun and shade.

The third bridge access comes at East Creek Road (**N42° 36.681' W88° 46.847'**). Past the bridge is a small, short area prone to tree fall and entanglements due to the tight bends and thick cluster of trees. Helpful volunteers maintain it, but change is the one constant on rivers and creeks. This is the only brief section on this trip that may require negotiating deadfall.

A relaxing straightaway follows for some 400 feet and takes you under a stately railroad bridge. If you time this right, you'll meet the train that typically passes at 3:30 p.m. each day, always a fun novelty while paddling.

The take-out is on river right 1,000 feet downstream from the railroad bridge, at a thoughtfully cleared-out section of grass. There's even a designated parking area here, too, attesting to the renewed interest in Turtle Creek recreational possibilities.

•THE•FUDGE•

ADDITIONAL TRIPS From its source at the spring-fed Turtle Lake south of the city of Whitewater, Turtle Creek has been artificially channelized for

8.5 miles to Comus Lake in Delavan; the effect is like paddling a canal that looks like a ditch. The creek environment here is attractive, but you won't see anything that you don't already experience in the three trips recommended in this book.

Alternatively, beginner-level paddlers looking for a safe taste of whitewater can find a couple of brief blasts—one easy, one challenging—on nearby **Swan Creek,** a tributary of Turtle Creek. The first set of rapids, Class I–II, is underneath and then again 25 yards downstream from the Washington Street bridge, one block south of Veterans Park and Comus Lake. Riffles will continue intermittently all the way to the dam.

Experienced whitewater paddlers might contemplate another run, this one below the dam, immediately west of Veterans Park. It's a thrilling rush of Class II–III rapids on river right. The run is only 800 feet, and paddlers must take out before the impassable low-clearance bridge at Richmond Road, but it is a raucous experience all the same.

CAMPING There is a public campground on Whitewater Lake in **Kettle Moraine State Forest–Southern Unit** (Hi-Lo Road, off Kettle Moraine Scenic Drive; 262-473-7501), as well as a private campground on Turtle Lake called **Snug Harbor** (W7785 Wisconsin Parkway, Delavan; 608-883-6999).

RENTALS **Delavan Paddle Sports** (109 Waterworks Drive, Delavan; 262-728-6397).

FOOD FOR THOUGHT In Delavan, I recommend **Brick Street Market** (116 E. Walworth Ave.; 262-740-1880) for soups, sandwiches, and fancy hors d'oeuvres; **Elizabeth's Cafe** (322 E. Walworth Ave.; 262-728-3383), for home-style diner fare; and **Fat Tuesdays** (337 S. Eighth St.; 262-725-6977) for delicious Cajun and creole.

SHOUT-OUT Take some time to explore the cute little historic town of **Delavan.** Upon entering it, you'll see gigantic giraffe and elephant statues, harkening to its former circus days, and it has one of the oldest brick-paved downtown main streets in the state.

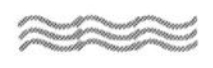

29 Turtle Creek B:
SOUTH O'RILEY ROAD TO SWEET-ALLYN PARK

•THE•FACTS•

Put-in/take-out South O'Riley Road/Sweet-Allyn Park in Shopiere. See "The Flavor" for an alternative put-in that will shorten your trip.

Distance/time 10 mi/Allow for 3.5 hrs

Gradient/water level 4 fpm/Below 200 cfs at USGS gage 05431486, you will scrape in the shallows, but this section can be paddled as low as 160 cfs.

Water type Quietwater, riffles, and light rapids

Canoe or kayak Either

Skill level Beginner

Time of year to paddle Anytime

Landscape A mix of agriculture and woods with some modest rock outcrops

---

OVERVIEW This little jaunt is the perfect summer-weekend paddle through a pleasant, tree-lined landscape, some tall banks, modest rock outcrops, mostly clear water, easy riffles, great wildlife, and quite possibly the prettiest bridge you'll ever see. You'll see turtles, muskrats, wood ducks, geese, frogs, clams, kingfishers, dragonflies, and many great blue herons.

SHUTTLE **9.1 miles.** From the take-out, turn right onto County Road J, then right again onto East Creek Road. Continue on East Creek Road past the WI 140 intersection. Turn right onto South Hofstrom Road—don't cross the railroad bridge—and continue on Hofstrom as it doglegs. After the intersection for South O'Riley Road on the right, stay straight—Hofstrom now becomes South O'Riley Road also—to the wayside parking area, on the right.

TAKE-OUT N42° 34.415' W88° 56.384' **PUT-IN** N42° 35.842' W88° 47.108'

•THE•FLAVOR•

PUT IN AT THE POPULAR AND SUPER-CONVENIENT wayside launch on South O'Riley Road, a couple hundred yards upstream of the bridge by the same name. The "creek" is

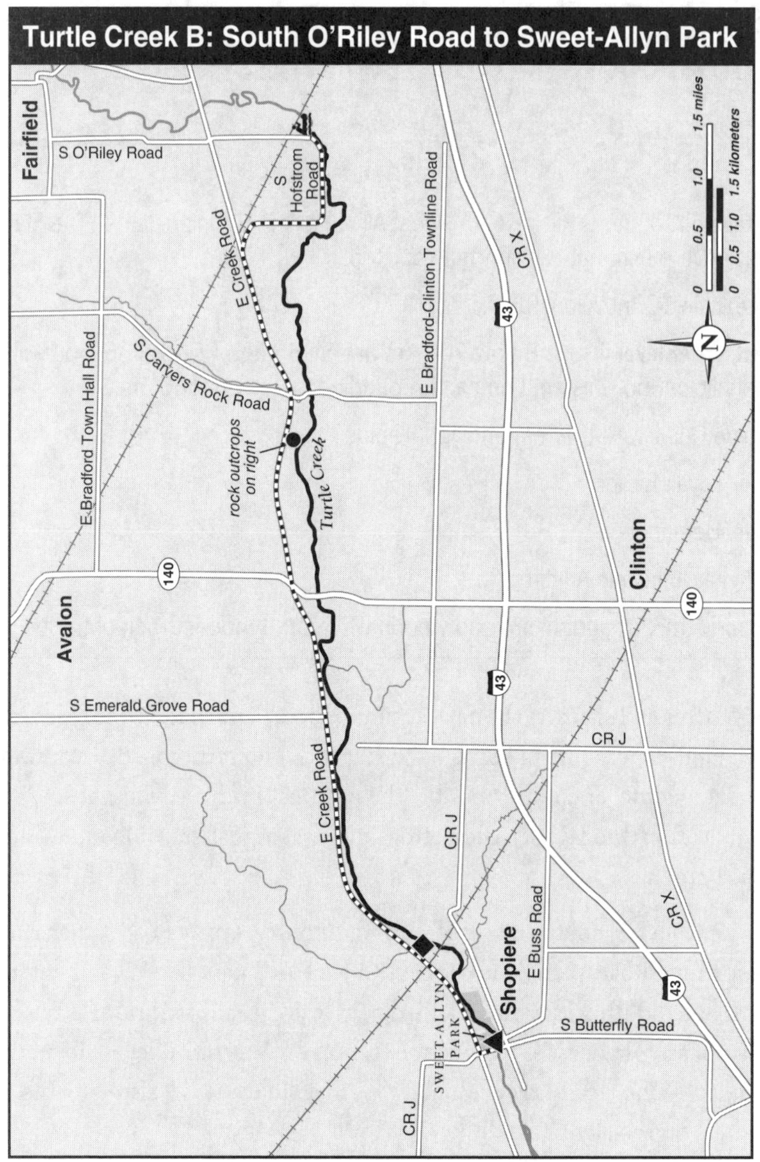

rather wide here at 90 feet, which will be typical for this trip. The water will be shallow as it always is, with a sand–gravel mix lining the streambed. Train-trestle enthusiasts may wish to paddle upstream 1,000 feet to take in a handsome bridge and then turn back around.

A third of a mile downstream from the launch, you'll see Little Turtle Creek enter on your left; keep to the right unless you want to explore the tiny tributary. After the first bridge, the banks open up on both sides as you pass farm fields. Much of this trip falls along an agricultural corridor, but the creek itself and the banks along it are for the most part preserved and natural. There are few, thanks to the width, yet the current is solid but not pushy. (These latter two facts do account for the occasional group of tubers—and I don't mean the vegetable kind.) There are no real meanders either, just long broad strokes past tree-lined banks, some of which are 20 feet high. (A smattering of islands along the way provides for different channels to explore if you want to break up what might otherwise be a monotonous journey.)

Following a bend to the left and then to the right, trees will reappear. The creek then heads north and west again past more beguiling islands. The landscape will continually alternate between cultivated fields and swaths of undeveloped trees and meadowy brush. South Carvers Rock Road is the second bridge you'll come upon, where you could begin this trip as an alternative to shave off 3 miles; put in on the downstream side of the bridge, on river right (**N42° 35.861' W88° 49.755'**).

Just past the bridge on the right, Spring Brook feeds the Turtle. The brook itself is much too narrow and shallow to paddle, but it leads just north to an attractive county park with limestone outcrops (see "The Fudge"). Just past the brook, a huge island splits the Turtle in two; follow the main channel on the right. Also on the right, you'll see some peek-a-boo outcrops ensconced in the woods. The next mile is quite lovely and undeveloped. There will be a bashful rock outcrop or two on the left bank as well. Lowlands and farms briefly follow this on both sides.

The bridge at WI 140 comes up next. On a hot weekend, you might see high school kids jumping into the Turtle from the bridge above. A mile downstream from the bridge, the landscape does become increasingly agricultural, but the creek remains "sleeved" in a tree corridor, so the scenery is only minimally compromised. Attractive tall banks on the left and a small hill or two on the right lend to the view as well. You can definitely afford to relax and open up that second beer in this stretch.

Eventually an iconic truss bridge comes into view at South Smith Road, where downstream right is a quaint county park. Soon you'll discern the gorgeous Tiffany Stone Arch Bridge. Built in 1869 for locomotives along the Union Pacific line, the elegant bridge is composed of limestone and reinforced concrete. At 387 feet long and about 70 feet tall, it comprises five arches and is one of only a few like it in the whole world. It's also the single oldest stone-arch bridge in Wisconsin, and it's truly magnificent. And for an added bonus, there's a light rapid below the bridge under the middle arch.

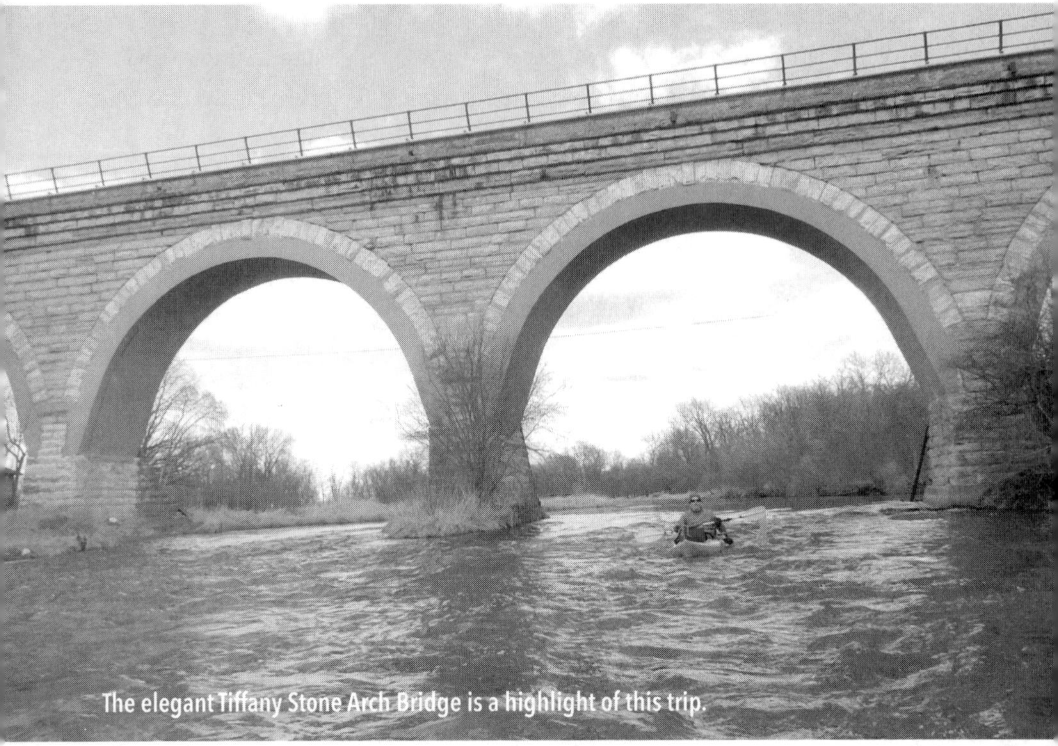

The elegant Tiffany Stone Arch Bridge is a highlight of this trip.

A couple more graceful bends to the right and then left follow the bridge in a pretty, wooded corridor, including some wispy weeping willows. You'll begin to see a few houses here and there. As the creek heads south, it will make a final subtle bend to the right past a small island and a set of fun riffles. The take-out is on the right, at the end of a walkway connecting the creek and parking lot at Sweet-Allyn County Park, where there are full facilities.

•THE•FUDGE•

ADDITIONAL TRIPS If you have time (it won't take long), stop by **Carver-Roehl County Park** (tinyurl.com/carver-roehlpark), just north of Turtle Creek at 4907 S. Carvers Rock Road. Located in a mesic forest with limestone cliffs sculpted by a babbling brook, it's a very pretty spot tucked away from the surrounding farms.

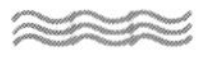

30 Turtle Creek C:

SWEET-ALLYN PARK TO DICKOP STREET IN ILLINOIS

•THE•FACTS•

Put-in/take-out Sweet-Allyn Park in Shopiere/Dickop Street just off WI 2 in South Beloit. See "The Flavor" for an alternative take-out and a mandatory portage.

Distance/time 11.5 mi/Allow for 4 hrs

Gradient/water level 6 fpm/Look for a minimum of 200 cfs at USGS gage 05431486. Ideal levels are 220–250 cfs.

Water type Quietwater, riffles, and several light rapids

Canoe or kayak Either

Skill level Beginner for kayakers, experienced for canoeists (due to a couple of strainers)

Time of year to paddle Anytime

Landscape Suburban backyards, urban roads, city parks, hilly woods

---

OVERVIEW The liveliest segment of Turtle Creek, this is a quintessential (sub)urban trip through a protected forest, hills, thrilling riffles, Class I rapids for miles on end, and great wildlife sightings. The action is nonstop, and the fun of it completely infectious. The only caveats are that this segment is often too shallow to run and is appropriate only for paddlers with some experience. But as long as you have solid boat control and there's been a good dose of rain, you will absolutely love this trip and will want to do it again and again. Turtles, hawks, muskrats, wood ducks, geese, frogs, green herons, great blue herons, Baltimore orioles, and bald eagles (in Beloit!) are some of the highlights.

PLANNING ADVISORY Sometimes debris collects at the upstream side of the Colley Road bridge in Beloit, a couple of blocks east of Oakwood and Calvary Cemeteries. The current here is strong, so it's wise to scout this beforehand.

CAR SHUTTLE **9.8 miles.** From the take-out, cross IL 2 and head east on IL 75 to the interstate. Head north into Wisconsin on I-94/I-39 and take Exit 183 to Shopiere Road/County Road S; then turn right at the top of the exit ramp. In Shopiere, turn left onto CR J, cross the creek, and then turn right into Sweet-Allyn Park.

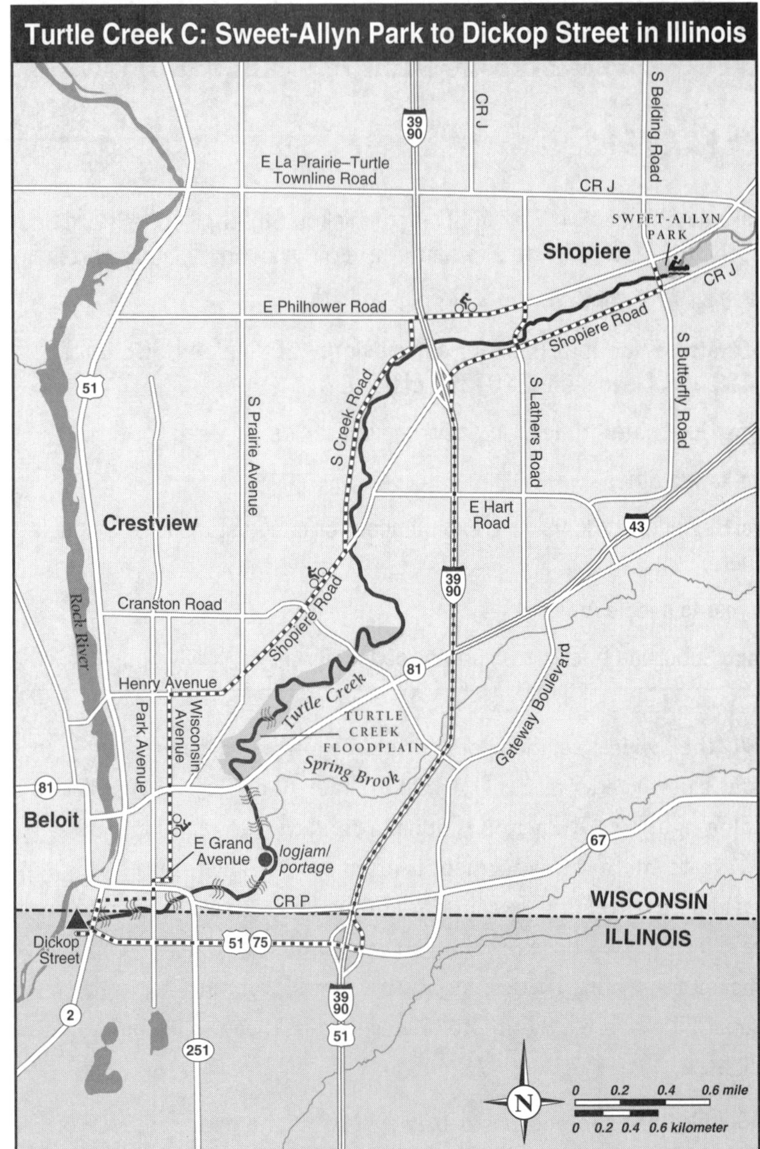

BIKE SHUTTLE 9.8 miles. From the take-out, turn left onto IL 2 and cross Turtle Creek into Wisconsin; just over the state line in Beloit, immediately past the McDonald's, turn right onto the bike path and head east. Turn left onto Park Avenue, right onto East Grand Avenue, and then left onto Wisconsin Avenue. After 1.6 miles, turn right onto Henry Avenue, then left at the Y onto Shopiere Road. After 1.6 miles, turn left on South Creek Road; then, after 2 miles, turn right onto East Creek Road. Cross the interstate and then turn right onto South Lathers Road, crossing the attractive truss bridge. Turn left onto Shopiere Road/CR S, then left again onto CR J, and then right into Sweet-Allyn Park.

TAKE-OUT N42° 29.652' W89° 02.336' **PUT-IN** N42° 34.411' W88° 56.378'

•THE•FLAVOR•

PUT IN AT THE ADORABLE SWEET-ALLYN COUNTY PARK, where there are full facilities as well as a convenient boat launch. You can examine the gravel-bed island in front of the concrete launch for a reliable old-school way of determining the water level for this trip. If it is totally submerged, you could be facing a pushy current and possible problems downstream; an entirely exposed island will mean a lot of frustrating scraping. A perfect paddling level is indicated by partial exposure.

The water here is representative of this trip: about 50 feet wide, only a couple of feet deep, with a gravel–sand bottom and turbid color. Riffles begin immediately and continue with only a few short breaks of flatwater for this entire trip. For the first mile, the left bank will be mostly undeveloped, while there are scattered houses on the right. Wildlife sightings are nonetheless excellent, herons and turtles particularly.

After a straightaway, the creek will turn left and then right into a set of riffles leading to a short but fun run of mild rapids at the attractive green truss bridge at South Lathers Road. Another straightaway follows as you pass beneath twin interstate bridges. Shortly downstream lies a tricky tangle of downed trees that, with good boat control, you can maneuver through without difficulty. Riffles will glide you down a mile of mostly undeveloped and lovely tree-canopied banks. Houses will begin to appear on the right, followed by Schollmeyer County Park, where there's a primitive but doable boat launch on the right (**N42° 32.965' W88° 59.377'**) that would shave off more than 3 miles of this trip.

On the right is a pretty pond you can access. On the left will be more houses before a pleasant wooded segment made all the more fun with riffles that take you to the Shopiere Road bridge. For a couple hundred yards, you'll pass by attractive houses on the right, while the left banks are woodsy and undeveloped. Soon the woods will enclose the right bank, too. There's a 30-foot-tall hill on the left and a good chance you'll see deer and bald eagles. This is a very pretty section of the creek, even though the din of highway traffic is not far off. Riffles will pick up again toward the bridge at Cranston Road.

Between the Cranston Road and Milwaukee Road bridges, the creek courses through a floodplain forest and the riffles graduate to light rapids. Other than a few houses, the surrounding landscape is positively intimate, preserved, and public. There are even a few rope swings for kicks. There is one tricky spot, however, where the creek drops in a subtle but powerful chute with two downed trees to avoid. The first fell from the right bank, so paddle to the left of it, then immediately pivot to the right to avoid the strong, sweeping current taking you to the second tree, which fell from the left bank. *You do not want to be pinned against this!* There's an opening to the far right that's easy to pass under without portaging these two obstructions.

Absolutely delightful Class I rapids prevail for the next few miles past the bridges at Milwaukee Road, Colley Road (see "The Facts" for an advisory here), and a railroad trestle. In December 2015, the Friends of Turtle Creek teamed up with the Beloit Fire Department Swift Water Rescue Team to remove a colossal logjam below the railroad trestle, making the final miles of the creek even more exhilarating and hassle-free. The best run of light rapids awaits past fun bends and twists around little islands that braid the main channel—now without portaging. There's a well-trod portage trail on the right; the banks are low here, so getting out and back in is easy. Below this logjam, the creek rewards you with its best run of light rapids past fun bends and twists around little islands that braid the main channel.

The creek will make a sharp right at the base of a hill. In its remaining 2 miles, it takes on the most urban character of the whole trip. Just the same, there's a green corridor of trees on both tall banks, and exquisitely resilient riffles just do not quit—up to and even past the take-out. First, you'll pass under the US 51 bridge, then invisibly sneak under the porous border into Illinois, pass under the Park Avenue bridge, and then pass under another random truss bridge.

Hang on, though: There's still a concrete wall, the IL 2 bridge, and another railroad trestle. The take-out is immediately downstream from *this* trestle, on the left; there's yet another trestle just downstream. (From here, it's 1,000 feet to the Rock River confluence, but there isn't a whole lot to see, frankly; plus, it's awfully slow-going and strenuous paddling upstream through the strong current back to the take-out.)

•THE•FUDGE•

ADDITIONAL TRIPS Again, I don't recommend continuing on to the Rock River. There is no adequate place to take out until Rockton Road, which is not an official access point and is situated below a dangerous low-head dam that you must portage, 4.6 miles downstream.

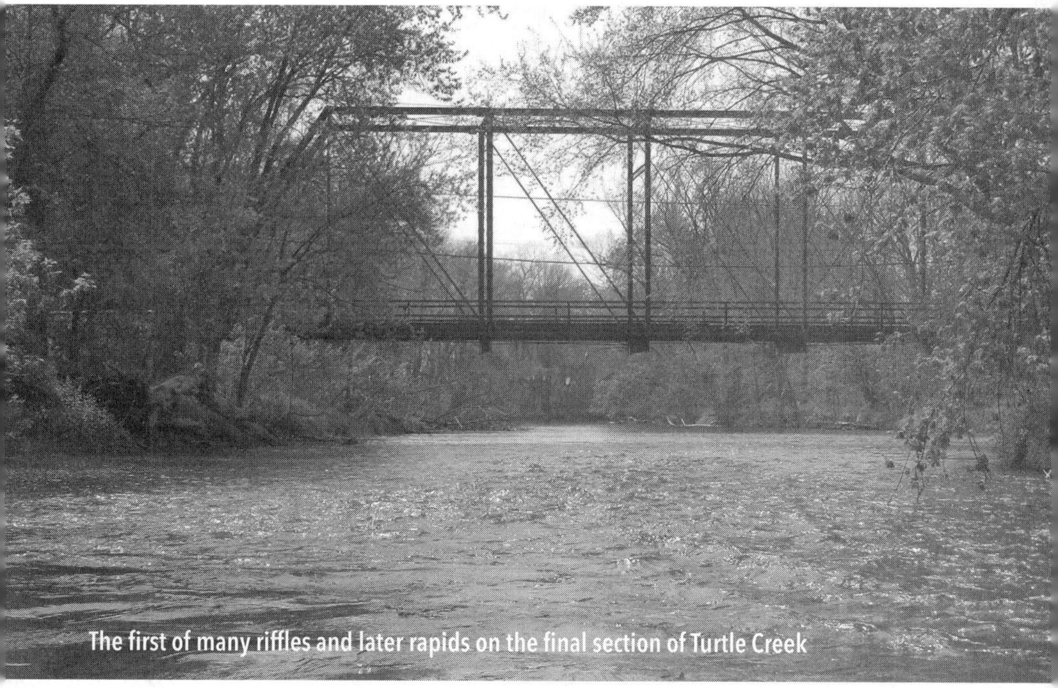

The first of many riffles and later rapids on the final section of Turtle Creek

CAMPING Primitive camping may be permitted by special request in select Rock County, Wisconsin, parks; call 608-757-5451 for more information. A better bet just a bit south is the **Hononegah Forest Preserve** (80 Hononegah Road, Rockton, Illinois; 815-877-6100).

RENTALS **Rocktown Adventures** (313 N. Madison St., Rockford, Illinois; 815-636-9066)

FOOD FOR THOUGHT Hungry paddlers have several great options in Beloit, just a few blocks north of the state line from the take-out. For delicious organic food, head to **Bushel and Peck's** (328 State St.; 608-363-3911). Just down the street is the fabulous **Mama Lou's Shrimp & BBQ Smokehouse** (315 State St.; 608-247-9421). For an unpretentious slice of mom-and-pop, check out **Jane's Cafe** (121 Dearborn St.; 608-365-7250). Or if you're just looking for a great homemade doughnut—and really, aren't we all?—treat yourself right at **Old Fashion Bakery** (1255 Park Ave.; 608-365-6461).

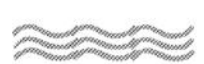

31 White River (Walworth County):
SHERIDAN SPRINGS ROAD TO BURLINGTON

•THE•FACTS•

Put-in/take-out Sheridan Springs Road by Buckby Road/Wagner Park in Burlington. See "The Flavor" for the recommended put-in for beginner paddlers.

Distance/time 12.4 mi/Allow for 5.5 hrs

Gradient/water level 9 fpm in the beginning, then 3 fpm/80 cfs at USGS gage 05548170 on Nippersink Creek in Genoa City

Water type Class I–II rapids first 4 miles, quietwater after

Canoe or kayak Kayak preferable

Skill level Experienced for the rapids, beginner afterward

Time of year to paddle Spring or after heavy rain

Landscape Wooded hills, sedge meadows, prairie, urban

OVERVIEW Beginning with a bang and ending with a whimper (albeit a pretty one), this trip offers something for adrenaline junkies and casual paddlers alike. The only catch is that the first 4 miles will be very shallow in low water. Wildlife includes beaver, deer, muskrats, redwing blackbirds, and great blue herons.

SHUTTLE 7.5 miles. From the take-out, head west on Chestnut Street, then turn left onto Mormon Road. Take Mormon all the way to its end and bear right onto Spring Valley Road/WI 36. Stay on WI 36 for 5 miles, crossing WI 11 as well as the White River State Trail. Turn left onto South Road. Turn right onto Sheridan Springs Road to the bridge.

BIKE SHUTTLE 7.5 miles. After bearing right onto Spring Valley Road/WI 36 from Mormon Road, bear left onto Spring Valley Road where WI 36 continues straight. After crossing the WI 11 overpass, turn right onto the White River State Trail. In Lyons, turn left onto Mill Street and then right onto Spring Valley Road. Bear left onto Sheridan Springs Road and follow it to the put-in.

Note: If you plan to do the trip as described, stop to scope out the big drop at Spring Valley Road during your shuttle.

TAKE-OUT N42° 41.097' W88° 17.160' **PUT-IN** N42° 37.895' W88° 23.028'

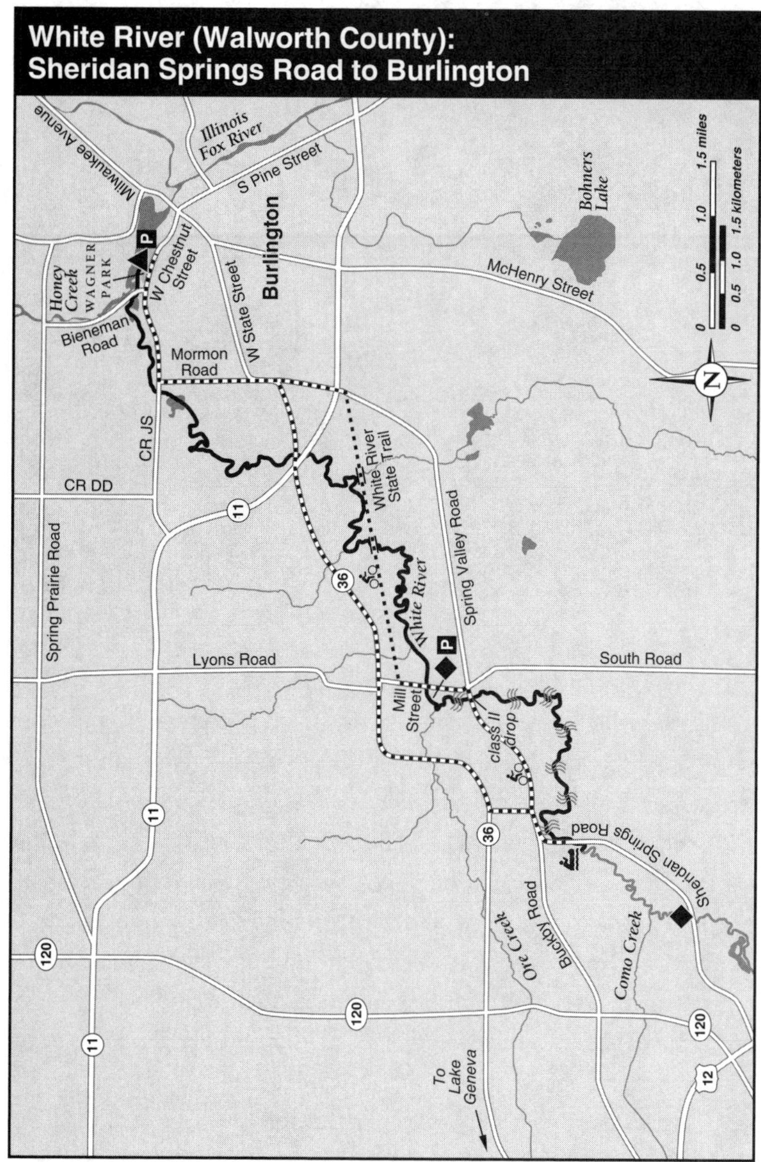

•THE•FLAVOR•

PUT IN ON THE UPSTREAM SIDE of Sheridan Springs Road, on river left. For the first few miles, the river is a wild ride of continuous riffles and a couple Class I ledges. There are some obstacles to dodge and engage, so you will need to be vigilant here. The setting is beautiful, with high wooded ridges surrounding you and random boulders. Only 30 feet wide, the river has a root beer hue to it, and the riverbed is mostly rocky.

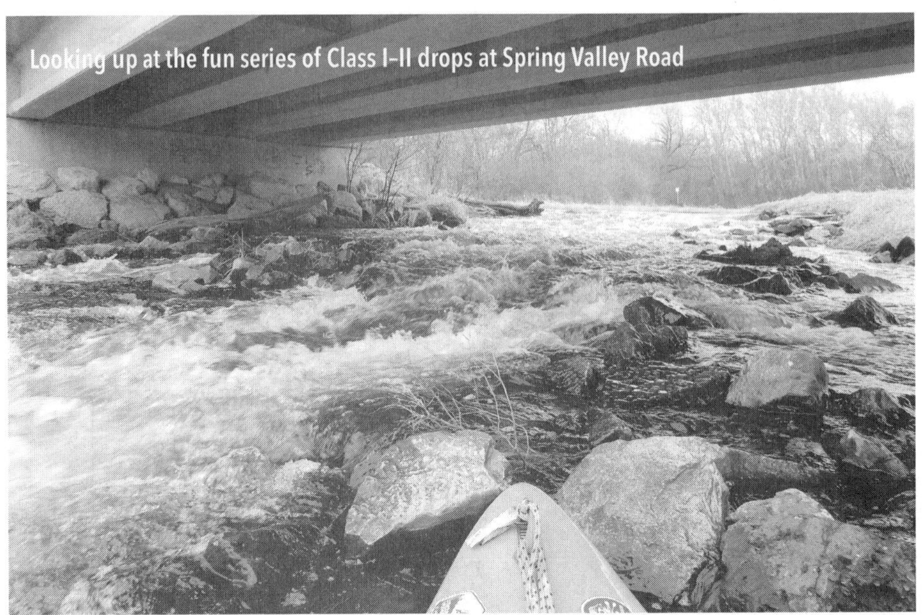

Looking up at the fun series of Class I–II drops at Spring Valley Road

After a sharp right-hand bend, the first ledge appears. This is followed by a straightaway, after which the river turns left and is followed by another ledge through a secluded wooded section. A large island splits the river in two channels; choose the right one. A series of riffly meanders follows, but soon the current slows. A series of meanders takes you past another hill on your left, after which the current slows again. Catch your breath before you hear the rush of water at the Spring Valley Road drop.

During your shuttle, you sensibly scouted the drop, right? There used to be a dam, but locals have arranged large rocks to create a fun but challenging Class I–II ledge, depending on water levels. (You can, of course, portage around this.) Line your path along the tongue of water in the center-left. One easy but fast dip leads to the bridge and then a larger drop directly underneath the bridge itself. At the bottom of the drop lies a deep pool and an opportunity to play in the hole at the base of the ledge.

Riffles continue downstream of the bridge in a meandering section with some deadfall to dodge. Houses come into view. At a sharp right-hand bend, Ore Creek feeds the river on the left. There's a small park on the right in Lyons where you can stop to have a snack, open that first beer, or use the bathroom. This is also where I recommend putting in if you're not up to tackling the rapids (**N42° 38.879' W88° 21.462'**).

For the next 7 miles, the river takes on a very different character, slowing as the surrounding landscape opens up to a prairie with occasional small hills in the near distance. When not straight, the meanders are mostly soft, easy curves, while a few random islands split up the channel. After a few tight turns and old oxbows, you'll come upon a rickety wooden footbridge. If the water is high, you'll probably need to portage it. Just past this is the much more modern and downright idyllic bridge on the White River State Trail, a beautiful path I highly recommend taking for the bike-shuttle option. A few tight zigzags lead to a pleasant straightaway where the river and bike trail run parallel to each other. This in turn will lead to a red truss bridge improbably in the middle of nowhere.

A few more oxbows follow, one shaped like a human ear where a feeder stream enters on the right. A narrow wooded corridor follows briefly, leading up to a highway bypass bridge. There are three bridges in all—two for WI 11, the third for WI 36. Just downstream from the bridges are some kinky deadfall obstacles you want to avoid.

The last section of this trip is especially pretty and historically fascinating. While the left side remains mostly prairie, the right side is wooded and punctuated by modest hills. Here, the river has widened to 50 feet. In one postcard moment, you'll see tall grass flanking the right bank with a stand of towering pines in the background. A long straightaway follows, leading up to the bridge at County Road JS.

Below the CR JS bridge, the river meanders a few more times and swells to more than 100 feet wide, the current virtually nonexistent. Houses will appear on the right. You'll pass under a bridge, after which Honey Creek enters on the left. There's a dam less than a mile downstream. Keep to the right-hand shore toward Wagner Park, on the right. There is no designated take-out, so pick whichever spot is most convenient to your car or bicycle.

•THE•FUDGE•

ADDITIONAL TRIPS You can put in 3 miles upstream at a different bridge on Sheridan Springs Road, on the outskirts of Lake Geneva. While this stretch doesn't have as steep a gradient, it is very scenic. Many paddlers begin here and take out at Riverside Park in Lyons for a 6.6-mile trip.

Alternatively, **Honey Creek** is a pleasant stream in and of itself. A pretty and riffly stretch lies between Bell School Road and CR D.

CAMPING **Richard Bong State Recreation Area** (26313 Burlington Road, Kansasville; 262-878-5600)

RENTALS **Tip a Canoe** (262-342-1012, tipacanoellc.com) or **Honey Creek Kayak Outfitters** (262-473-9057, honeycreekkayakoutfitters@gmail.com), both in Burlington

FOOD FOR THOUGHT For great Mexican food in Burlington, check out **El Burrito Loco** (557 Milwaukee Ave.; 262-767-1172). For great Italian food, check out **Napoli Restaurant and Pizzeria** (132 N. Pine St.; 262-763-8390).

SHOUT-OUT You may have wondered why a road was named "Mormon" during your shuttle. If you paid even closer attention, you would have seen the **Mormon House** on the side of the road. A plaque outside it explains the history behind the house, which is extremely interesting and worth investigation.

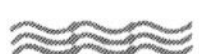

32 Yahara River B: DUNKIRK DAM TO ROCK RIVER

•THE•FACTS•

Put-in/Take-out Dunkirk Dam at County Road N/County Road H at Rock River. See "The Flavor" for an alternative take-out.

Distance/time 14.1 mi/Allow for 6 hrs

Gradient/water level 3.6 fpm/Consult USGS gage 05430175. A range of 400–450 cfs is perfect—at 500+ cfs, the riffles wash out and the water becomes turbid; at lower than 400 cfs, you will scrape.

Water type Riffles, quietwater

Canoe or kayak Either

Skill level Beginner

Time of year to paddle Anytime

Landscape Farms, forest, floodplains, high ridges

OVERVIEW The magnificent final stretch of the Yahara River features swift riffles, clear water, sweeping ridges, gnarled oak trees, great wildlife, and minimal development. This trip feels like you're truly away from it all, even though it's only half an hour south of Madison. Look for bald eagles, mergansers, sandhill cranes, herons, fish, deer, mink, hawks, and turkeys.

SHUTTLE **11.3 miles.** From the take-out, turn right and head north on CR H. Turn left onto CR M. Just after 4 miles, turn right on Riley Road. Cross Badfish Creek, then stay straight on Riley at the WI 59 intersection. Turn right on Stebbinsville Road,

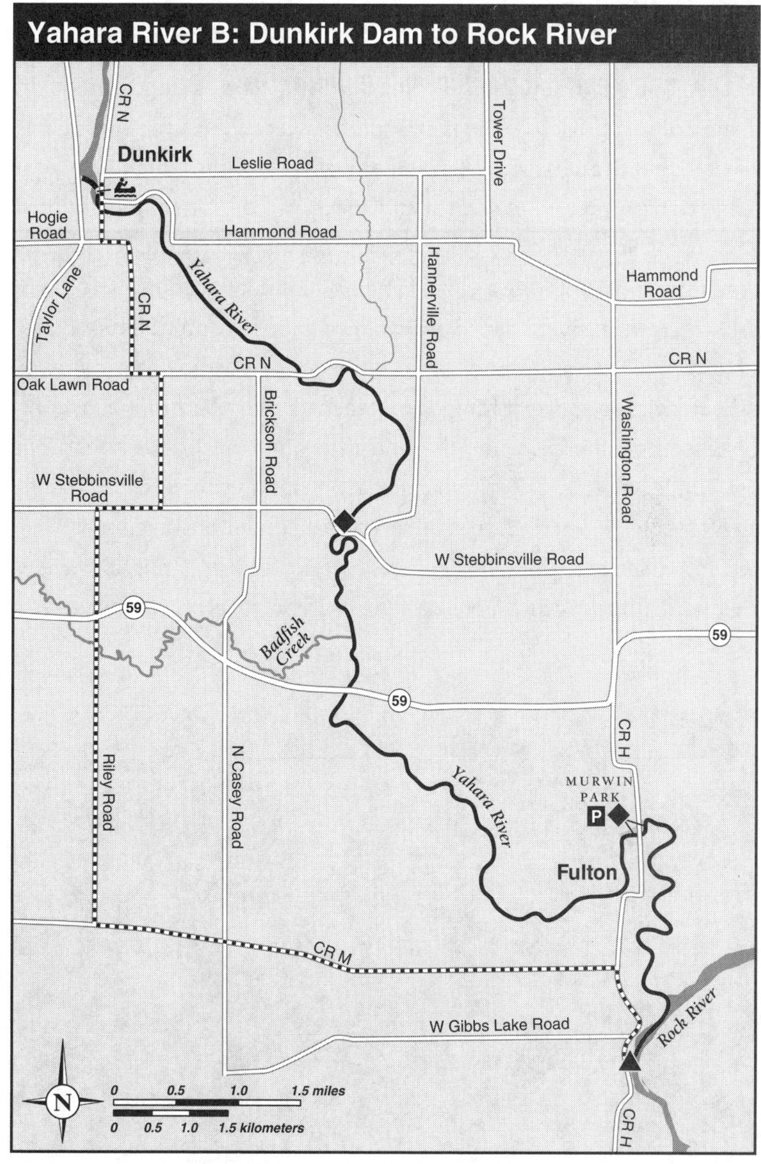

then left on McGinnis Road. Turn left on CR N and follow as it doglegs right, then left, then right again. Cross the Yahara River, then turn into the parking area for the Dunkirk Dam, on the left.

TAKE-OUT N42° 47.108' W89° 07.763' **PUT-IN** N42° 52.831' W89° 12.620'

•THE•FLAVOR•

PUT IN BELOW THE POWERHOUSE OF THE DUNKIRK DAM, a handsome old building clad in cream-colored brick. (If this is closed off, you can put in upstream of the dam and paddle 300 feet to an earth embankment just west of the dam, portage, and carry down the hill to the water below on the downstream side. Or simply put in at the CR N bridge, 70 yards downstream.)

Already the river environs feel wild and enchanted. For some 40 miles upstream of Dunkirk, the Yahara River has fed and drained the Madison Chain of Lakes, as well as a number of marshes and ponds, and has been impeded by four dams. However, below the Dunkirk Dam, everything changes: The Yahara becomes a river again. The current is swift, the water clear, and the landscape quite pretty. The river drops 30 feet in the first 5 miles; no rapids form, but the river has a number of fun riffles to run. Averaging 80 feet wide, there should be no concern about obstructions.

In this first section, the river features a series of long straightaways with only a few kinks and turns until Stebbinsville Road. But the banks are steep and the

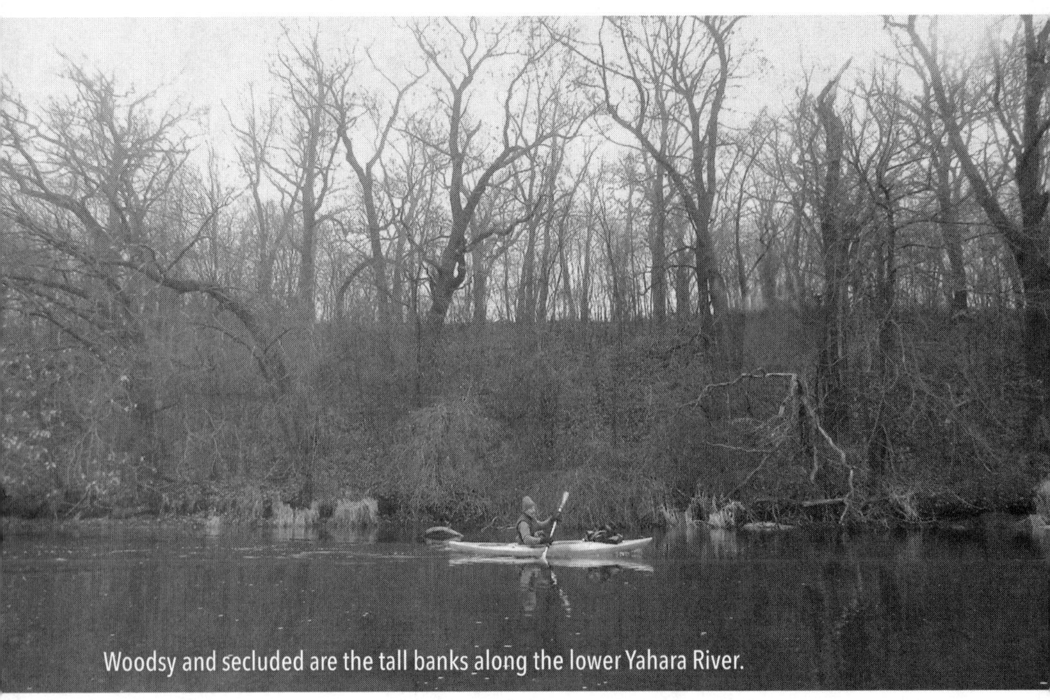

Woodsy and secluded are the tall banks along the lower Yahara River.

environment wild-feeling. An invigorating run of riffles greets you below Stebbinsville, where an island splits the river in two. The river bends like a horseshoe before zigzagging southward. After passing the confluence of Badfish Creek on your right (see Trip 18, page 104), the Yahara sweeps along a lovely tall ridge on your left approaching the WI 59 bridge. This first 6-mile leg of the trip is truly beautiful with riffles, clear water, islands, gorgeous old gnarled oak trees straight out of a Brothers Grimm tale, a sandy bottom, gravel bars, small boulders, undeveloped banks, tall ridges, and a palpable sense of intimacy. What else could you want?

If you don't have the whole day to paddle, you could take out at WI 59 on the left, upstream of the bridge (**N42° 49.577' W89° 10.337'**)—incidentally, this is where the USGS gage is located—but plenty more fun and beauty await downstream. The river swells below WI 59 for about half a mile before tapering again. Riffles flicker here and there while the landscape alternates between woods and open farmland, many of which are tobacco fields. (Years ago, Wisconsin was a major tobacco-production state, and the majority of the farms were in Dane and Rock Counties along the Yahara River corridor.) A long shoot of swift riffles takes you past the Caledonia Road bridge as the river heads south then east. The banks will have lowered here, but, since the current is swift, this is an especially fun section.

Approaching the town of Fulton, the river heads north abruptly into its second and last horseshoe bend. The best riffles of this second half of the trip take you toward Murwin Park, a fine resting point or final destination; there is plenty of parking, plus water, restrooms, and picnic tables. But it's worth sticking it out for the final 3 miles.

Just past the parking area on the downstream side of the CR H bridge at Murwin Park (the first parking area is on the upstream side), a strong current takes you along a tall, sandy bank. After this are a trailer and carport on your right. The river meanders around a wild-feeling floodplain, and the current will begin to slow (though there are still some riffly segments) before its confluence at the Rock River. Both here and then on the Rock River, you will see signs of high-water marks on the trees—ghostly white lines wrung around the trunks, many as tall as 4 feet. After a short straightaway, the Rock River looms directly before you, huge and flat—turn right. You're on the Rock for only half a mile. Stay to the right of an island and you'll see the parking area along CR H on your right. If the water is high enough (almost always in spring), you can paddle through the floodplain on your right up to the parking area.

•THE•FUDGE•

ADDITIONAL TRIPS Putting in upstream of Dunkirk is not recommended since the dam impounds the river all the way up to Stoughton and both banks are lined by houses. A short 5-mile trip can be paddled from Lake Kegonsa to downtown Stoughton by putting in at La Follette County Park off Williams Drive and taking out at Riverside Drive at the dam. Including two large bays and ponds, the trip is mostly marshy, with developed shoreline, and there is virtually no current.

For more information on the stretch of the Yahara River connecting the Madison Chain of Lakes, see Appendix A: Madison Metropolitan Area Trips, page 318.

CAMPING **Lake Kegonsa State Park** (2405 Door Creek Road, Stoughton; 608-873-9695)

RENTALS **Rutabaga Paddlesports** (220 W. Broadway, Madison; 608-223-9300); **Stoughton Canoe Rental** (2598 CR B, Stoughton; 920-728-0420)

FOOD FOR THOUGHT Each year in September, nearby Edgerton hosts **Chilimania,** a chili and salsa cook-off that's a lot of fun and would be the perfect reward after a great day of paddling. For more information, see chilimania.com.

For restaurant recommendations in Stoughton, see Trip 18, Badfish Creek (page 104).

OPPOSITE: Paddling on the second half of the Mukwonago River *(see Trip 24, page 132)* is easy after the riffles and rapids.

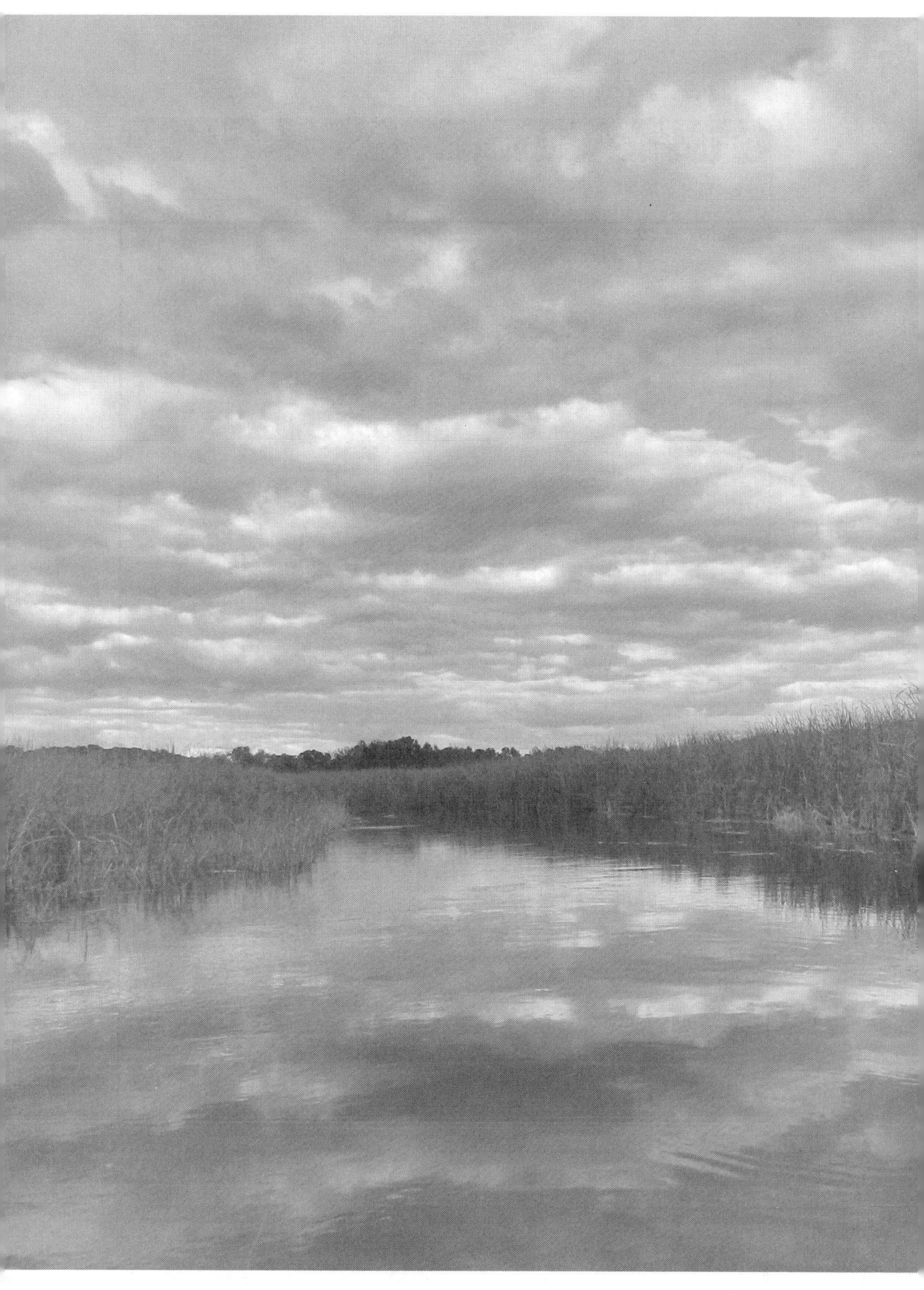

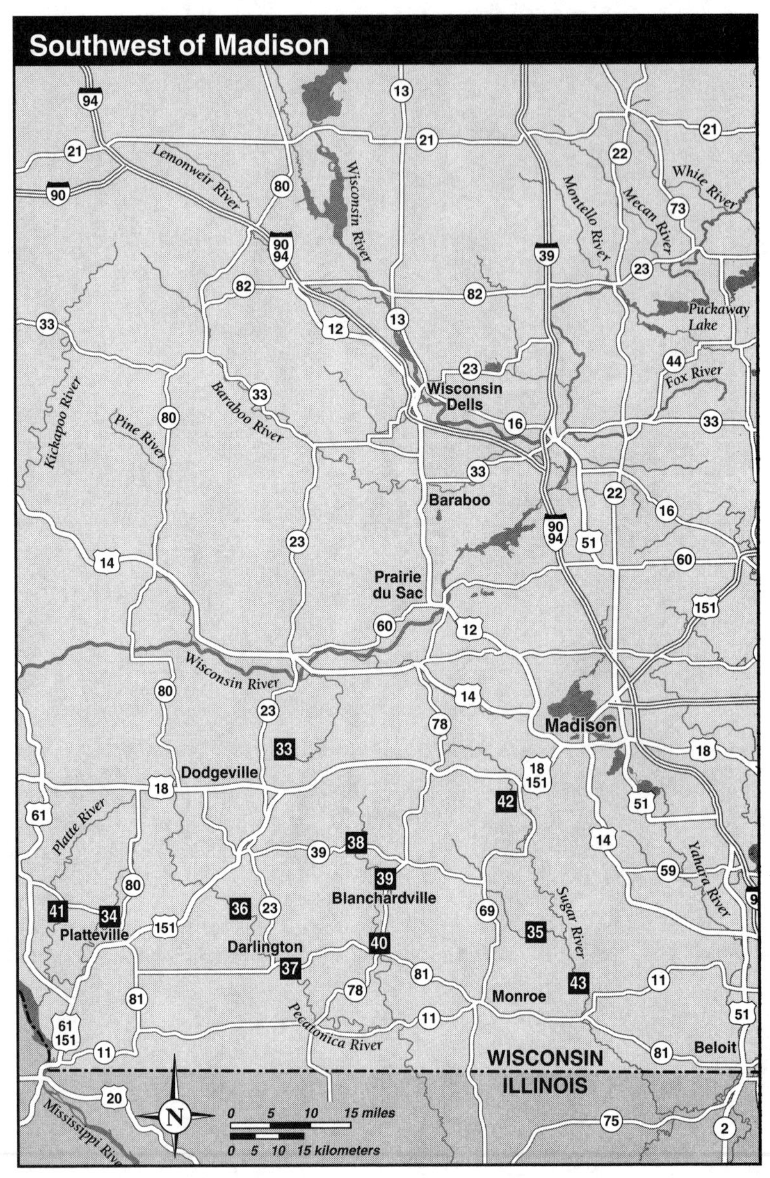
Southwest of Madison
Lemonweir River
Wisconsin River
Montello River
Mecan River
White River
Puckaway Lake
Fox River
Kickapoo River
Pine River
Baraboo River
Wisconsin Dells
Baraboo
Prairie du Sac
Wisconsin River
Madison
Dodgeville
Platte River
Blanchardville
Platteville
Darlington
Sugar River
Yahara River
Monroe
Pecatonica River
Beloit
WISCONSIN
ILLINOIS
Mississippi River
0 5 10 15 miles
0 5 10 15 kilometers

part three

Southwest of Madison

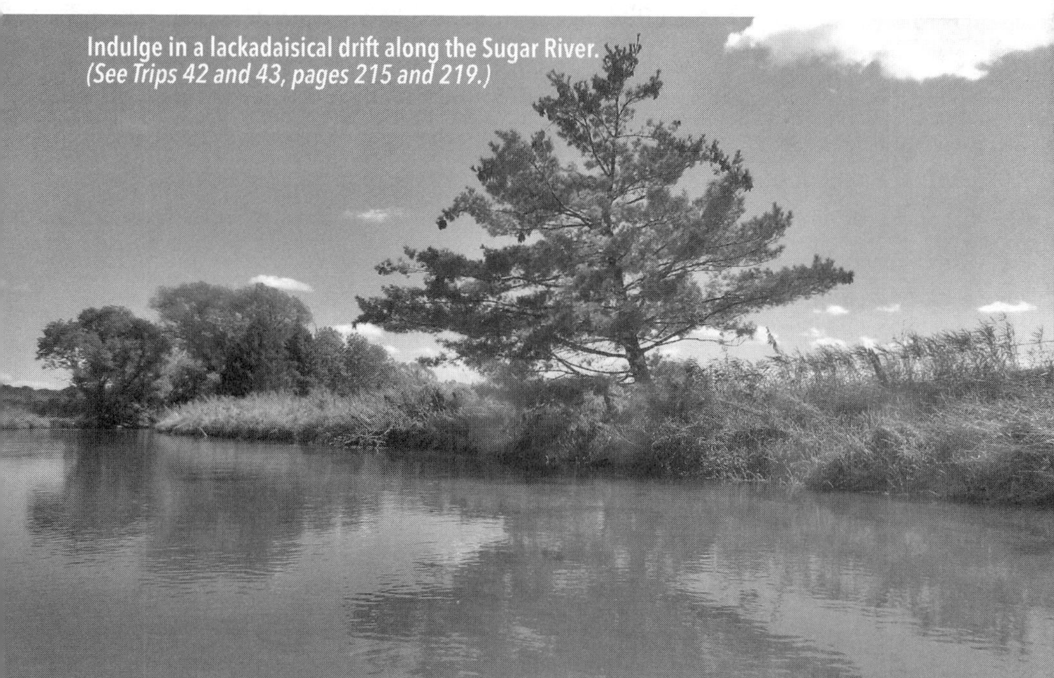

Indulge in a lackadaisical drift along the Sugar River.
(See Trips 42 and 43, pages 215 and 219.)

33 Governor Dodge State Park:
COX HOLLOW AND TWIN VALLEY LAKES

•THE•FACTS•

Put-in/take-out The accesses for each lake are located at official boat launches; follow park signs.

Distance/time *Cox Hollow Lake:* 2.2-mi round-trip/Allow for 2 hrs; *Twin Valley Lake:* 4-mi round-trip/Allow for 2.5 hrs. Distances and times take into account a hike up the bluffs.

Gradient/water level N/A

Water type Lake paddling

Canoe or kayak Either

Skill level Beginner

Time of year to paddle Anytime, though the park is busiest in summer

Landscape Beautiful Driftless hills enclosed within a state park

---

OVERVIEW Offering two beautiful lakes surrounded by ancient Driftless bluffs and cliffs for the price of one admission, this extraordinary state park is worth a day of your time—or more. Multiple hiking and mountain biking trails, in addition to three campgrounds (one of which is hike-in), provide for ample opportunities of quality outdoor time. You'll see geese, turtles, frogs, loons (in spring), turkey vultures, fish, ospreys, muskrats, sandhill cranes, great blue herons, coots, ruffed grouses, woodpeckers, clams, and oh so many snails.

Note: You must buy a Wisconsin State Parks vehicle-admission sticker to enter the park ($8 per day or $28 per year). For general information about the park, call 608-935-2315 or visit tinyurl.com/govdodgestatepark.

SHUTTLE N/A **PUT-INS/TAKE-OUTS** N43° 00.809' W90° 06.893' (Cox Hollow Lake), N43° 01.915' W90° 05.225' (Twin Valley Lake)

•THE•FLAVOR•

EACH OF THESE LAKES OFFERS SOMETHING SPECIAL and spectacular; I strongly recommend paddling both. Alas, there is no practical way to portage from one to the

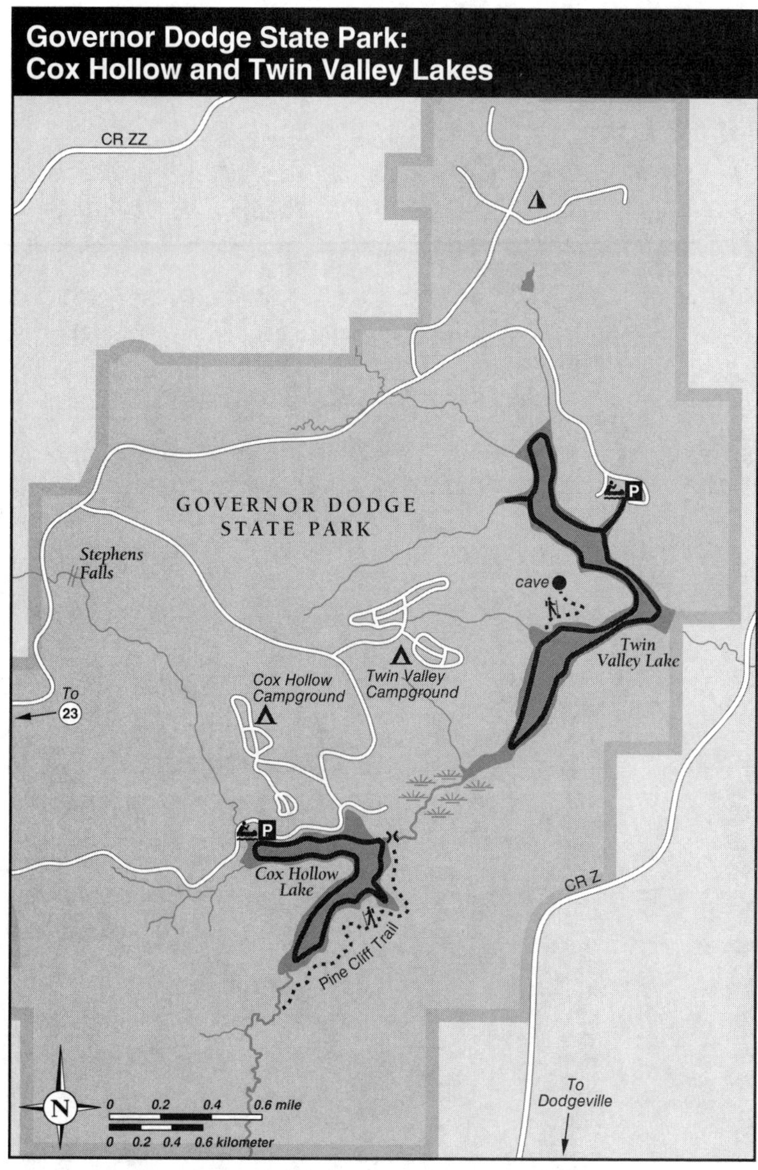

other, even though the two are essentially connected. Combined, they can be paddled in the same amount of time that an ordinary river day trip would take. There are no individual road names inside the park, so pick up a map upon entering and follow the signs directing you to the lake(s). Cox Hollow Lake is closer to the entrance of the park, so this tour begins there. Both tours follow a counterclockwise circuit. Each boat launch has water, restrooms, and plenty of parking.

Cox Hollow Lake

Put in at the official boat ramp and head to the right. Initially, you'll come upon two small recesses: one a cattail marsh, the other a wetlands area with flowers and tall grass, both at the western edge of the lake, at the base of two bluffs. (There's a gorgeous craggy outcrop atop a tall bluff called Enee Point behind the wetlands less than 500 feet to the west of the boat ramp that you can't see from the water but is worth a look-see while on land.)

To the east, a small bluff lines the right shore as you head westward, first with patches of moss, rocks, and swaths of pine. As you round the peninsular corner of this bluff and now head south, you'll see a breathtaking cliff on your left, part of Pine Cliff

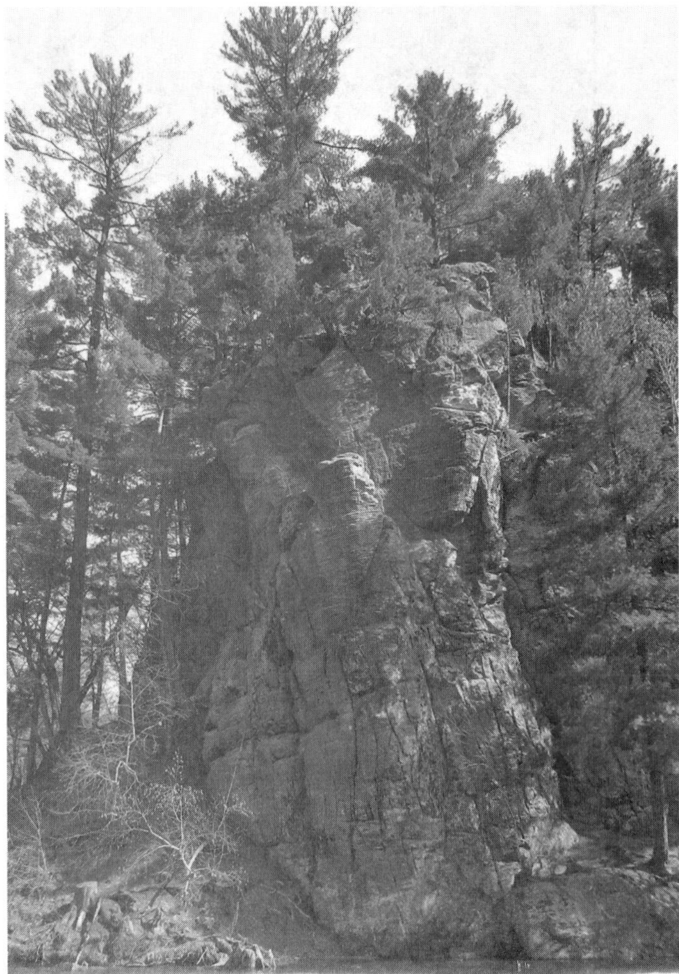

The majestic Pine Cliff at Cox Hollow Lake

State Natural Area, a sheer vertical wall 100 feet high (more on this in a moment). Undulating bluffs beckon the eye toward the south, going on seemingly forever.

A much larger cattail complex thrives at the southern edge of the lake. Turning back around and now heading north, you'll see that the bluff on the right still bears the scars of a tornado that swept through this part of the park in the summer of 2014; large boulders lie at the bottom of the bluff, seated in the lake, surrounded by a carpet of pine needles. Just after this, you'll come upon the base of Pine Cliff, seeping directly into the water and rising as high as a skyscraper (or so it seems). Just to the left of it, you can lodge your boat and clamber up the steep slope to the top of the rock. This is not an official trail, so hike carefully and with low impact upon the environment. This is a protected natural area, because all three types of pine native to Wisconsin—red, white, and black—are found here. The ledge at the top is narrow, offering glimpses of the lake below and bluffs beyond. A veritable rock garden with various levels of terraces can be climbed up and down, some of them leading to open views of the Driftless valley that are simply stunning.

Back on the water, a recess to the right (east) leads to an eponymous hollow, followed by a grassy berm on the right and a dam to its left. You can safely paddle up to the dam and look below a concrete wall to the small waterfall it creates. (The creek here is far too tiny to paddle to Twin Valley Lake.) The beach and pavilion follow on the right.

As you paddle westward now and back to the boat launch, you'll see a random grassy area with picnic tables. Behind it lies a magnificent rock face resembling a stage or theatre. Make a mental note to check this out once you're done; called Deer Cove Rockshelter (see next section), it's about 300 feet east of the boat launch. Follow the tall right bank back to the launch.

Twin Valley Lake

Put in at the official boat ramp and turn right. Behind you is a recess with the first of innumerable beautiful views of the Driftless valley. A patch of cattails and maybe a hidden painted turtle lie to your right. As you move northwest, the beach and pavilion also will be on your right. Here, as elsewhere, the color of the water varies with the sun and wind, sometimes clear, other times jade green. Occasional logs and whole trees can be discerned beneath the surface. The right shore rises to the top of a big bluff, where exposed outcrops and boulders are embedded in the hillside, part of the official Woodland Trail.

As you paddle southward, a different bluff looms straight ahead. It's not called Twin Valley for nothing; you're ensconced within a nook of huge bluffs as far as the eye can see. A peninsula juts into the lake from the right, the top tip of which is crowned with a gorgeous limestone rock outcrop like a Christmas tree ornament, daubed in yellowy green. Rounding the peninsula, keep close to the shore, for soon you'll see a path leading into the woods where two large stones provide a convenient place to dock your boat.

The path is short though a bit hardscrabble, and it may not be suitable for all, since the ascent is about 100 feet. At the top there is a beautiful rock outcrop to the right, while the trail continues to the left; follow it. In a very short distance, you'll walk up to another set of rock outcrops. One is a cave you should plan to explore, but you'll need a headlamp and/or flashlight. The cave is absolutely thrilling for those who aren't claustrophobic or afraid of bats. On a hot summer day, the cool cave offers incomparable relief, and you may even see it breathe, too.

Back on the water, cattails line the right shore with a pretty meadow beyond. (I don't recommend heading to the meadow, however. There's not too much to see beyond a marsh environment, and it's a slog through thick, silty mud.)

Turning back around, now facing north, you'll see two magnificent outcrops pointing away from each other, resembling sentinels at a watchtower. These bluffs are half a billion years old. By contrast, the Grand Canyon is as "young" as 60 or 70 million years (depending on which geologist you ask). The Driftless Area is an incredibly old, haunting place. The right shore is similar to the Woodland Trail, a hillside studded with rock. Another grassy berm conceals a dam in a recess to the right, after which one last rocky hill bulges toward the water. The slope will diminish, gradually yielding to a sun-exposed savanna, and an assembly of aluminum canoes on the right leads you back to the boat launch.

•THE•FUDGE•

ADDITIONAL TRIPS In lieu of alternative paddling trips, you'll find miles of hiking, biking, and horseback-riding trails within the park's 5,350 acres. Whether you're here for a day or a weekend, take a moment at least to stop by **Stephens Falls**, a 15-foot waterfall reached by a half-mile hike. In spring or after a hard rain, you can walk behind the falls; otherwise, it's simply a pretty trickle. Near the Cox Hollow Lake boat launch is a magnificent hike along the **Deer Cove Rockshelter Trail**, where a huge overhang of dolomite limestone was home to American Indians 10,000 years ago.

CAMPING There are three campgrounds in the park: two for each lake, plus a backpack walk-in site at the north end of the park (608-935-2315).

RENTALS Rowboats and canoes can be rented at the park.

FOOD FOR THOUGHT For some of the best dang barbecue you'll find in southern Wisconsin, stop by **Bob's Bitchin' BBQ** in downtown Dodgeville (167 N. Iowa St.; 608-930-2227). Or tease your sweet tooth across the street at **Quality Bakery** (154 N. Iowa St.; 608-935-3812) or **The Cook's Room Café & Espresso Bar** (138 N. Iowa St.; 608-935-5282).

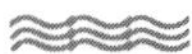

34 Little Platte River:
QUARRY ROAD TO COUNTY ROAD O

•THE•FACTS•

Put-in Quarry Road, off WI 81 in Platteville/CR O in Cornelia

Distance/time 12.3 mi/Allow for 4 hrs

Gradient/water level 11.5 fpm/Look for a minimum of 4' and 160 cfs at USGS gage 05414000 (Platte River). Even this will result in minor scraping. Unless you are a skilled whitewater paddler, significantly higher levels (6' and above) will be dangerous due to barbed wires and hairpin turns at limestone walls.

Water type Riffles, Class I–II rapids

Canoe or kayak Kayak preferred but can be canoed

Skill level Experienced

Time of year to paddle Early spring or just after a hard rain

Landscape Driftless limestone bluffs, rolling hills, farms

OVERVIEW An exhilarating trip that does not quit, the Little Platte is a creek-like river with constant riffles and rapids, spectacular limestone bluffs, outstanding wildlife, and nearly no development. Tricky to catch with enough water and dangerous when high, the Little Platte does not easily give up its secrets. But when it's running right, this simply is one of the best. You'll find muskrats, river otters, owls, great blue herons, green herons, bald eagles, dragonflies, deer, cows, and bulls.

CAR SHUTTLE **8.5 miles.** From the take-out, head east on CR O, then turn left on US 151. Take the CR D exit and turn left at the off-ramp. Where CR D and US 151

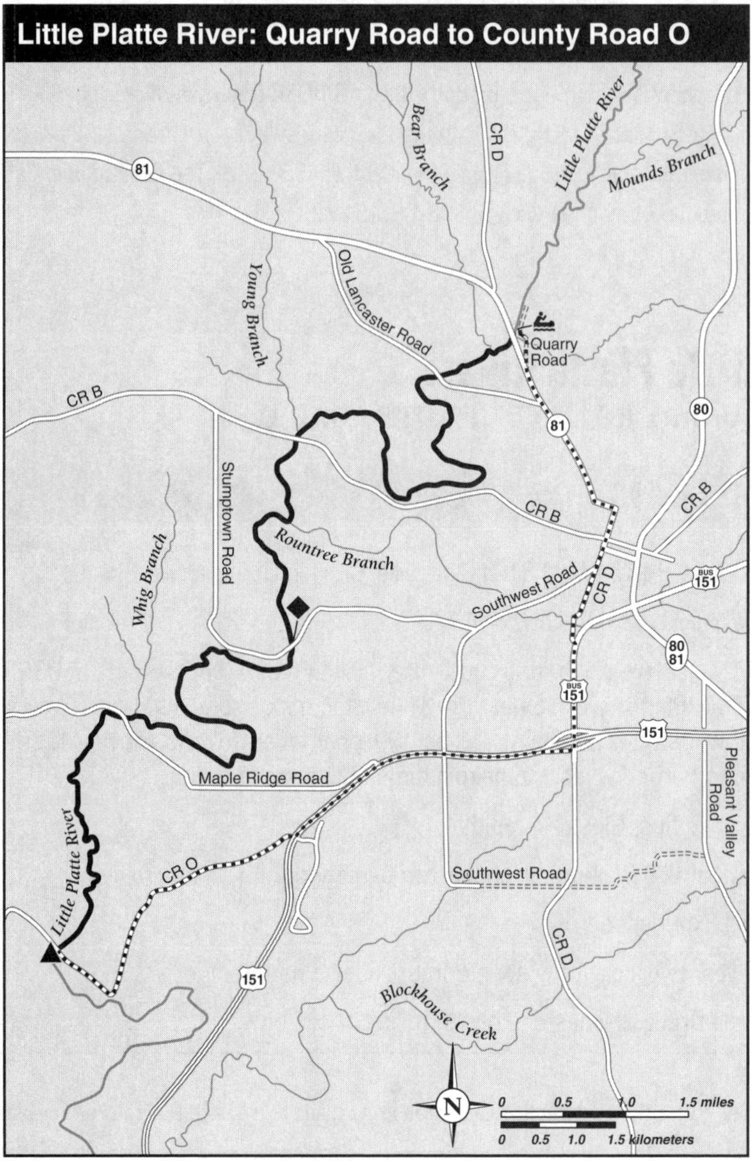

Little Platte River: Quarry Road to County Road O

Business split, turn left to stay on CR D. Follow it into downtown, then turn left on WI 81/CR D/Lancaster Street. Quarry Road will be on your right, just before the bridge, but it is easy to miss.

BIKE SHUTTLE **8.5 miles.** A nice bike trail runs parallel to US 151. From the take-out, head east on CR O and carefully cross US 151 at the intersection. At the stop sign, turn left onto Classic Lane, which leads to the trail. The trail ends conveniently at the CR D exit. Turn left onto CR D and into town as above.

TAKE-OUT N42° 41.381' W90° 33.860' **PUT-IN** N42° 45.406' W90° 29.656'

•THE•FLAVOR•

PUT IN OFF QUARRY ROAD, where a makeshift path leads to the river; just be sure to park your car out of the way so that others can pass. The river is delightfully narrow, only 20 feet wide. The first moments will be tranquil and lush with soft, small hills. Passing under the Old Lancaster Road bridge, you might spook a swarm of swallows. As the river begins to meander, riffles will announce each bend. Soon you will see an outcrop along the right bank at a sharp left bend. This has been a nice warm-up for what lies below.

At the end of a long straightaway, the river makes an abrupt right-hand turn. Directly in front of you is a limestone wall, and if you don't anticipate the turn in time, the light rapid will take you head-on toward the rock. *Remember:* Streams are always at their deepest on the outside bends, especially when lined with rock formations. If you need to slow down, intentionally run aground on the inside bend, where it will be shallow. Big boulders lie in the streambed here and there, fun obstacles to dodge in the swift current. Meanwhile, limestone outcrops continue to edge into and along the river, increasing in height as they do.

This is a quintessential Driftless stream, and the setting seems tucked away in another time and place. Also true of Driftless streams, cow pastures are plentiful, which for a paddler means two things: the likelihood of barbed wires and cows or bulls standing in the water. Of the former, at last count there were four individual strands of barbed wire. (They're often in pairs of two.) Usually wires will be flagged with a piece of tape to be more visible, and usually there's more clearance to pass underneath unscathed at either of the banks where the wire is more taut. Of the latter, be cautious and patient, because it's not always easy in a strong current. Cattle are apprehensive of strangers, and eventually they will get out of your way, but you don't want to be perceived as a threat, since you're outnumbered and vastly outweighed.

The river will flirt with CR B but then turn north away from the bridge before heading west and under it. In spring and after heavy rains the rest of the year, you will likely see weeping sedges draped and dripping off limestone shelves. Shortly after CR B, the river will gently turn to the right, and you'll see a covered bridge over a small

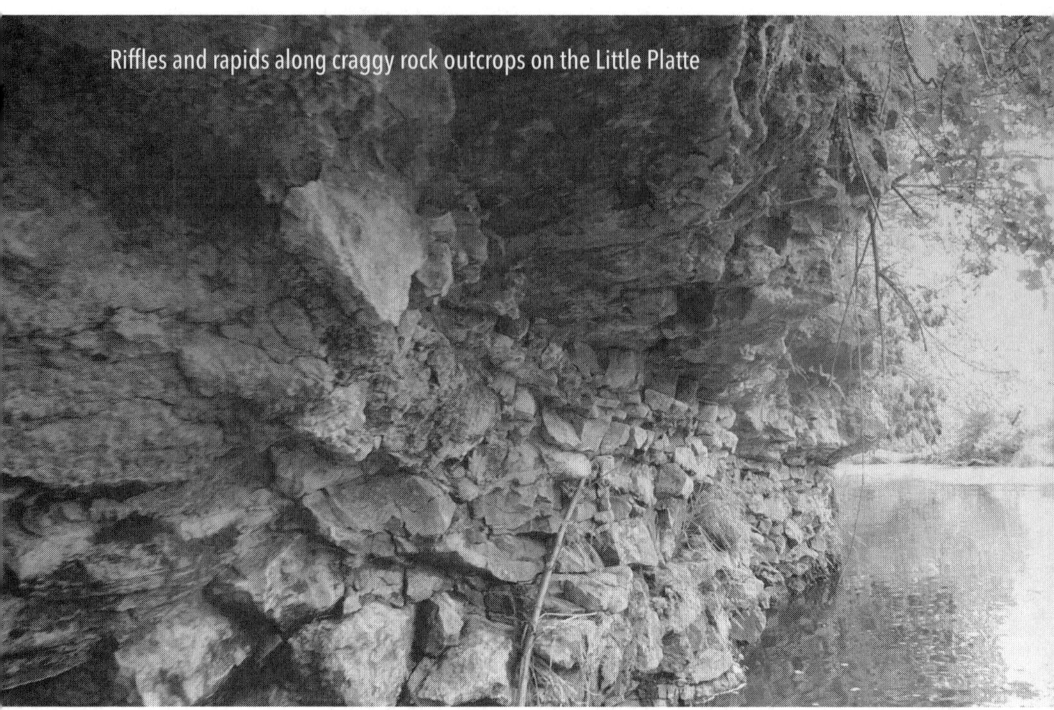
Riffles and rapids along craggy rock outcrops on the Little Platte

creek. After a riffly left bend, the river tumbles down a couple ledges. In average water levels, these will rank as Class I, but in higher conditions, this can be a favorite play spot for whitewater paddlers. Gorgeous undulations in the rock wall line the river here in a secluded section, and you might even spot a playful otter.

Where the river opens up some, a pretty panorama of Driftless hills envelops you. But then woods enclose again, and the setting is more intimate. You're never far from a farm, but you'll swear sometimes that you're surrounded by wilderness. A straightaway takes you to the Stumptown Road bridge, where some whitewater-only paddlers take out. The river will again abruptly bend to the right before following a farm; don't be surprised to encounter more cattle cooling off in the water. A set of power lines towers above you in a shallow spot, but then the stream deepens again as the river sweeps past another bluff. Here, you might inspire a deer to leap across the stream or dart deep into the woods. A small waterfall cascades down a series of rocks.

The next, and penultimate, bridge is at Maple Ridge Road. The final few miles are more agrarian and thus more open than the rest of the trip, but the current remains riffly. A long, graceful straightaway takes you to the bridge at CR O. This will not be the easiest take-out; the best spot is on the downstream side of the bridge, on river left. You'll drag or carry your boat up a small but slightly steep hill about 15 feet high to the road.

•THE•FUDGE•

ADDITIONAL TRIPS Downstream, it's 5 miles to the next bridge at Church Road, but the sound of US 151 increasingly creeps in. From there, it's another 8.5 miles to the confluence with the Platte River and then another 3 miles to the Mississippi River. While pretty in its own right, this stretch is less riffly and has fewer rapids and outcrops than the trip outlined here. Above Quarry Road, the river usually is too shallow to paddle and doesn't do much to capture the imagination.

CAMPING **Nelson-Dewey State Park** (12190 CR VV, Cassville; 608-725-5374); **Grant River Recreation Area,** on the Mississippi River south of Potosi (3990 Park Lane, off WI 233; 608-763-2140); and **Mound View Park** in Platteville (East Madison Street and Broadway; 608-348-6111)

RENTALS **Grant River Canoe & Kayak Rental** in Beetown (608-794-2342, grantrivercanoerental.com)

FOOD FOR THOUGHT For great food and pretty good beer, stop at **Steve's Pizza Palace** in downtown Platteville (175 Main St.; 608-348-3136).

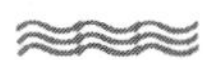

35 Little Sugar River: SCHNEEBERGER ROAD TO ALBANY

•THE•FACTS•

Put-in/take-out Schneeberger Road/North Water Street

Distance/time 7.6 mi/Allow for 3.5 hrs

Gradient/water level 1.3 fpm/There is no gage; water levels are generally adequate year-round.

Water type Quietwater and flatwater; lake-like paddling the last mile

Canoe or kayak Kayak preferred

Skill level Beginner, with caution—there are some obstructions, and you'll need good boat control.

Time of year to paddle Anytime

Landscape Sedge meadow, hardwood floodplains, prairie, hills

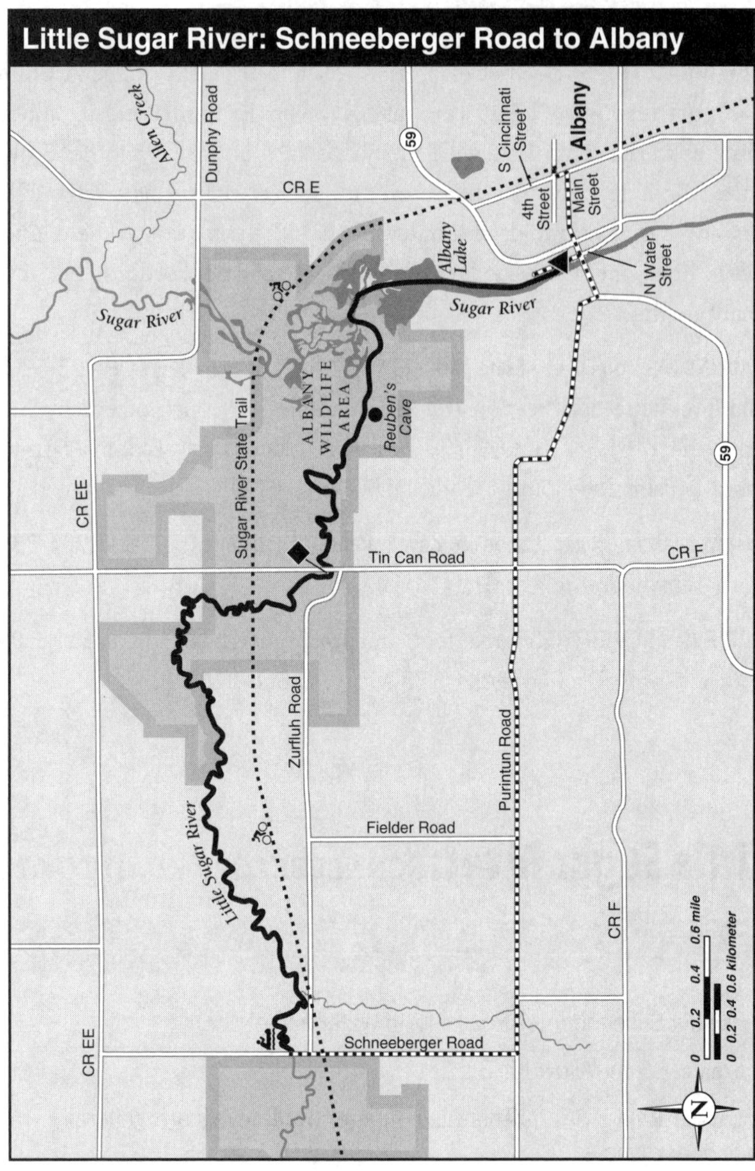

OVERVIEW The Little Sugar is a hidden gem of a stream that requires maneuvering around many obstacles but rewards your efforts with miles of protected wildlife area, pretty views of gentle hills, some rare rock outcrops, and even a small cave. This trip offers an outstanding paddle-and-pedal shuttle option, and you're bound to see such creatures as sandhill cranes, wood ducks, hooded mergansers, hawks, painted turtles, softshell turtles, muskrats, beavers, plovers, bald eagles, and owls.

CAR SHUTTLE 5.2 miles. From the take-out, head south on Water Street, then turn right onto WI 59. Turn right onto North Taylor Street, which will become Mineral Street, and then turn right again onto Purintun Road. Follow Purintun 3.7 miles to Schneeberger Road, and turn right. Park on the west side of the bridge.

BIKE SHUTTLE 5.8 miles. You'll need a Wisconsin State Trail pass; see tinyurl.com/witrailpassfees. From the take-out, head south on Water Street, then turn left onto WI 59. Turn left on Cincinnati Street and then take a quick right onto Fourth Street. Turn left onto the Sugar River State Trail and follow it 5 miles. Turn right at the Zurfluh Road intersection and then right again onto Schneeberger Road.

TAKE-OUT N42° 42.607' W89° 26.383' **PUT-IN** N42° 43.653' W89° 30.691'

•THE•FLAVOR•

PUT IN AT SCHNEEBERGER ROAD on the upstream side of the bridge, river left. The area is very woodsy, so be sure to check for ticks and watch out for any poisonous plants. For the first mile, you'll likely encounter some low-clearance fallen trees. Depending on how limber your torso is, it may behoove you to portage. After an initial series of meanders, the river will follow a gradual curve to the left and then enter an abrupt right-hand bend. On the right bank lie the curious ruins of a shooting gallery, right here in the middle of a floodplain woods (but no adjacent house or shack). Head back to the put-in if you hear even the faintest twang of twin banjos!

The river takes many turns, but because the current is gentle, negotiating them is not too much of a workout. It's only 25 feet wide, so you'll often encounter a downed tree to dodge here and there; many of these can be ridden over, so long as you don't mind the occasional bump and slide. The water's hue falls between shale and lime green, and the bottom is beautifully sandy. You'll paddle past plenty of logs just below the surface, reminiscent of a shipwreck. The number of submerged logs and intermittent trees growing out of the water contributes to this trip's aesthetics.

This section of the river is fun, as it keeps you on your toes; it's a good section in which to hone your boat-control and river-reading skills. Most of the time, it's generally simple to follow the main stream, with the ambiguous exception of an island about 3 miles downstream from the put-in—take the right channel. While the left bank remains wooded and generally flat for this whole trip, the right bank gives way to the occasional view of pastures, rolling hills, and eroded sand walls.

Eventually you'll head south, rather than east, and paddle underneath a bridge of the Sugar River State Trail. Soon, the river will widen as much as 80 feet as a meadowy ridge looms directly before you. This is one of the prettiest stretches on this trip, so relax and soak up the scene. Just below, you'll paddle parallel to the only road bridge on this trip, at Tin Can Road. In the next 2 miles, the landscape will gradually rise and become rocky. Also, you'll be entering the heart of the Albany Wildlife Area, some 1,700 acres large.

Unless you're paddling during a hunting season, you'll hear far more cranes trumpeting than gunshots. The surrounding solitude is what makes this river trip so special. Shortly after a horseshoe loop, you'll see outcrops on the right dipping down to the water's edge. The palette here is truly exquisite: lime green, kelly green, moss green, muddy brown, burnt orange. Inside one of these outcrops lies the former cave dwelling of Reuben Folsom, an eccentric hermit who was an expert wolf hunter and Paul Bunyan–type legend of Green County. Time has reduced "Reuben's Cave" to little more than a slivered recess, but it's still pretty cool to think of this wayward curmudgeon sleeping in this cave with his dog after a long day on the hunt for wild wolves.

The rock formations will continue for another 0.5 mile before yielding to a long corridor of gnarled oaks on the left bank. Before you know it, the Sugar River itself

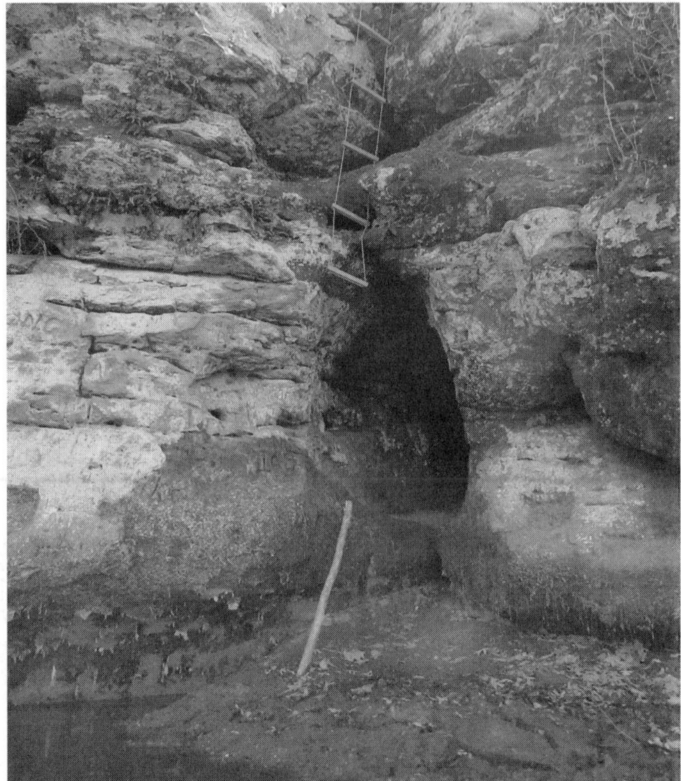

Reuben's Cave along the Little Sugar River: a good place for hermits (or hobbits)

appears, perfectly perpendicular to the Little Sugar River. The former seems gigantic compared to its diminutive tributary. Turn right and follow what's left of the current before it washes out in the sluggish impoundment caused by the dam 1 mile downstream. The good news is that, while deep and slow, the river here still looks like a river and not a lake.

Keeping to the right still, thread your way through a couple of marshy islands. On your left, you'll see a short row of houses lining the shore, surrounded by tall pines and a sweep of weeping willows. After this, both banks rise to up to 80 feet, a rarity along the Sugar River. The right bank reveals a house or two, but the left bank remains undeveloped until town. After the left bank tapers to the water level, you'll see a baseball field on the left and then a dirt parking area signaling the take-out. There's a public boat launch here at a concrete ramp.

•THE•FUDGE•

ADDITIONAL TRIPS Even though access is adequate and additional parcels of the Albany Wildlife Area coincide with the river, I don't recommend putting in upstream of this trip's parameters. Constant obstructions in the water make the paddling more work than play, and the landscape offers nothing mentionable that you won't already have seen on this trip. Likewise, continuing below the Albany Dam is not recommended due to the plethora of tubers on hot weekends, not to mention the generally dull landscape.

CAMPING AND RENTALS **Sweet Minihaha Campground** (N4697 CR E, Brodhead; 608-862-3769). For rentals only, try **S&B Tubing** (100 E. Main St., Albany; 608-862-3933).

FOOD FOR THOUGHT For a charming and unique experience complete with a pretty patio out back and fancy food, try **Franklin Grove Etc.,** an antiques shop and tearoom on the west bank of the Sugar River at the intersection of the CR C bridge (N7302 CR X, Albany; 608-862-1161). Or treat yourself to some pizza at **Gabriella's** (102 Water St., Albany; 608-862-7499), just down the road from the take-out.

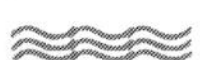

36 Pecatonica River A:
COUNTY ROAD O TO DARLINGTON

•THE•FACTS•

Put-in/take-out County Road O/Wells Street. See "The Flavor" for an optional take-out.

Distance/time 14.2 mi/Allow for 5.5 hrs

Gradient/water level 3 fpm/There should always be enough water, but consult USGS gage 05432500. The ideal range is 350–400 cfs, but the river is prone to springtime flooding, so also check with local outfitters.

Water type Quietwater with a couple of riffles and one light rapid at the very end

Canoe or kayak Either

Skill level Experienced

Time of year to paddle Anytime, but early spring and late autumn allow for better views of the hills. Also, a popular canoe race from Calamine to Darlington takes place the second weekend of June.

Landscape Limestone and sandstone outcrops, Driftless hills, farmland, urban downtown

---

OVERVIEW Virtually nonstop hills with outcrops in the Driftless Area, a few easy riffles, and one fun rapid, this trip even includes a beautiful truss bridge, a historic courthouse, and an appealing bike-shuttle option. Just expect to get a little muddy. Wildlife highlights include bald eagles, sandhill cranes, muskrats, minks, redwing blackbirds, woodpeckers, hawks, and horses.

CAR SHUTTLE **10.6 miles.** From the take-out—which is essentially the Piggly Wiggly parking lot—head north on Wells Street, then turn left onto Ann Street. Turn right onto Main Street, up the hill, and follow signs for WI 23. Turn left onto Short Cut Road into Calamine. Cross the river and then turn right onto CR C. Turn right onto CR O and head down the hill to the bridge. Park roadside.

MOUNTAIN BIKE SHUTTLE **10 miles.** You'll need a Cheese Country Trail sticker ($15); to order, go to tricountytrails.com and click "Trail Stickers" on the left. From the take-out, head north on Wells Street, then left onto Ann Street. Cross Main Street to the Cheese Country Trail, a dedicated trail. *Don't attempt this on a road bike*—the trail is compact

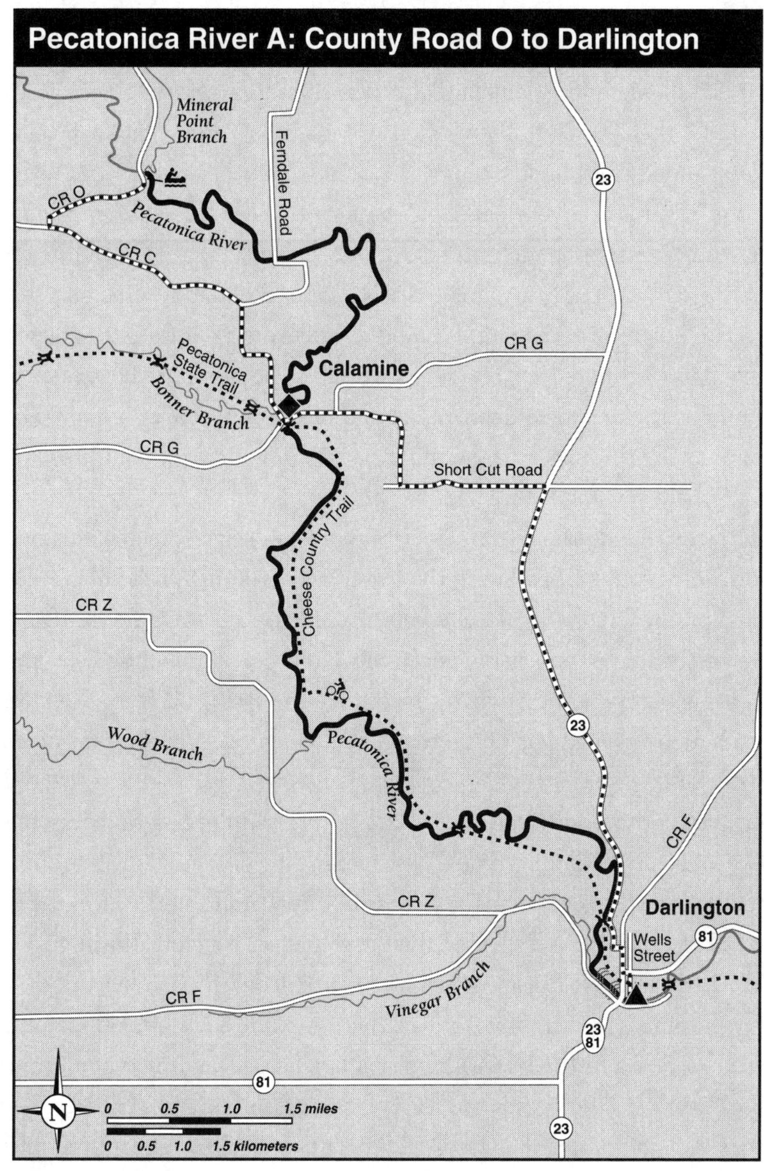

dirt and rutted from ATVs. It's a pretty trip, though, and it runs parallel to the river, thus sparing you a number of hills. You can stay on the trail by bearing right before the Calamine bridge and then turning left onto CR O to the bridge. Or you can bear left at Calamine, get off the trail, and take CR C to CR O as detailed in the car shuttle.

TAKE-OUT N42° 40.618' W90° 06.976' **PUT-IN** N42° 46.079' W90° 11.467'

•THE•FLAVOR•

PUT IN AT CR O, where the Mineral Point Branch merges with the Pecatonica River, making a 40-foot-wide stream. There's plenty of roadside parking, plus a small wayside. For the least muddy and least steep access, walk along the river downstream of the bridge about 25 yards on river right. Don't be surprised if you startle a muskrat or two.

I've seen at least three definitions for *Pecatonica,* a word of Algonquian origin: (1) "place of many canoes," (2) "crooked river," and (3) "muddy." The last seems the most credible; Pecatonica, thy name is mud. Expect to get a little dirty on this trip—it's going to happen. There are a few tree obstacles to be negotiated between Ferndale Road and Calamine. If you're determined and dexterous, you'll probably be able to squeeze and sneak through these without having to get out of your boat. Having a handsaw will help you and future paddlers also.

The river bends to the left at the base of a large ridge. The angled slope of the ridge soon yields to outcrops lining the water on the right. While not as showy as those found on the Grant and Platte Rivers, these are quite a sight nonetheless, especially here on the underappreciated Pecatonica. In the next mile, the "Pec" meanders past the base of a sandstone bluff to the left. It's set back a bit from the river but is 70 feet high and crowned with pine trees. You'll begin seeing the first of umpteen glimpses of the Cheese Country Trail on the left as well. For the next few miles, the river flows past continuous ridges and bluffs, several with peek-a-boo outcrops.

Before reaching Calamine, you'll pass under three bridges: The first one is Ferndale Road; the other two are along the Cheese Country Trail. Shortly after the first trail bridge, you'll see in the near distance a quarry at the top of a bluff. The huge pyramidal mounds of gold sand give the appearance of a surreal desert oasis, a stark contrast to the evergreen pine trees and mud-brown river. A random slalom course of deadfall in the water leads up to the quarry bluff; it's not difficult, but it is something to be mindful of. The river then passes the bluff on the left in one of its prettiest stretches.

Exposed sand leads to the Cheese Country Trail, and then beautiful outcrops of sandstone bask in the western sun. After this, you'll likely encounter clusters of deadfall and logjams. These spots will be tricky in a canoe, but in a kayak you should be able to negotiate without having to portage. There's also a random riffle before the next trail bridge. Soon you'll see two buildings atop a ridge on the right, signaling Calamine.

The river meanders before making a beeline to the wonderful metal truss bridge at CR G. (The creator and curator of MilesPaddled.com describes it as "painted in a green that only bridges this old are.") If you wish to take out, there's a landing on river right, upstream of the bridge (**N42° 44.469' W90 10.149'**). Take a moment whether you take out or continue on the water to Darlington; there's a small gravel island between this bridge and the next trail bridge. The scene is iconic. If you wait long enough, you might well hear the timeless clip-clop of horses and the rickety clatter of an Amish buggy crossing the bridge. There are many Amish farms in Lafayette County, and many of their veggies, jams, and pies are sold at local farmers' markets.

Below Calamine, you'll still see ridges in the near distance, and farms with barns are the only development, but the next few miles will be characterized by long straightaways. The pace is tranquil. You won't find the same outcrops, but there are plenty of hills. You should face no obstructions here, in part because the river has broadened to 50 feet in width but mostly thanks to volunteers who keep the Calamine–Darlington segment clear for the annual canoe race in June. After a long straightaway, the river meanders toward the next trail bridge, below which lie some fun riffles.

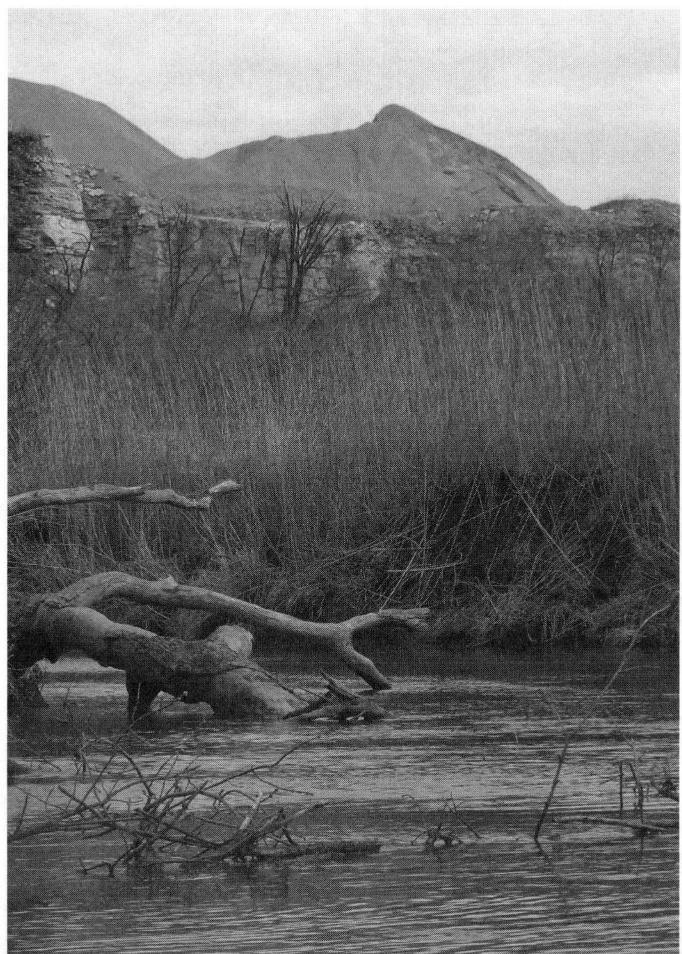

Ethereal pyramids of quarry sand near the Pecatonica River

Eventually, alas, you'll see a cell tower and then a water tower, both foreshadowing Darlington. The river will run parallel to WI 23 heading into town. Black Bridge Park will be on your left, with an inconspicuous landing upstream of the next and last Cheese Country Trail bridge. Below the bridge is a fun riffle. Expect to see folks fishing on the left bank.

The final mile of this trip is fun and pretty. On the left, you'll see the stately Lafayette County Courthouse as well as a walking/biking path. (The courthouse has the unique distinction of being the only one in the entire country funded solely by one individual.) A huge bluff looms before you, at the base of which the river sharply turns left and runs through about 10 seconds of light Class I rapids, where there used to be a dam. Darlington's nickname is "The Pearl of the Pecatonica"—a cute play on words, as the river used to be a prized location for clamming.

Once the rapids settle down, you'll notice a small park on the left where you can camp or take out. (It's more of an RV park, and downtown is only a block away, but it will do in a pinch.) Or simply continue on a few hundred yards, past the WI 81 bridge. You'll see a landing on the left below a gentle riffle. It's easy to take out here, and it's a very short walk to your bike or car.

•THE•FUDGE•

ADDITIONAL TRIPS You can try your luck putting in on Mineral Point Branch about 1 mile farther north on CR O, or on Oak Park Road about 2 miles west of CR O, where the bluffs are ruggedly beautiful but access will be an issue. The next trip describes what happens downstream from Darlington.

CAMPING **Yellowstone Lake State Park** (8495 Lake Road, Blanchardville; 608-523-4427) and **Pecatonica River Trails Park** (400 Washington St., Darlington; 608-776-4970)

RENTALS **Husie's Bar and Grill** (211 S. Main St., Blanchardville; 608-523-4085)

FOOD FOR THOUGHT The **Red Rooster Cafe** in Mineral Point (158 High St.; 608-987-9936) is an old-time diner and former pharmacy where you can order a soda with phosphates at an actual counter. If you've never had one, ask for the pasty. For more-gourmet tastes and excellent beer, check out the **Brewery Creek Inn,** also in Mineral Point (23 Commerce St.; 608-987-3298).

SHOUT-OUT Think about camping for this paddle, because you'll want to spend a day in **Mineral Point,** a delightful little village that's one of the oldest towns in the state. Rough-hewn buildings line the hill-slanted Main Street. Also in Mineral Point is the fascinating **Pendarvis** (pendarvis .wisconsinhistory.org), a nationally registered historic site of Cornish cabins and cottages from the time when lead mining put Wisconsin on the map.

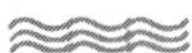

37 Pecatonica River B:
ROLLER COASTER ROAD TO WALNUT ROAD

•THE•FACTS•

Put-in/take-out Roller Coaster Road in Darlington/Wells Landing on Walnut Road in Red Rock

Distance/time 7 mi/Allow for 3 hrs

Gradient/water level 1.3 fpm/There should always be enough water; consult USGS gage 05432500.

Water type Quietwater

Canoe or kayak Either

Skill level Beginner

Time of year to paddle Anytime, but early spring and late autumn allow for better views of the hills.

Landscape Agricultural, sandstone rock outcrops, Driftless hills

---

OVERVIEW This pretty, remote trip surrounded by Driftless hills and farms offers two outstanding features: spectacular sandstone outcrops and a mile-long bluff with a bald-eagle rookery (you'll also see sandhill cranes, muskrats, and hawks). A pleasant current and no serious obstructions add to the delight.

CAR SHUTTLE 4.3 miles. From the take-out, head west on Walnut Road, then turn right onto Red Rock Road. Turn right onto Roller Coaster Road and follow it north, then east, to the bridge.

BIKE SHUTTLE 3.6 miles. You'll need a Cheese Country Trail sticker ($15); to order, go to tricountytrails.com and click "Trail Stickers" on the left. From the take-out, head west on Walnut Road, then turn right onto the Cheese Country Trail, which will run parallel to Red Rock Road for most of the shuttle. Turn right onto Roller Coaster Road to the bridge.

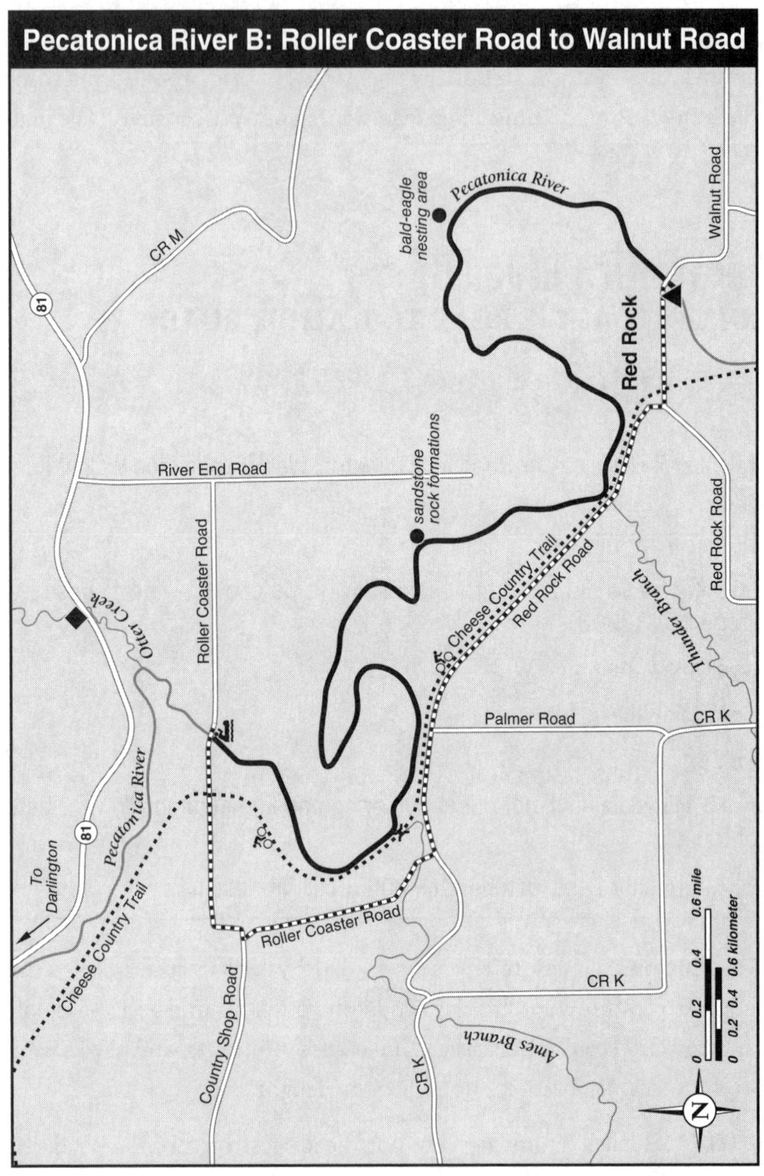

TAKE-OUT N42° 38.543' W90° 02.392' **PUT-IN** N42° 40.089' W90° 04.406'

•THE•FLAVOR•

PUT IN AT ROLLER COASTER ROAD on the downstream side of the bridge, on river left. This is a rugged access point with a steep incline leading down to the river. It's quite doable, but if you are in doubt, put in farther upstream (see "Additional Trips"). The river here is 50 feet wide and very deep. Now and again, it will bulge as wide as 70 feet, but what you see at the put-in is typical for this segment of the Pecatonica. The river and banks are plumb muddy; there's just no getting around that reality. However, while there will be downed trees, even logjam clusters, there should be no river-wide obstructions requiring you to portage.

Tall banks will line the river for most of this trip and conceal the agricultural landscape, but there's almost always a bluff or ridge in the foreground and background framing the view. Right away, the setting is intimate and hidden. While somewhat wide and straight, the enclosing banks and uplands make the experience feel remote. After passing a set of electrical wires, the river will make a big left-hand bend at the base of a bluff. As the river continues curving to the left, you'll see on your right a Cheese Country Trail bridge spanning a small creek.

The river will make a gradual S-curve north and east at a point where the landscape briefly flattens. At the top right-hand curve of the *S*, the left bank begins to rise, and it's here the show begins. Small rocks line the left shore, giving rise to grasses, shrubs, spindly trees, and a teasing glimpse of outcrops like sunlit slits cut into the earth. Heading east now, the left bank rises higher still. A bluff will begin to lean back away from the water, but the outcrops will be more exposed in finer striations. A sharp left-hand turn will precede a short straightaway, along which more rock formations await.

Now, the river will bend to the right, and, much like a magician commanding "abracadabra," a wall of gorgeous sandstone outcrop suddenly lines the water. The wall follows a crenellated outline with several crevices and concave recesses; each bulges in tritone hues of ancient slate, beige-orange, and rich, mossy green. Rising some 30 feet high and crowned with conifers, this underscored curtain of sandstone calls to mind the Dells on the Wisconsin River or the bluffs on the Kickapoo River. After the showy sandstone, a meadow of lovely oak trees (also on the left) and the foundation of a long-abandoned bridge provide a fine denouement.

The river next flows south, briefly east, and then northeast. Once again, the landscape seems to flatten, but only briefly. The surroundings are more subdued as the river courses through the heart of pastureland. As before, you'll pass by another Cheese Country Trail bridge; at the next bend to the left, you'll begin to see the incremental rise of a tall ridge off to the left. There's a very good chance you'll see some eagles, too, or at least glimpse their many large nests.

As the river makes some gentle meanders to the north and east in a gradual horseshoe bend, you'll pass a rookery on the left where the ridge spills all the way down to the water. You may even see some fluffy white tufts of molted eagle feathers floating on the surface of the water or snagged on a stick. It's impressive to see so many of these majestic birds congregating. After rounding this ridge, the river will lead to the take-out bridge in a lazy straightaway. A wonderfully convenient landing is located on the downstream side of the bridge, on the right.

•THE•FUDGE•

ADDITIONAL TRIPS Continuing downstream from the take-out, while certainly doable, is not recommended, as the bluffs recede and the landscape becomes monotonously agrarian.

Putting in upstream, you have three options, depending on how many additional miles you wish to paddle as well as your environmental druthers:

1. You can put in at **Black Bridge Park,** along WI 23 just north of downtown Darlington, which would add almost 5 miles to this trip. The advantages here are a good, if muddy, landing with plenty of parking, plus a short set of riffles followed by 50 yards of light rapids as you enter town with pleasant views of the courthouse.

2. If you wish to skip the swift current, put in at the take-out for **Pecatonica River A** (page 190) at a designated boat launch by the parking lot

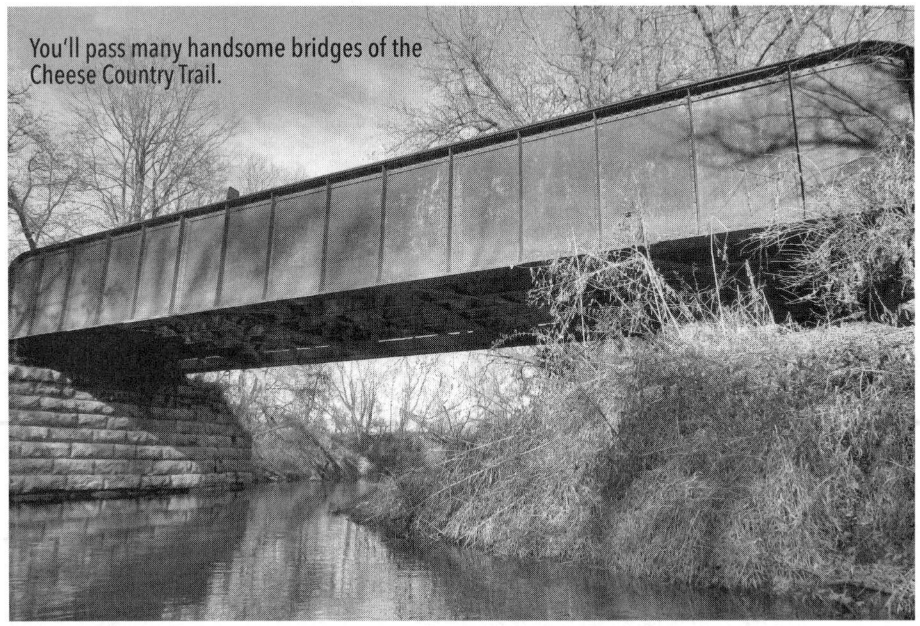

You'll pass many handsome bridges of the Cheese Country Trail.

for the grocery store, adding 4 miles to this trip. The disadvantage of these first two put-ins upstream is dull paddling from downtown Darlington to Roller Coaster Road, where 10-foot-high muddy banks surrounded by farm fields are all that one sees and the roadside noise of WI 81 is constant.

3. You could also put in **Otter Creek** just south of WI 81 and 1 mile north of the Roller Coaster Road put-in. Access is doable. From here, Otter Creek flows into the Pecatonica 0.5 mile downstream. The creek is narrow and shallow, however, and obstructions might be an issue. That said, at the confluence is a fun set of riffles that whisks you past an attractive bluff all the way to Roller Coaster Road. Of the three, this one is my personal favorite.

CAMPING **Yellowstone Lake State Park** (8495 Lake Road, Blanchardville; 608-523-4427) and **Pecatonica River Trails Park** (400 Washington St., Darlington; 608-776-4970)

RENTALS **Husie's Bar and Grill** (211 S. Main St., Blanchardville; 608-523-4085)

FOOD FOR THOUGHT See Pecatonica River A, page 190.

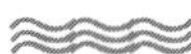

38 Pecatonica River East Branch A:
HOLLANDALE TO BLANCHARDVILLE

•THE•FACTS•

Put-in/take-out WI 39 bridge in Hollandale/Water Street at dam in Blanchardville. See "The Flavor" for an alternative take-out.

Distance/time 10.3 mi/Allow for 4 hrs

Gradient/water level 2.4 fpm/Look for a minimum of 170 cfs to avoid scraping. Consult USGS gage 05433000.

Water type Quietwater with some riffles in the first 4 miles

Canoe or kayak Either

Skill level Beginner

Time of year to paddle Spring and autumn to better appreciate the rock formations sans foliage

Landscape Pastures, oak savannas, prairie, Driftless bluffs

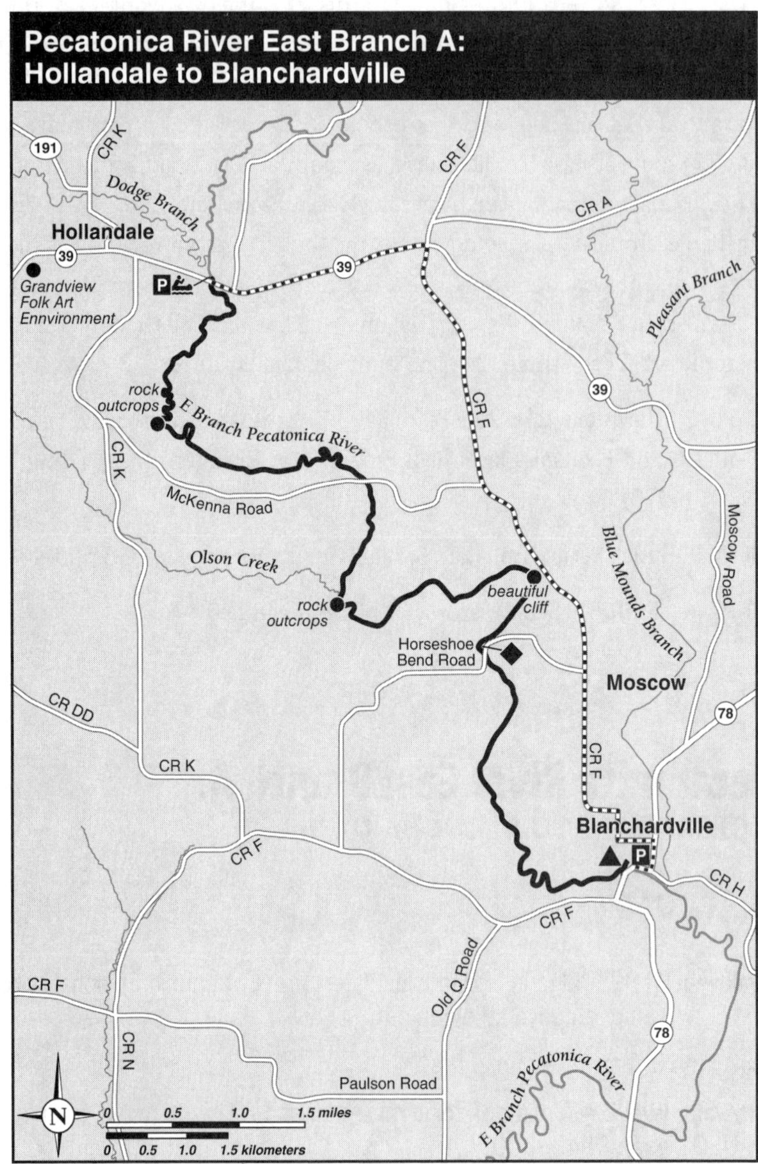

OVERVIEW This just might be the best-kept secret for paddling in the Madison area, despite good access points in two towns and stunning scenery between. Combining oak savannas, tallgrass prairies, and bucolic pastures with pine-crowned cliffs, pockmarked boulders, and gorgeous sandstone outcrops, this section of the east branch will keep you coming back. You'll see bald eagles, kingfishers, hawks, geese, and cattle.

SHUTTLE 7.2 miles. From the take-out, head east on County Road F, then bear left to stay on CR F where it splits at WI 78 and then again as it doglegs. At the WI 39 intersection, turn left. Cross the river and turn right into the designated parking area.

TAKE-OUT N42° 48.686' W89° 51.731' **PUT-IN** N42° 52.285' W89° 55.256'

•THE•FLAVOR•

PUT IN BENEATH THE BRIDGE AT WI 39. There is a nice parking area just to the west of the bridge; from there, a path leads to the water, where it's easy to launch. The river wends its way through pastureland, carving 10-foot-tall mud banks. On your right, you'll see some crumbling remnants of a former land bridge. Only 20 feet wide here, this is creek paddling at its best. The river heads to a small attractive ridge on your left from which it bounces westward. Lush tallgrass prairies surround both banks as you pass tiny islands and gravel bars. You may encounter an impassable fallen tree here, requiring you to portage around it on the right.

The first bluff soon appears; hooking to the left, you will paddle alongside this ridge for the next mile. The water is clear, the bottom sandy, which is not always the case when on the Pecatonica. (The river will continually alternate between sand and

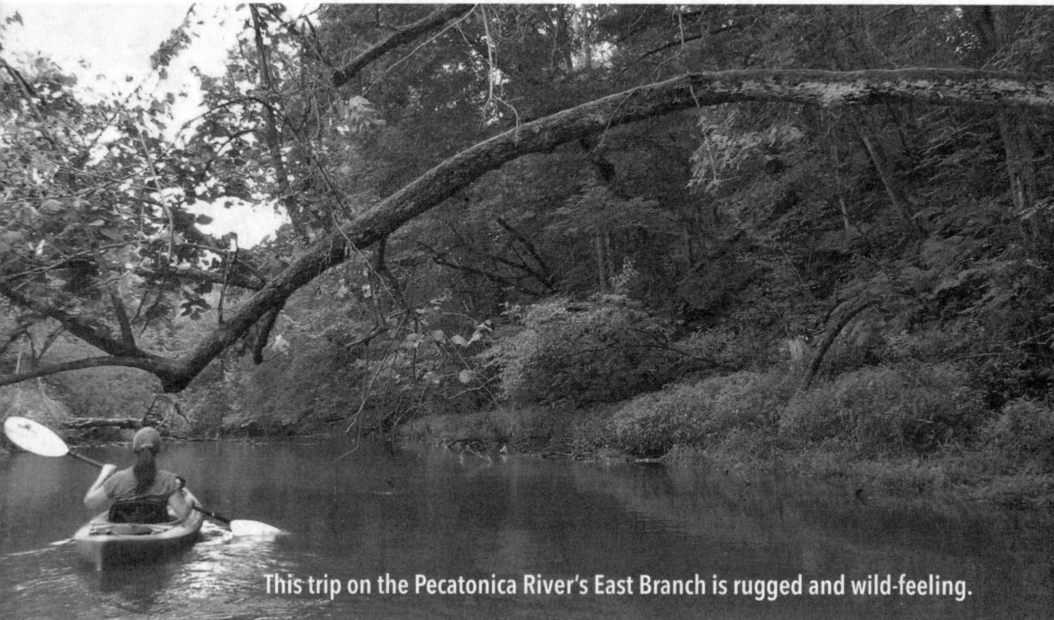

This trip on the Pecatonica River's East Branch is rugged and wild-feeling.

mud throughout this trip.) This scene is quite lovely, with lush pine trees, boulders embedded in the bluff, Driftless limestone outcrops, and cool mossy slopes. Look for an osprey platform on the right. There may be another downed tree requiring a second portage on the right across grassy banks. The river will turn abruptly to the left and the current will pick up some. Thread your way carefully through the sawed-off clearance of a fallen tree from the left bank by keeping close to the left. On the other side of the tree, you'll find more outcrops and the remnants of a wooden pier.

The first bridge at McKenna Road is found at the 4-mile mark. Get ready to find your socks knocked off, because the best bluffs come in this next section. The first is found about a mile downstream of the McKenna bridge. The geology here is woodsy and forest green, with buxom boulders embedded in the hillside, moss draping many of them. The river passes along the base of a bluff for 100 yards, allowing generous time to take in one craggy overhang and mysterious fissure after another. Overhanging trees from the right bank drape gracefully over the river. On the right lies a huge chunk of rock in the stream. The river then bends to the left and heads northeastward. The paddling is easy, and the feel is one of supreme intimacy.

Following a long straightaway with a bluff looming in the distance, the river will twice bend to the right, and suddenly the most dazzling rock formations will be found

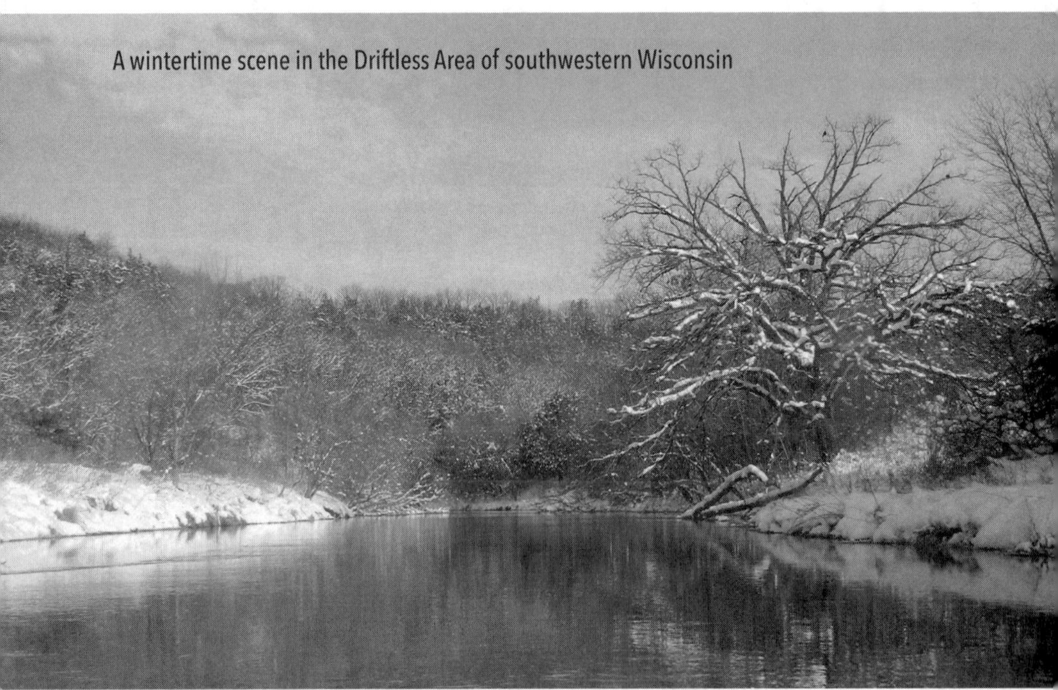

A wintertime scene in the Driftless Area of southwestern Wisconsin

on the left. Whereas the preceding ridges were gently sloping dolomite limestone, here a wall of St. Peter sandstone drops straight into the water. Above, the top of the cliff hovers 100 feet high and lines the river for 75 yards before the Horseshoe Bend Road bridge. The tall pine trees at the top of the bluff look like bonsai figurines. This is the most dazzling section on this trip and arguably anywhere on the Pecatonica River, either branch. Take your time here and savor the impressive sight. One can take out on river left at the upstream side of the bridge at Horseshoe Bend Road for a beautiful 7.5-mile trip (**N42° 48.686' W89 51.730'**).

After Horseshoe Bend Road, the river heads southward in a couple of long straightaways. A bend to the east provides a welcome diversion from the sun. Soon you will see a white church atop a hill in front of you. This is your cue to get ready to take out soon. You will hear the waterfall-like dam before you eye the horizon line or the bridge just downstream. A small park and fishing area on river left is where you want to take out; look for the picnic table and telephone pole.

•THE•FUDGE•

ADDITIONAL TRIPS Unfortunately, no good options exist upstream because of horrendous logjams. There are some absolutely stunning sandstone outcrops and beautiful bluffs, and a few upstream bridges allow for surprisingly adequate access, but chronic low water levels and nasty obstructions prohibit putting in upstream of WI 39.

CAMPING **McKellar Park** (on the riverfront in Blanchardville, just east of downtown; blanchardville.com/community/mckellar-park) and **Yellowstone Lake State Park** (8495 Lake Road, Blanchardville; 608-523-4427)

RENTALS **Husie's Bar and Grill** (211 S. Main St., Blanchardville; 608-523-4085)

SHOUT-OUT Just a few miles west of the put-in lies **Nick's Grandview** (7351 WI 39, Hollandale; 608-967-2322), an outdoor sculpture garden that's open to the public. It's a little on the hokey side, featuring a combination of outsider art and art that's just outside. There are more than 40 sculptures, most life-sized, all made by hand, embedded with shards of china, glass, beads, buttons, sea shells, anything shiny. Some are historic, others prehistoric. Some take their cues from fairy tales and mythology, others from Nick Engelbert's imagination. It's definitely worth checking out.

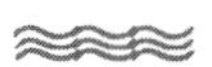

39 Pecatonica River East Branch B:
BLANCHARDVILLE TO ARGYLE

•THE•FACTS•

Put-in/take-out County Road H boat launch/Argyle boat launch off WI 78

Distance/time 16 mi/Allow for 6 hrs

Gradient/water level 1 fpm/There should always be adequate water for this section. Recommended levels are 4–5 feet high with 100–200 cfs at USGS gage 05433000. Due to the low gradient, paddling this trip when the river is high (but not dangerously so) helps move things along.

Water type Quietwater

Canoe or kayak Either

Skill level Beginner

Time of year to paddle Anytime, but autumn is quite lovely

Landscape Farmland, Driftless hills, prairies, meadows

OVERVIEW Here is a tranquil, slow-paced trip featuring oak savannas, tallgrass prairie, lowland forests, southern sedge meadows, and notable outcroppings. Expect to see bald eagles, great blue herons, kingfishers, snakes, muskrats, turtles, frogs, hawks, bulls, and pigs.

SHUTTLE 8.7 miles. From the take-out, head east on WI 78, then turn left at the WI 81 intersection to stay on WI 78. Continue north on WI 78 to Blanchardville. Turn right onto CR F and cross the river; the dam will be on left. The road will head east. Stay straight where CR F and WI 78 veer to the left; you are now on CR H. The put-in will be on your right 600 feet after CR F/WI 78—if you cross the bridge over Gordon Creek, you've gone too far.

TAKE-OUT N42° 42.112' W89° 52.240' **PUT-IN** N42° 48.555' W89° 51.357'

•THE•FLAVOR•

PUT IN AT THE BOAT LAUNCH WHERE GORDON CREEK, a popular trout stream, flows into the Pecatonica. There are no facilities here, but there's room for a few cars, and the access to the river is excellent, which cannot be said of other spots downstream.

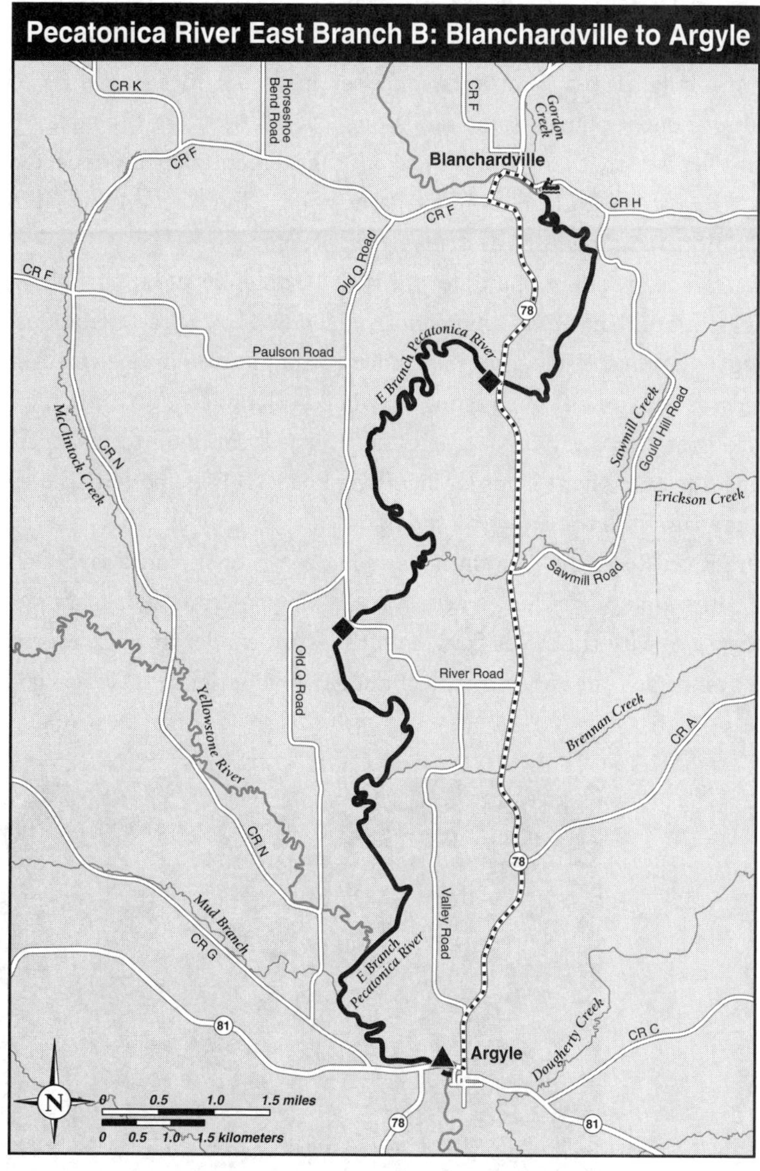

Unfortunately, the first 3 miles are not noteworthy, but the river is wide and slow, so obstructions should never be an issue.

(Alternatively, you could put in at the first bridge at WI 78 [**N42° 47.140' W89° 51.682'**], but access can be frustrating: The hill from the road down to the river is steep and uneven, punctuated by loose boulders, thorns, and weeds. Watch out for snakes and nasty spiders, too! It is doable, though, and it cuts 3.3 miles off this otherwise long trip.)

It gets better after WI 78. A short straightaway follows the bridge before the river begins to meander. Hills begin in earnest, and the environs alternate between oak savanna, tallgrass prairie, forests, and open meadows, together with peek-a-boo cliffs and rock outcroppings, some sandstone, others limestone. There are portions where the river is more than 50 feet wide, but there are intimate sections, too, where it tapers and conveys a much more reclusive feeling. The surrounding landscape is lush and gentle, what might be described as "Driftless light."

There are many outcroppings for the next 10 miles, most lining the river, some of which are more than 50 feet high and studded with pine trees tenaciously clung onto scraggly fissures. You'll also pass under a wrought-iron bridge where someone has placed a sawed-in-half couch acting as twin Barcaloungers. Ah, life in the country. Another long straightaway follows, but the river will continue to meander around hills, bluffs, and outcrops as it approaches River Road. (This is a potential access point, just downstream from the bridge on the right.)

After River Road, the Pecatonica flows in a series of straightaways. On a sunny day, this is the kind of paddling where you kick up your bare feet, snap open a cold beer, and just go with the sweet flow. After the last meander through a forested section, the river begins one very long straightaway. On your right, you'll see a golf course

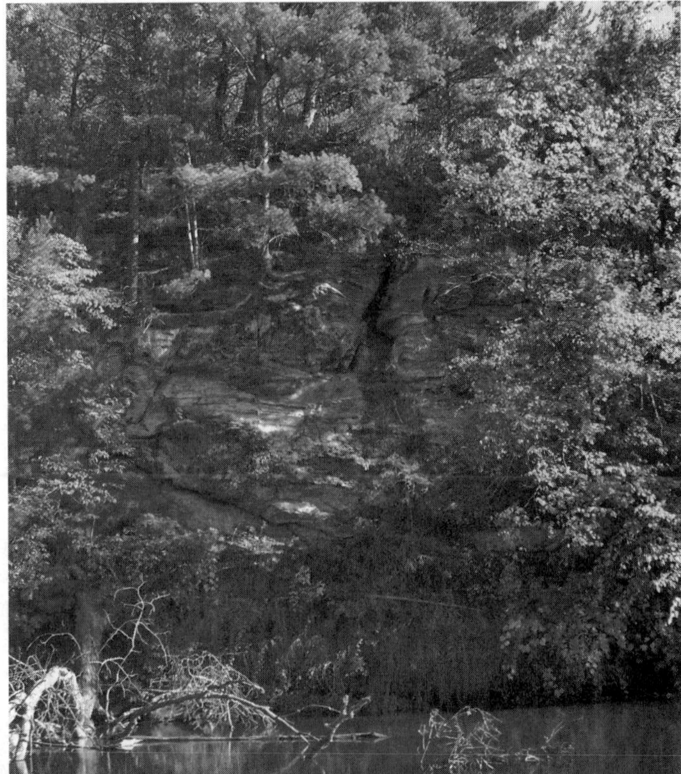

The East Branch of the Pecatonica River is studded with sandstone outcrops.

and then the confluence of the Yellowstone River, after which you'll see signs of town. Due to the depth and width created along this section by the dam's impoundment, you might encounter a motorboat here (but not elsewhere upstream). After one final bend to the left, you'll see houses and buildings. The take-out is on the right at the official Argyle boat launch; there's a concrete ramp and a floating dock.

•THE•FUDGE•

ADDITIONAL TRIPS See the previous and next profiles for trips upstream and downstream of this one.

CAMPING **Blackhawk Memorial Park** (CR Y south of Argyle; 608-776-4830); **McKellar Park** (on the riverfront in Blanchardville, just east of downtown; blanchardville.com/community/mckellar-park); and **Yellowstone Lake State Park** (8495 Lake Road, Blanchardville; 608-523-4427)

RENTALS **Husie's Bar and Grill** (211 S. Main St., Blanchardville; 608-523-4085) and **Yellowstone Valley Canoe Rental** in Argyle (608-543-3220 or 608-214-7229)

40 Pecatonica River East Branch C:

ARGYLE TO BLACKHAWK MEMORIAL PARK

•THE•FACTS•

Put-in/take-out River Street below dam in Argyle/Blackhawk Memorial Park

Distance/time 7.8 mi/Allow for 3 hrs

Gradient/water level 0.5 fpm/There should always be enough water to paddle this trip; ideal levels are 150–200 cfs at USGS gage 05433000.

Water type Quietwater

Canoe or kayak Either

Skill level Beginner

Time of year to paddle Anytime

Landscape Driftless hills, farmland, woods, tallgrass prairie

Pecatonica River East Branch C: Argyle to Blackhawk Memorial Park

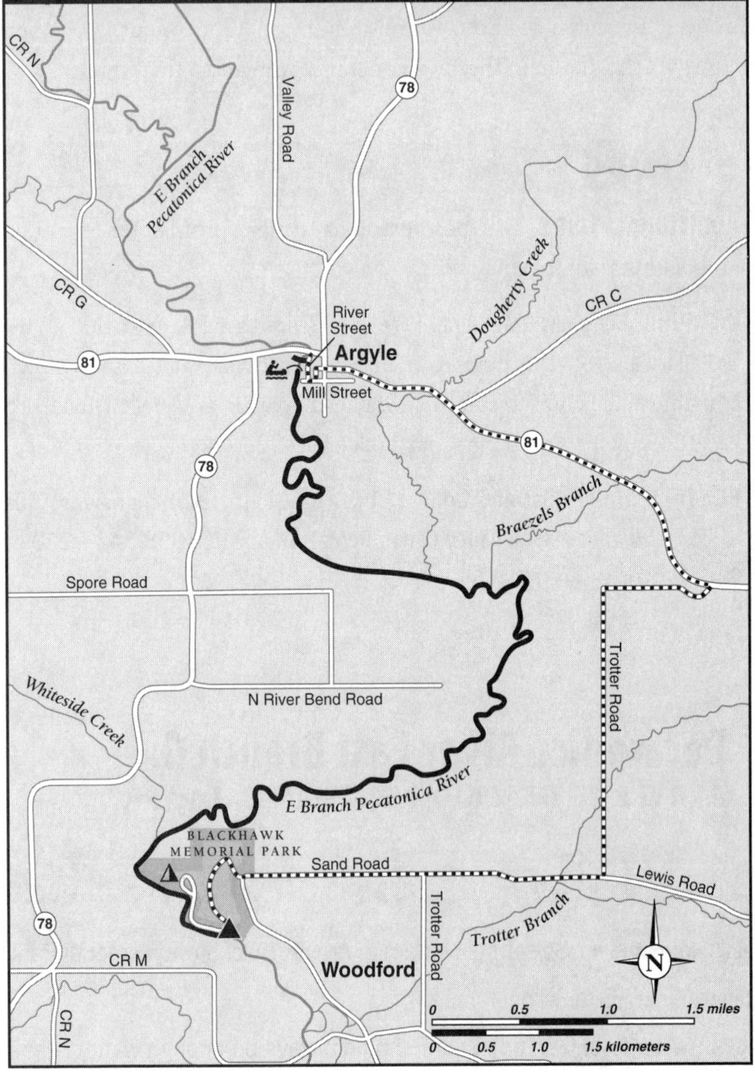

OVERVIEW Less showy than the two previous trips upstream, this next section of the Pecatonica River's east branch is still very pretty and leisurely as it saunters past gorgeous oak trees, bluffs, hills, and tallgrass prairies. A pleasant (though historically unsettling) county park provides for paddling up to your campsite. Wildlife includes bald eagles, sandhill cranes, turtles, wood ducks, mergansers, fish, pheasant, and cows.

SHUTTLE 7.53 miles. From the take-out, head out of the county park and turn left onto Sand Road. Take Sand east (it will become Trotter Road). Turn left onto Trotter Road at the Lewis Road intersection at the base of a hill. Follow Trotter north and bear right at a perpendicular right-hand bend. Turn left onto WI 81 and follow it west into town. Where WI 81 turns right, stay straight instead on Monroe Street. Turn left onto South Street at the next block, then right onto Mill Street, then right again onto River Street. The boat launch is on the left.

TAKE-OUT N42° 39.410' W89° 52.691' **PUT-IN** N42° 41.984' W89° 52.180'

•THE•FLAVOR•

PUT IN AT THE BOAT LAUNCH ON RIVER STREET, near the water-treatment plant downstream of the dam. There is no concrete ramp; it's just a muddy easement. About 40 feet wide, the river will meander lazily around eroded banks with rolling hills in the background, a common vignette in Driftless southwestern Wisconsin.

After a mile you'll come upon one of the prettiest scenes on this trip, as the river caresses the base of a small bluff like a silk scarf across a neck: a veritable holler with attractive slopes folded in a few different directions. The bluff doesn't spill directly into the river but is rather tucked away some 20 yards off to the side. One can imagine Tolkien characters from Middle-Earth scratching out a patch of grass or poking through some rock rubble to the light of day. In the long straightaway that follows, a hill on your right, covered in a flaxen-colored tallgrass, leads to water—one of several such scenes on this trip. Pockets of scrub oaks will be found here and there as well.

A few sharp turns follow, but since the current is virtually nonexistent, they're not a problem. Before sweeping across a second bluff, you'll see a wide oxbow on the left; don't turn into it (unless you're curious to explore backwater), as it is the river equivalent of a dead-end alley. A lovely hill extends on the left, and you'll pass under wires. As there are no bridges on this trip until the take-out, consider the wires the landmark signifying the halfway point (it's actually a little past halfway).

Now the river lazily wavers. On the left is an easy-to-miss access, but I don't recommend it since there's plenty of pretty left on this trip. There will be some deadfall to dodge around in this section, but all of it should be negotiable without requiring you to portage. Soon both banks of the river are enclosed with lush trees as you enter the heart of Blackhawk Memorial Park.

The river will flow now alongside a beautifully barren hill, nearly treeless, the earth swollen and rolling, calling to mind the Scottish lowlands (or maybe it's just the influence of a town named Argyle). Campsites lie on the left bank, some of which you could paddle directly to if you were to camp overnight. The main boat launch for the park will be on the left.

•THE•FUDGE•

ADDITIONAL TRIPS There's a 9.4-mile trip from Woodford to the confluence at the main branch of the Pecatonica, plus 3 more miles to the official boat launch at WI 11 at Browntown, just below a Cheese Country Trail bridge that spans two streams. This trip has intermittent rock outcrops plus one set of random riffles, but it's monotonous and otherwise nondescript.

CAMPING **Blackhawk Memorial Park,** at the take-out (CR Y; 608-776-4830); **Yellowstone Lake State Park,** northwest of Argyle (8495 Lake Road, Blanchardville; 608-523-4427)

RENTALS **Husie's Bar and Grill** in Blanchardville (211 S. Main St.; 608-523-4085) and **Yellowstone Valley Canoe Rental** in Argyle (608-543-3220 or 608-214-7229)

SHOUT-OUT Take time to explore the history behind Blackhawk Memorial Park, the site of a skirmish associated with but not actually a part of the 1832 Black Hawk War.

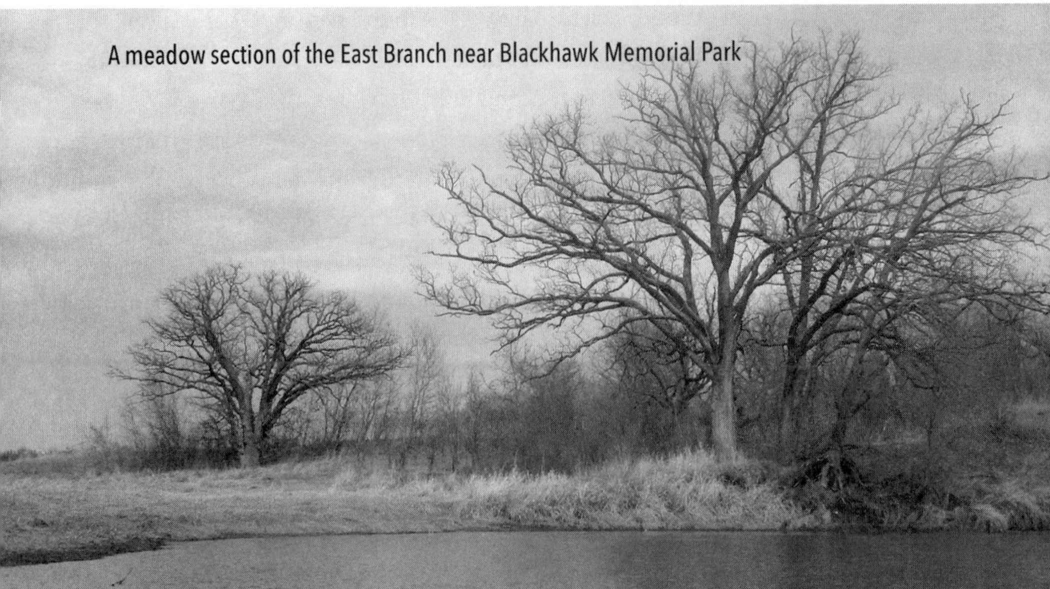

A meadow section of the East Branch near Blackhawk Memorial Park

41 Platte River: PLATTE ROAD TO BIG PLATTE ROAD

•THE•FACTS•

Put-in/take-out Platte Road in Harrison just south of Ellenboro/Big Platte Road in Tennyson

Distance/time 8.3 mi/Allow for 3–4 hrs

Gradient/water level 9.5 fpm/100–180 cfs on USGS gage 05414000

Water type Riffles with a few Class I rapids

Canoe or kayak Either

Skill level Experienced

Time of year to paddle Anytime

Landscape Rolling hills, Driftless bluffs, rock outcrops, and farmland

---

OVERVIEW The very best of the venerable Platte, this trip is quintessential Driftless, with sweeping bluff vistas, clear water with swift riffles and nice rapids, and nearly no development but the occasional farm. This is the only trip in this book that technically falls just outside of the 60-mile periphery, but it's oh so worth the extra little drive time! You'll see bald eagles, ducks, kingfishers, crows, hawks, deer, sheep, killdeer, horses, bulls, turkey, turtles, and coots.

SHUTTLE 5.5 miles. From the take-out, head north on Big Platte Road. Make a sharp left at Quarry Road to stay on Big Platte Road and continue north. Turn right on County Road B, then left on Platte Road. Cross the river over the bridge. Bear right onto Platte Road. The put-in is at the next bridge. *Note:* If you're unfamiliar with this area, it's best to consult a map and even allow a little time to get lost, as these country roads can be a bit confusing.

TAKE-OUT N42° 41.968' W90° 38.317' **PUT-IN** N42° 45.770' W90° 36.798'

•THE•FLAVOR•

PUT IN AT PLATTE ROAD ON RIVER RIGHT. There is no official landing, but you should be able to discern a footpath to the water. Access is a little steep and muddy, but these are paltry admission costs considering the big beautiful bluff looming directly in front

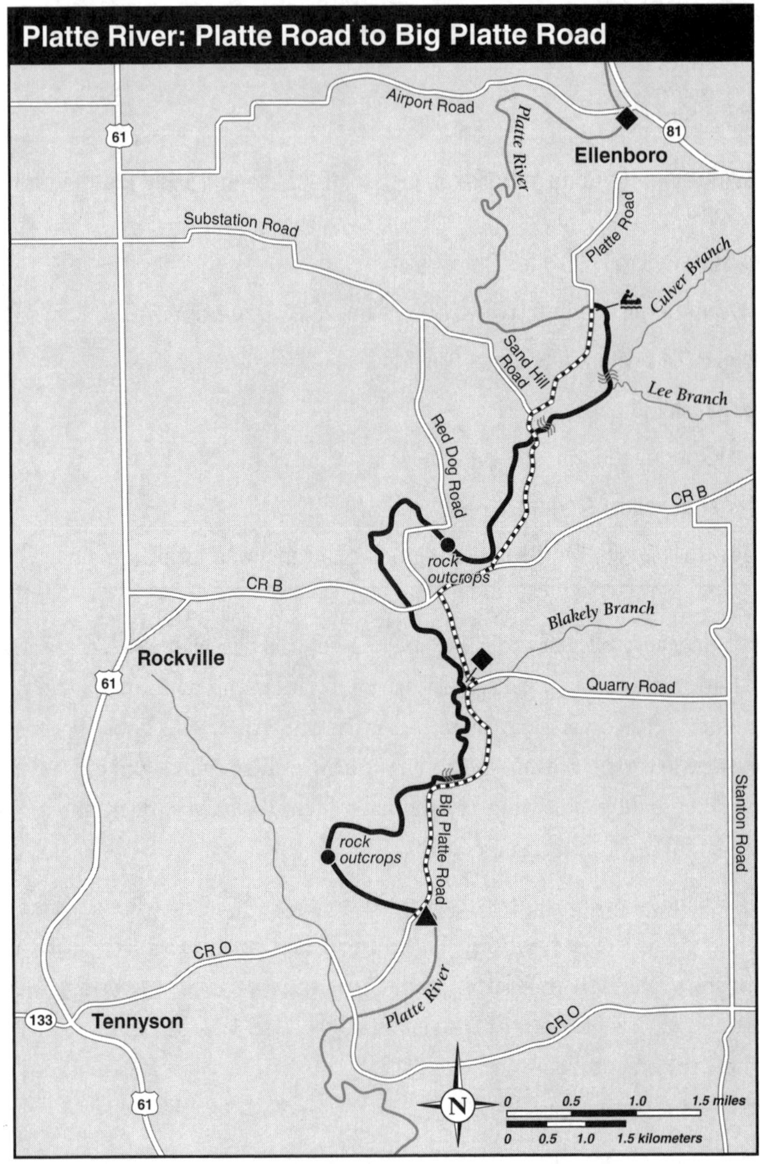

of you downstream, preceded by a short riffle (and there are many such vignettes on this trip). As you approach the Baker Ford Road bridge, an outcrop lines the left bank. Here, as elsewhere, the hue of the water may alternate between muddy brown, clayish gray, clear, and sometimes a light shade of jade. Look for a cluster of swallows' nests in a nook beneath the bridge.

Below the bridge is a long stretch of riffles in a straightaway that sweeps you beside a lovely bluff on the left. Something else you'll see in abundance on this trip are horizon lines—not the dramatic type signaling a dam or large ledge, but a clean delineation between flatwater and riffles/light rapids. Leaving the shadow of the bluff momentarily, the scene switches to pastoral. You'll see another small drop with a light rapid, and then another. Deep pools of cool, colored water lie below crumbling rock walls on the left. In quick succession, you'll pass under a set of power lines and the rustic bridge on Platte Road.

Below the Platte Road bridge, a few intermittent islands provide a variety of channels to choose for possible exploration. A lower bluff will divert the river to the left. In the long straightaway that follows, you will glide down more riffles, past crops on your left. Nestled beneath a tree, yet perilously close to the eroding banks, are the remains of an old car that's been there for decades.

Shortly after a second set of power lines, the river bends to the left approaching Platte Road. Don't worry, though: Another bluff bounces the river away from the road and toward an exceptionally scenic series of exposed limestone, swift riffles, and giant boulders in the streambed, leading to bridges at Red Dog Road and then CR B beyond. In between the latter two bridges, the landscape is more agrarian but by no means featureless. While shallow, the water should be supremely clear.

Immediately downstream from where Big Platte Road jackknifes and the river sweeps around a hill and down some fun riffles, you'll see a series of stairs on the left where locals have created an excellent access. Look for bald eagles and beavers as the swift current threads its way past various small islands. Rock rubble from a nearby quarry lines the banks for a short distance, creating a solid run of easy but fun Class I rapids. Shortly after this is a third set of power lines. Another rocky wall lines the left, past which is a beautiful, tall bluff leading directly into the river on the left with more boulders and riffles. The only barbed wire on this trip is unfortunately placed right at a light rapid. It can be easily portaged. Additionally, be mindful of strainers where the river bends and the current picks up.

At a sharp turn to the left, a glorious bluff lines the river on the right with several exposed rock formations and even a few ledges. What's more, there are some shallow gravel bars on which you can beach and picnic. Or you can lodge on the bluff itself and climb up to some large rock formations with beguiling fissures that resemble a cave. The view from up top is splendid. The bridge at Big Platte Road is only 0.5 mile from here, so take your time. Take out on the downstream side on the right.

•THE•FUDGE•

ADDITIONAL TRIPS Putting in upstream in Ellenboro at Airport Road adds 4 very pretty miles. This can be its own short day trip or tacked on for a longer day on the Platte. It too has many riffles and some nice rock formations and bluffs, plus the water is a striking jade. Airport Road offers a good put-in, too. As of April 2016, there were no strands of barbed wire, but this is subject to change, of course.

Putting in at Big Platte Road and taking out at Indian Creek Road offers a separate trip, around 8 miles. Perfect for beginners, there are fewer riffles and rapids (with the exception of one small, half-foot ledge) but lots of glorious bluffs, outstanding wildlife, and even more seclusion. Indian Creek Road is a designated launch only 1.5 miles upstream from the Mississippi River. Paddling to the confluence and back is easy due to the slack current.

CAMPING **Nelson-Dewey State Park** (12190 CR VV, Cassville; 608-725-5374); **Grant River Recreation Area,** on the Mississippi River south of Potosi (3990 Park Lane, off WI 233; 608-763-2140); and **Mound View Park** in Platteville (East Madison Street and Broadway; 608-348-6111)

RENTALS **Grant River Canoe & Kayak Rental** in Beetown (608-794-2342, grantrivercanoerental.com)

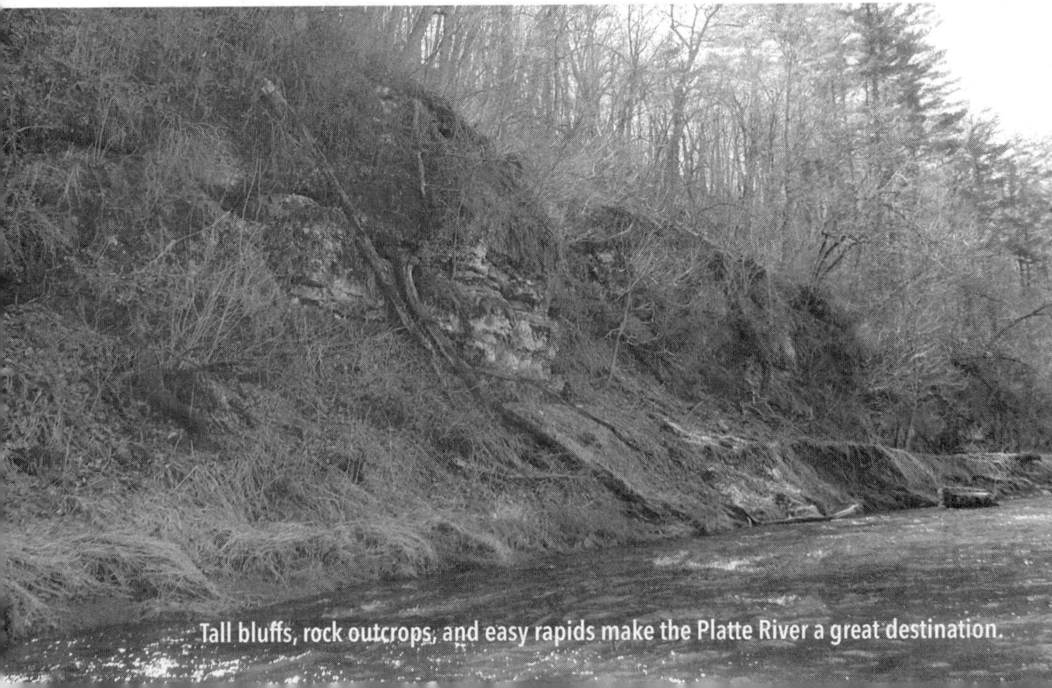

Tall bluffs, rock outcrops, and easy rapids make the Platte River a great destination.

SHOUT-OUTS Check out the **National Brewery Museum** and **Potosi Brewing Company,** just to the west in Potosi (209 S. Main St.; 608-763-4002). Nearby is the bizarre but irresistible **Dickeyville Grotto** (305 W. Main St., Dickeyville; 608-568-3119). The former has incredible memorabilia for the best beverage ever, while the latter offers a surreal visual experience of religious kitsch bordering on madness.

42 Sugar River A: VERONA TO PAOLI IN DANE COUNTY

•THE•FACTS•

Put-in/take-out Riverside Road/Canal Street

Distance/time 5 mi/Allow for 2.5 hrs

Gradient/water level 3.5 fpm/Consult USGS gage 05435950. Below 50 cfs, you will be scraping the bottom.

Water type Mostly quietwater with one 2-foot drop near the end, followed by delightful riffles

Canoe or kayak Kayak preferred but canoe will suffice

Skill level Experienced

Time of year to paddle Anytime

Landscape Small rolling hills, pastures, protected public land

---

OVERVIEW This trip along a charming stretch of the Sugar, nestled in the soft hills and farms of southwestern Dane County, features clear water, riffles, pretty stands of oaks, a fun rapid, and the button-cute hamlet of Paoli—plus blue-winged teals, great blue and green herons, deer, killdeer, kingfishers, fish, cows, and bald eagles.

SHUTTLE **5.5 miles.** From the take-out, turn right onto Range Trail, then left onto Sunset Drive. Turn right onto WI 69, then left onto Riverside Road. The put-in is on Riverside Road on the upstream side of the bridge, river left.

TAKE-OUT N42° 55.783' W89° 31.465' **PUT-IN** N42° 57.513' W89° 33.523'

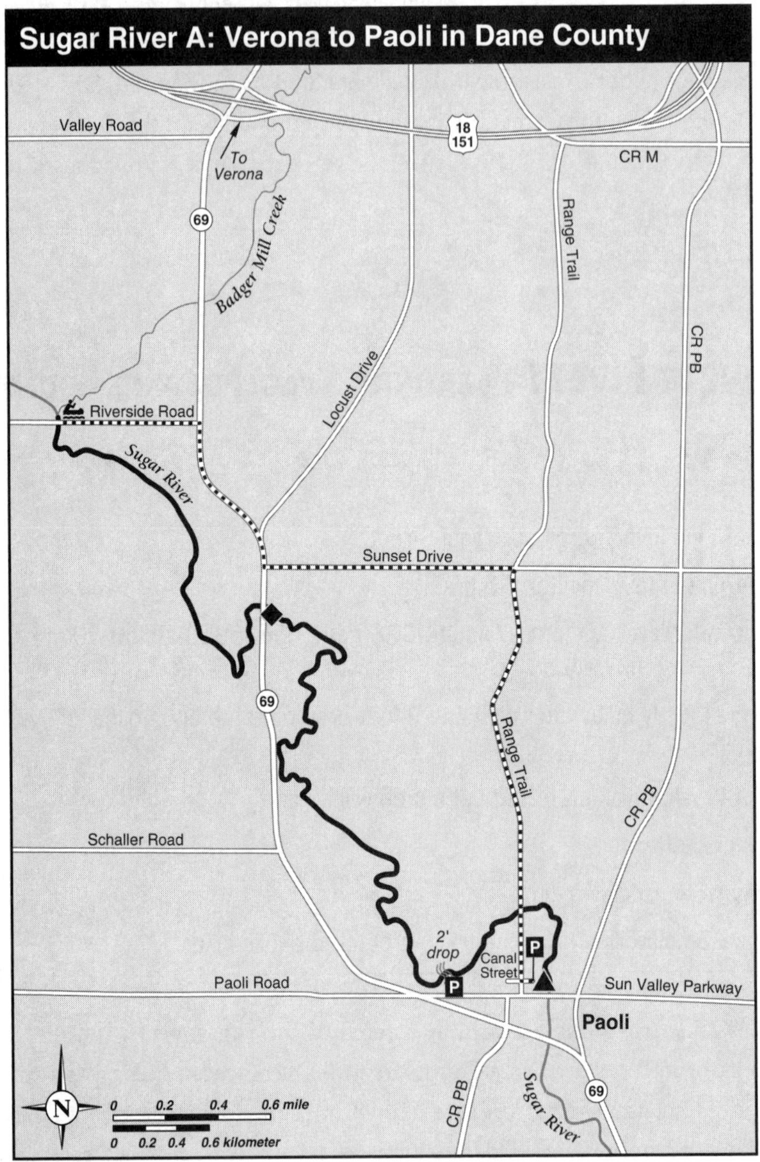

•THE•FLAVOR•

ONE OF THE NICEST PARTS OF THIS LITTLE TRIP is how much variety there is in only 5 miles. True, most of the paddling is alongside pastures, but there are glimpses of where the last glaciers ended and the Driftless Area begins. Especially nice are the many old oaks, handsomely macabre in their gnarled isolation. The river does meander, but it has moments of straightaways, too, sometimes tree-canopied, other times in savanna settings of unbroken sunshine.

Shortly after a pretty corridor of leafy tree canopies, you'll come across two strands of decrepit barbed wire. They're easy to discern from afar and to duck under, especially when the current is pretty slow. On this trip, these two strands should be the only barbed wire. This first mile, where the river is about 30 feet wide, alternates between a wooded corridor and a sun-drenched open sprawl of pastureland. The water is clear, the bottom sandy, and the current generally reliable. There are obstacles to dodge, but usually none so formidable as to be dangerous. Conditions can change overnight, of course, especially on a narrow river, but you should be able to negotiate these obstructions without having to portage.

The banks of the river rise gently, many lined with handsome oaks. Don't be surprised to see cattle or a bald eagle's nest atop a tree. The gentle hills of the Sugar River Valley please the eye and tease the imagination. The river jackknifes before passing under WI 69. (On the downstream side of the bridge, on river right, is an alternative access: **N42° 56.940' W89 32.647'**.) Following WI 69 is an exceptionally pretty stretch through woods where the river meanders but also picks up a little speed by way of small riffles. Here and there, you'll see big chunks of broken concrete; these are recent remnants of nasty footbridges that impeded the river and required portaging. Dane County has purchased tracts of land along the river to Paoli and, together with groups like Capitol Water Trails and the Upper Sugar River Watershed Association, has made the river paddler-friendly through considerable cleanup efforts.

As you approach Paoli, buildings begin to appear, the first of which is a large white garage off a way to the right. One of the thrilling highlights of this trip is an 18-inch ledge where there used to be a dam. Predictably, you'll hear the sound of the rushing water well before you come upon it. Also, there's a sign that reads DAM, SWIFT WATER alerting you beforehand. A well-marked portage trail on the right allows you to circumvent the drop or allows you to run it, get out, and run it again as many times as your heart desires. It's a sweet little drop that gets the adrenaline surging but isn't dangerous. Surfing below the drop is a whole lot of fun, too.

Riffles will take you along a pretty backdrop of woods and steep banks for the next 0.5 mile to the bridge at Range Trail and then another 0.5 mile to the charming takeout behind the beautifully restored old mill building in downtown Paoli. Take out 20 feet upstream of the County Road PB bridge at the backyard of the old mill off Canal Street. There's no designated launch, but the lawn is only half a foot higher than the water, so taking out is easy. A short walk across the lawn leads to the gravel parking area on Canal Street.

•THE•FUDGE•

ADDITIONAL TRIPS Putting in farther upstream is tricky. There are public-access landings on Bobcat Lane north of US 18/US 151 and on Valley Road south of the highway. To run the upper stretch from Bobcat Lane without getting frustrated and stuck in shallows, the river will need to be above 3.3 feet at the gage. There is a rapid between Bobcat and Valley. There is another problem, though: As of 2013, there still are barbed wires and a questionably legal cattle gate on the segment of the river between Valley and Riverside. Incidentally, Bobcat to Valley is 2.3 miles, and Valley to Riverside is 1.8 miles, so tacking both on would make for a 9-mile trip to Paoli. These upper stretches can be run, but they come with baggage.

Continuing on the river past Paoli is a mixed bag. It's only 4 miles to the next bridge, at CR A in Basco, but for half of that distance the river runs parallel to WI 69, and the traffic is distracting. There are two fences to duck

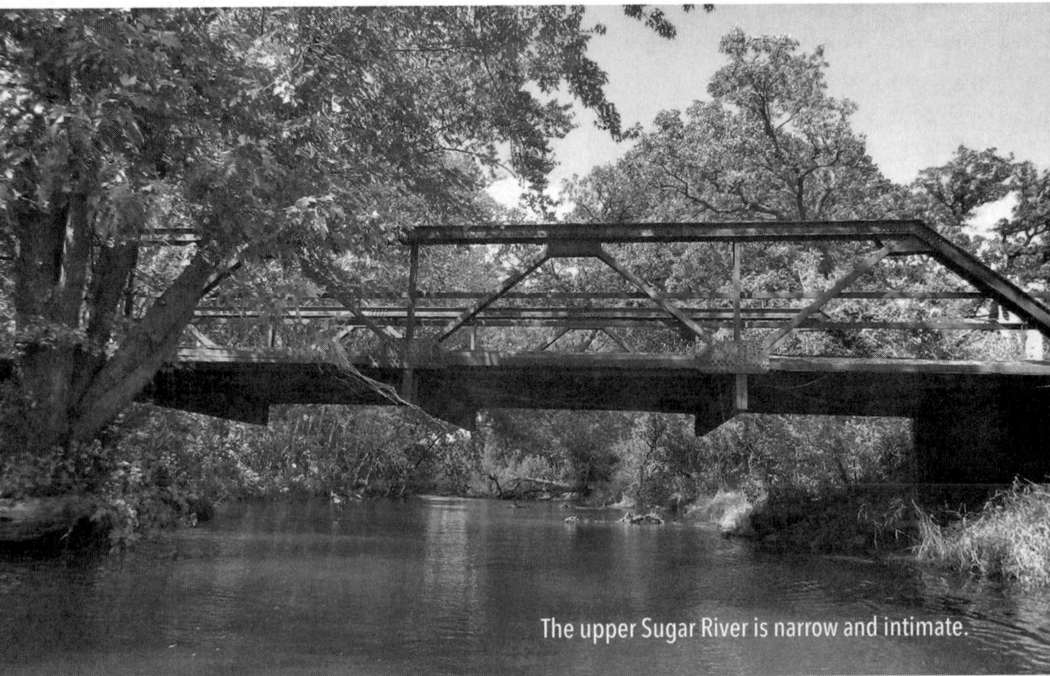

The upper Sugar River is narrow and intimate.

under as well. But then woods enclose, and the scenery is intimate and truly pretty. Riffles are plentiful, but some downed trees can intimidate the casual paddler. But for those who don't mind a bit of dodging and ducking, Riverside to Basco is a delightful 9-mile day trip.

CAMPING **Blue Mound State Park** (4350 Mounds Park Road, Blue Mounds; 608-437-5711) and **Lake Farm County Park** (3113 Lake Farm Road, Madison; 608-224-3730)

RENTALS **Sugar River Sports** (7008 Little Lakes Road, Belleville; 608-424-6045) and **Rutabaga Paddlesports** (220 W. Broadway, Madison; 608-223-9300)

FOOD FOR THOUGHT At the mill by the take-out is **The Hop Garden Tap Room** (6818 Canal St.; 608-516-9649), and just across the river is **Paoli Schoolhouse Shops & Café,** in an actual red schoolhouse (6857 Paoli Road; 608-848-6261). In Verona, try **Wisconsin Brewing Company** (1079 American Way; 608-848-1079), and in Belleville, try **Sugar River Pizza Company** (1019 River St.; 608-424-6777).

SHOUT-OUT There are many cute shops and many studios of fabulously talented artists to explore in Paoli.

43 Sugar River B: BRODHEAD DAM TO AVON BOTTOMS

•THE•FACTS•

Put-in/take-out Decatur Park off Park Road/Avon Bottoms Wildlife Area (17305 W. Beloit–Newark Road). See "The Flavor" for two alternative access points.

Distance/time 14.7 mi/Allow for 6–8 hrs

Gradient/water level 2 fpm/Reliable throughout the season; see USGS gage 05436500.

Water type Quietwater

Canoe or kayak Either

Skill level Beginner

Time of year to paddle Anytime, though spring and autumn are particularly nice

Landscape Hardwood forests, prairie, a couple bluffs, sedge meadows, and bottomlands

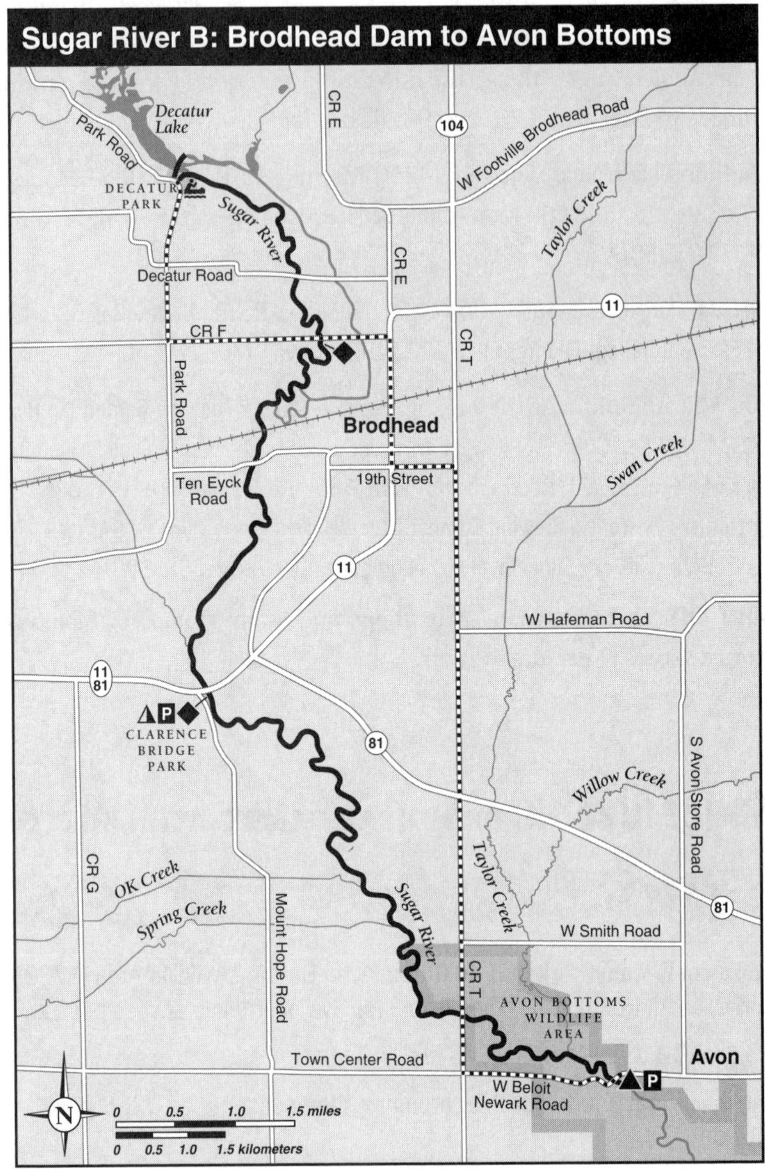

OVERVIEW A delightfully isolated stretch with a lot of sweet scenery, this longish trip can be broken into two parts by using the convenient access at Clarence Bridge Park. You can also camp at the wayside park at this access for an overnight excursion. Wildlife includes great blue herons, kingfishers, muskrats, bald eagles, turkey vultures, hawks, frogs, and sandhill cranes.

SHUTTLE 10.5 miles. From the take-out, go west on Beloit–Newark Road, then turn right onto County Road T. Continue north on CR T past the WI 81 intersection. Turn left onto 23rd Street or 19th Street into town, then right onto First Center Avenue/ WI 11 (the main thoroughfare in historic downtown Brodhead). Turn left onto Fourth Street/CR F and cross first the millrace (see below) and then the main branch of the Sugar River. Turn right onto Park Road and then right again into Decatur Park.

TAKE-OUT N42° 32.542' W89° 20.483' **PUT-IN** N42° 38.668' W89° 24.538'

•THE•FLAVOR•

THOUGH AT FIRST RUGGED, THIS TRIP'S FINISH IS SERENE. The put-in at Decatur Park is not for the faint of heart, or hoof, as it requires schlepping your boat and gear down a steep slope, but it's definitely worth the effort. At the base of the bluff, you'll feel like you're in another world: The dam itself is pretty cool, the outcropping is gorgeous, and the feeling of being away from it all is palpable.

For the first 3 miles, you'll see no signs of development but for a couple bridges and the peripheries of farms. What's novel about this is that on the other side of the river is the town of Brodhead, yet from the channel of the river you'd have no idea that the town exists. In the early 1860s, a 3-mile-long millrace—basically a canal to divert water—was hand dug to operate a gristmill. The effect was twofold: A de facto island was created in the river, and Brodhead became the second city in Wisconsin to generate its own electric power. You can paddle the millrace itself, but it's flatter, slower, and more developed than where this trip begins (see "Additional Trips").

If toeing your way down the bluff at Decatur Park isn't your cup of tea, CR F provides for an excellent alternate put-in (**N42° 37.560' W89° 23.233'**). A mile of totally unspoiled landscape is found below CR F until the Crazy Horse Campground appears on the right. Immediately after this, a picturesque metal railroad bridge comes into view and then the Ten Eyck Road bridge. There's nothing interesting about the bridge itself, but it does signal the first signs of development, mostly cabins and shacks on river left (one of which features a rather impressive wooden sculpture of a life-sized grizzly bear holding an actual keg of beer on its shoulder). Thick woods reappear and the cabins recede. Small islands and occasional downfall that is easy to maneuver provide navigation choices to help spice things up.

You'll begin to see a gentle rise of the right bank and some very modest crumbling rock exposed. Once you see the huge WI 11 bridge, look to the right and up (and maybe a little bit behind you): A very pretty, very cool, *very old* outcrop slopes down to the river on a sharp angle. This and the rocky bluff at the put-in are some of the only geological notorieties on the Sugar River. Just below the WI 11 bridge on the right is Clarence Bridge Park (**N42° 35.179' W89° 24.349'**), which makes for a great stopping or pausing point; plus, it has free camping and a portable toilet, but no potable water.

After the bridge, the Sugar River Raceway is off to the right. Because this go-cart track is lively and loud in summer, it's wise to plan your trip when races are not being held. You'll be out of earshot of the track within minutes, after which there are few signs of civilization. Sandbanks begin to appear together with iconographic deadfall in the water that is easy to maneuver around but enhances the authenticity of the river's character.

The Sugar meanders a bit for the next few miles, but mostly in broad strokes. There are some wide sections, but the average width is 60 feet. Adding to the charm, the bottom becomes increasingly sandy and less muddy. You'll pass under a low-clearance (but not dangerous) abandoned railroad bridge, but otherwise there's nothing out here but stretches of unspoiled scenery. This is the Sugar River at its best. Paddling this section in autumn will reward you with spectacular displays of fall foliage. In spring, wildflowers are downright raucous.

Finally, you'll first pass under the CR T bridge, where you could take out, but it's more sensible to paddle 2 additional miles down to the Beloit–Newark Road bridge, because along the way you'll get to see the Swenson Wet Prairie State Natural Area, which encloses both banks of the river and marks the northern boundary of the vast Avon Bottoms Wildlife Area. These areas are home for both cerulean and yellow-throated warblers as well as the majestic yellow-crowned night heron. Taylor Creek comes in from the left and is worth an upstream exploration if you have the time and inclination. Just downstream from the Beloit–Newark Road bridge on the left is the take-out, at a dedicated landing with an adjoining parking area.

•THE•FUDGE•

ADDITIONAL TRIPS I don't recommend putting in upstream, where the river often hosts motorboats and Jet Skis. Plus, you'd have to portage around the dam. Alternatively, you can paddle the millrace by putting in either at **Head Gates Park,** at the confluence of Norwegian Creek, or 1.5 miles downstream at **Putnam Park,** off CR F. I recommend the former, as it is less developed and allows you to paddle upstream on Norwegian Creek to a lovely covered bridge that is part of the Sugar River State Trail.

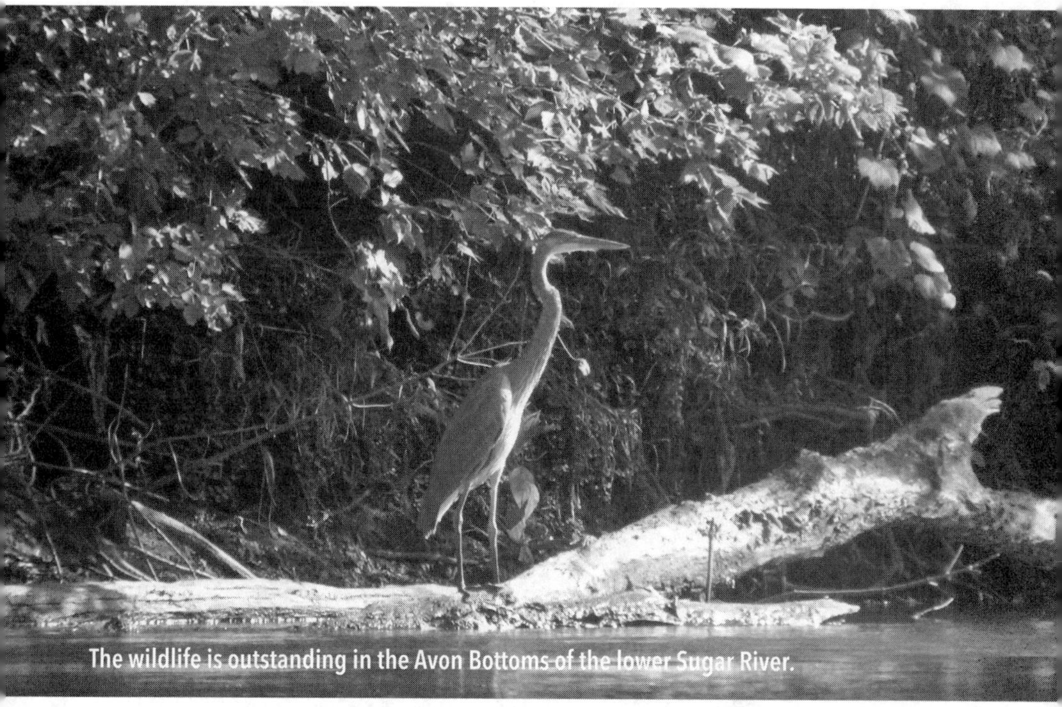

The wildlife is outstanding in the Avon Bottoms of the lower Sugar River.

CAMPING Primitive camping is allowed at no charge at **Clarence Bridge Park,** between Mt. Hope Road and the river at WI 11/WI 81.

FOOD FOR THOUGHT For great pizza and classic Italian food, check out **Villa Pizza Inn** (1011 First Center Ave., Brodhead; 608-897-8066).

SHOUT-OUT Brodhead is home to the **1st Brigade Band,** whose original 1860s incarnation entertained the crowds in Freeport, Illinois, that had gathered for the historic debate between Stephen Douglas and Abraham Lincoln over the issue of slavery. Four years later, the members of the band found themselves stationed in Shenandoah, Virginia, during the Civil War. Revived in 1964, the band performs antebellum and war-era music around the country (visit 1stbrigadeband.org for more information).

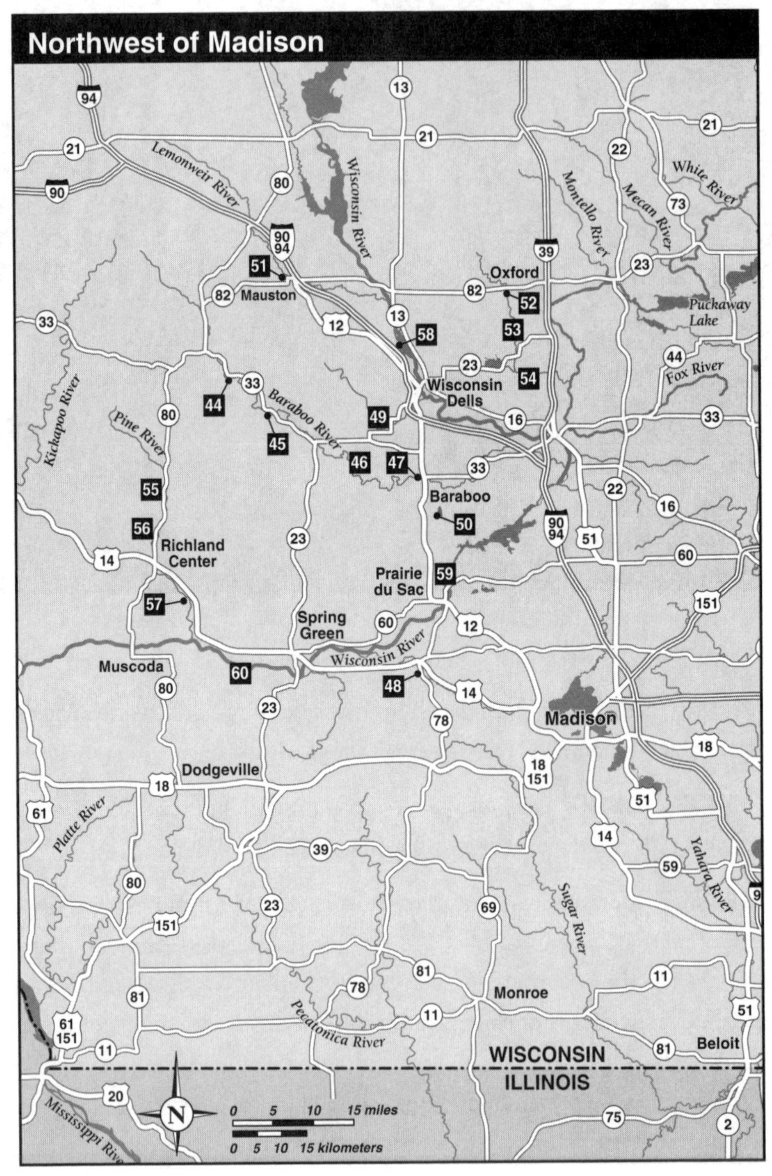
Northwest of Madison
Mauston
Oxford
Wisconsin Dells
Baraboo
Richland Center
Prairie du Sac
Spring Green
Muscoda
Madison
Dodgeville
Monroe
Beloit
WISCONSIN
ILLINOIS
Lemonweir River
Wisconsin River
Montello River
Mecan River
White River
Puckaway Lake
Fox River
Baraboo River
Kickapoo River
Pine River
Platte River
Sugar River
Yahara River
Pecatonica River
Mississippi River
0 5 10 15 miles
0 5 10 15 kilometers

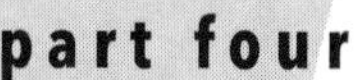

part four

NORTHWEST OF MADISON

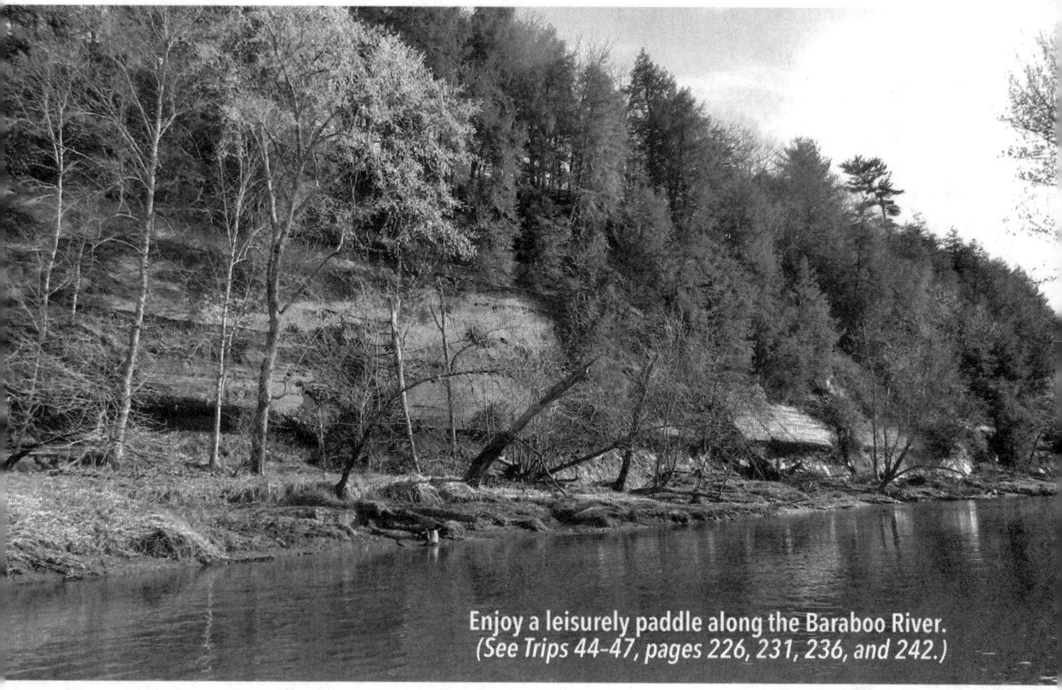

Enjoy a leisurely paddle along the Baraboo River.
(See Trips 44–47, pages 226, 231, 236, and 242.)

44 Baraboo River A: WONEWOC TO LA VALLE

•THE•FACTS•

Put-in/take-out WI 33 wayside at Strawbridge Road/West Main Street boat launch

Distance/time 12.5 mi/Allow for 5 hrs

Gradient/water level Under 1 fpm/Should be fine year-round; consult NOAA gage in Reedsburg.

Water type Quietwater

Canoe or kayak Kayak

Skill level Experienced

Time of year to paddle Anytime, though spring is quietest and autumn is awfully pretty.

Landscape Rugged Driftless sandstone bluffs, hardwood bottomlands

---

OVERVIEW This is, hands down, the most beautiful section anywhere on the Baraboo River—and that's saying something. Gorgeous rocky bluffs, absolute intimacy, spectacular wildlife, and the most scenic bike-shuttle trip in this book are just a few of the delights you'll discover on this seldom paddled section. Wildlife you may encounter include sandhill cranes, geese, wood ducks, deer, teals, turkey vultures, bald eagles, muskrats, walleyes, turtles, hawks, and great horned owls.

CAR SHUTTLE **7 miles.** Simply take WI 33 west toward Wonewoc and turn left into the Wisconsin 400 State Trail area at Strawbridge Road.

BIKE SHUTTLE **6 miles.** You will need a Wisconsin State Trail pass here (see tinyurl.com/witrailpassfees). Simply take the Wisconsin 400 State Trail west toward Wonewoc. It's a gorgeous bike ride, and it directly connects the take-out with the put-in.

TAKE-OUT N43° 34.970' W90° 08.064' **PUT-IN** N43° 38.391' W90° 12.674'

•THE•FLAVOR•

PUT IN ANYWHERE ON RIVER LEFT that's the least muddy, as there is no official launch. There's a convenient (and mostly clean) lowering in the bank just to the east of the natural spring. The beauty of this spot will strike you before your boat even touches

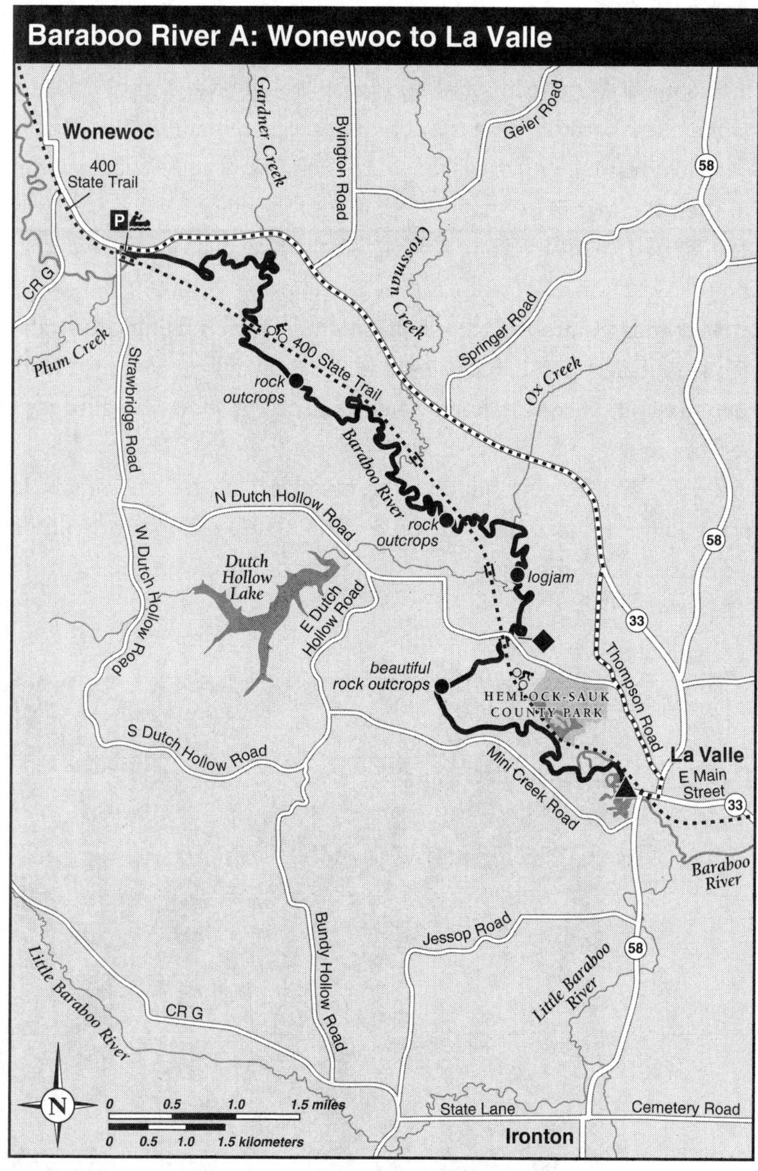

the water: an iconic rusty red railroad bridge from the 1890s (today converted into a state trail) crossing the river just upstream of an impressive display of a bulging sandstone bluff lined with pine trees.

For the first 2 miles the river courses through a meadowy lowland with sneak-peek glimpses of sandstone bluffs off in the distance. Here, as elsewhere, the river will be deep and brown, slow moving, and 50 feet wide. There will be a clutter of trees to maneuver around, duck under, and occasionally ride over, but you should not have to portage until much later on (though conditions always change, of course). You'll soon encounter clusters of festooned straw and grass looking like shaggy little monsters caught on branches. Each of these is a sobering measurement of how high the river can rise when it's cresting. Woods will begin to enclose and you'll paddle under a footbridge and then the first of several 400 State Trail bridges. It's been a pleasant few miles, but, once you see a charming red barn with silver silos ensconced in a hillside nook off on the right bank, get ready for the real show.

The river bends left around a magnificent sandstone bluff lining the water, about 50 feet high at its tallest point. The colors are simply exquisite: muddy brown, mossy green, lichen gray, sunburned red on a canvas of rock. A short straightaway follows, with some trees to dodge to the next bluff (also on the right). This bluff is less rocky than before, more of a sloping hill down to the river, but here there's an indented holler much taller than upstream. The setting is entirely intimate and undisturbed. It's truly beautiful and absolutely worth the occasional inconvenience of tree debris.

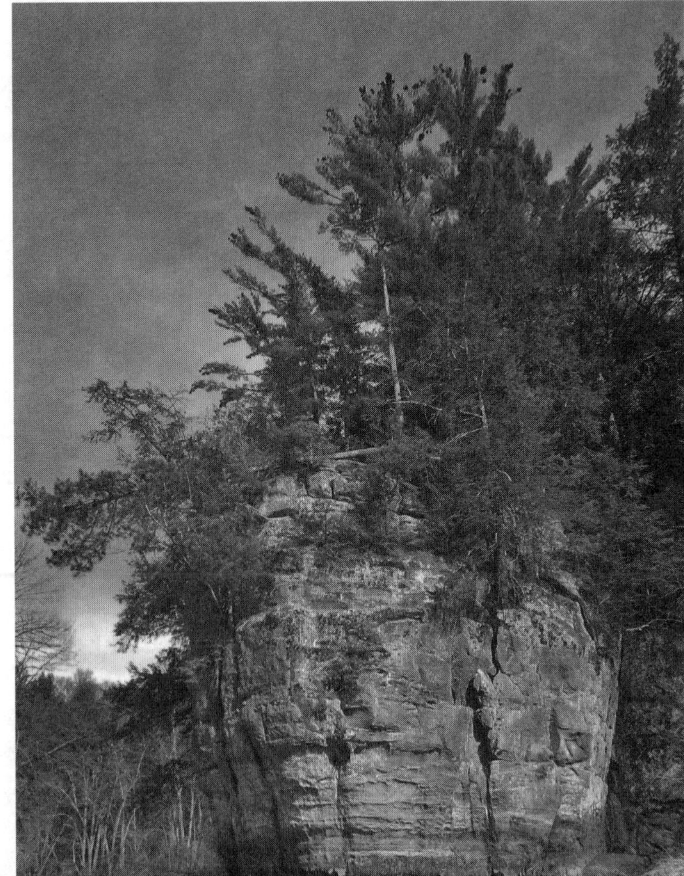

The 4 miles of the Baraboo River upstream of La Valle are sublime.

While the background remains ruggedly undulating, the immediate foreground flattens out some as the river runs parallel to the 400 State Trail for 1 mile. You won't cross it until later downstream, but you will paddle under a curious mini–truss bridge. The river will leave the valley for a moment and take cover under the shade of woods before returning to the sun-drenched expanse. As it does, you'll meander around the base of a stunning 100-foot-tall bluff. This is a particularly pretty stretch, as you'll see the rock face itself from several perspectives, as well as a lush woodsy hillside.

You'll cross under a 400 State Trail bridge as the river veers east and away from the bluff into thick bottomlands, where, alas, you will encounter obstructions that you'll have to negotiate. The first of these is just a stubborn old dead tree blocking the river from bank to bank, leaving no room to sneak through, under, or over. You'll have to get out of your boat and portage around this on the banks. Unfortunately, the banks are muddy and steep. Look for the most accessible spot, usually on river right.

There's another obstruction just downstream, so don't get too cozy yet. In fact, you may wish simply to take your boat for a short walk at this point, as there are a few other obstructions shortly downstream, each of them requiring you to portage. The river will meander toward the east before coming back around to the west and south. To avoid the umpteen disruptions, simply walk due south, until the river comes back out of the woods on your left. Reenter wherever it's most convenient. The distance for this would be about a third of a mile. The alternative is putting up with a few more portages.

This nasty section will end, I promise, and you'll soon see the Dutch Hollow Road bridge. You can certainly take out here to shorten this trip, but I really, strongly, firmly discourage it, as the most beautiful section of this already lovely trip lies shortly downstream. Now there are pretty views of another rippling sandstone bluff up- and downstream from the bridge. Then you'll paddle under the last 400 State Trail bridge on this trip. Shortly thereafter, a spectacular rock wall lines the left bank, seeping springs from its fissures, the water glimmering in the western sun. The river will bend to the left around a jutting exposure basking in the sunset and then through a miniature gorge. Here, a long, tall ridge crowned with hemlocks and studded with random outcrops lines the right bank, while the left is all piney green. The angular rock outcrops snag your attention again and again.

The final few miles are pretty as a picture. Still hilly in the background, the landscape does flatten out some in the foreground of a pastoral setting. Off to the left, you'll see a red barn flanked thrice by silos. The banks will rise to 8 feet, now sandy, not muddy. There's a good chance you'll see horses grazing in the meadow on the left. Also on the left is a quick glimpse of another 400 State Trail bridge, to the right of which is an outcrop, which is also the southern tip of the haunting Hemlock-Sauk County Park (see "Additional Trips").

The river will then take one final dip into woods before entering the hamlet of La Valle. You'll see a row of houses straight before you. The river will turn right, after which you'll see some cool sandstone shelves on the left bank. In the final straightaway, you'll spot a hill in the background shortly before the boat ramp appears on the left in between two bars.

•THE•FUDGE•

ADDITIONAL TRIPS While not visible from the river, just a couple of miles upstream of the take-out is **Hemlock-Sauk County Park.** A slough only 12 feet deep, the still waters are punctuated with dead or dying trees still upright, a northern cousin of a cypress bayou, and the whole park is surrounded by sandstone bluffs. It's an otherworldly sight that can be paddled in its own right or just hiked around.

Another popular trip upstream begins at WI 33 in **Union Center,** with two take-out options: at County Road FF in Wonewoc (5.5 miles) or where this trip begins at the wayside park (8.5 miles). The highlight of this trip is "Third Castle," a colossal sandstone cliff 150 feet high.

CAMPING **Wonewoc Legion Park** (North Road/CR G; 608-464-3114) and **Chaparral Campground** (316 Dreamland Drive, Wonewoc; 608-464-3200)

RENTALS **Beyond Boundaries** (113 Center St., Wonewoc; 608-464-7433) and **Chaparral Campground** (see above)

FOOD FOR THOUGHT It doesn't get much more convenient than having your choice of two bars on each side of a take-out: **The River Mill** (305 W. Main St., La Valle; 608-985-7723) and **Fishy's Bar and Grill** (100 Commercial St., La Valle; 608-985-7710).

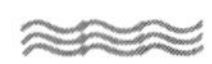

45 Baraboo River B: LA VALLE TO LAKE REDSTONE

•THE•FACTS•

Put-in West Main Street boat launch or North River Street across WI 58 bridge

Take-out Boat launch off Douglas Road at Big Creek confluence

Distance/time 4 mi river paddling, 2+ mi lake paddling/Allow for 3 hrs

Gradient/water level 1.5 fpm/Should be fine year-round; consult NOAA gage in Reedsburg.

Water type Class I–II rapid at put-in, quietwater and lake paddling afterward

Canoe or kayak Either

Skill level Beginner

Time of year to paddle Anytime, though spring is quietest and autumn is lovely

Landscape Hardwood floodplains followed by exposed sandstone bluffs, semi-developed lake

---

OVERVIEW There's something for everyone in this expedition: a thrilling Class I–II rapid, beautiful sandstone rock outcrops, a huge waterfall, and a pretty lake with an array of rock formations not unlike Wisconsin Dells. Plus, there's an excellent bike shuttle, along with sandhill cranes, geese, wood ducks, deer, teals, turkey vultures, bald eagles, muskrats, walleye, turtles, hawks, and great horned owls.

CAR SHUTTLE **3.1 miles.** From the take-out, turn right and head east on Douglas Road, then turn right onto County Road V. Turn right onto WI 33 and follow it into town, where it becomes Main Street. The boat launch is at the end of West Main Street.

BIKE SHUTTLE **3 miles.** You will need a Wisconsin State Trail pass here (see tinyurl .com/witrailpassfees). From the take-out, turn right and head east on Douglas Road, then turn right onto CR V. Turn right onto the Wisconsin 400 State Trail. You'll cross under WI 33 through a fun mini-tunnel, then come across it again at an intersection. Leave the trail and turn left onto WI 33, which becomes Main Street in town. The boat launch is at the end of West Main Street.

PLANNING ADVISORY Before you put in, you should decide whether you wish to run the rapid underneath the Center Street/WI 58 bridge in town, located only 400 feet downstream from the boat launch. The rapid is a lot of fun as long you're comfortable

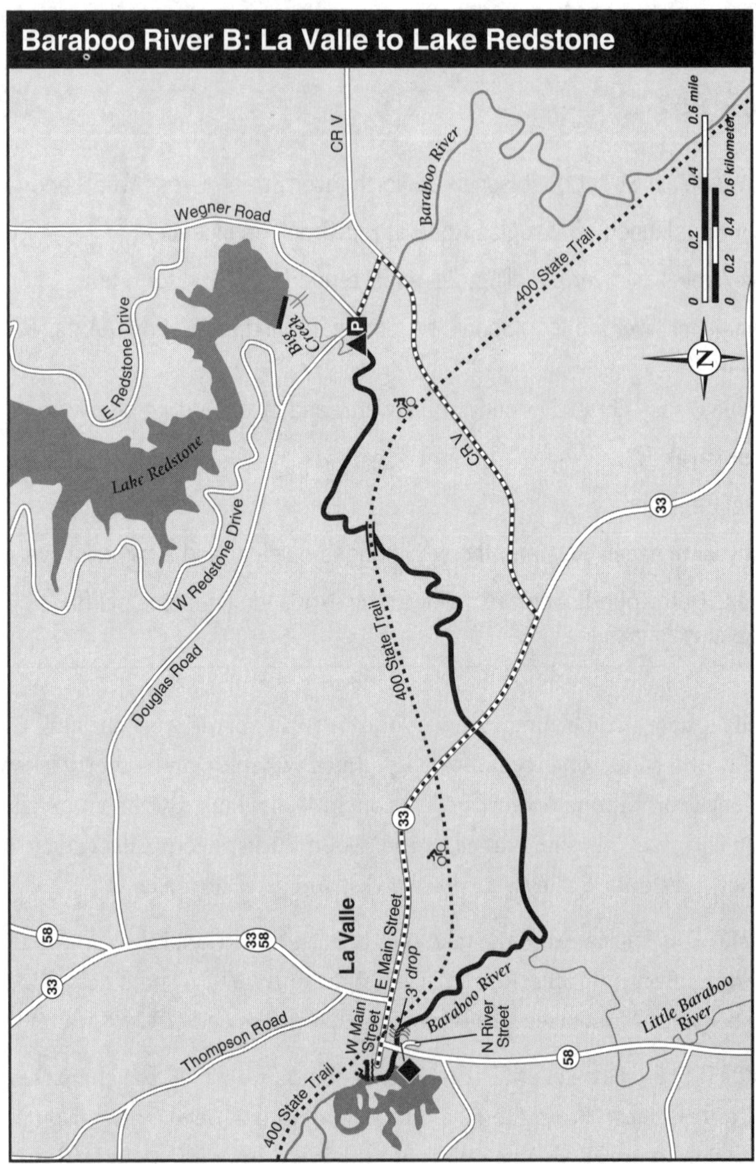

with a Class I–II drop, but if you wish to skip it, turn left off of West Main Street and cross the bridge before you reach the boat launch. Take the first left off the bridge onto North River Street, then turn left again at the Y to reach an alternate put-in. This is also a good scouting spot if you're still trying to decide where to start.

TAKE-OUT N43° 35.021' W90° 05.402' **PUT-INS** N43° 34.971' W90° 08.064' (boat launch), N43° 34.908' W90° 07.912' (North River Street below the rapid)

•THE•FLAVOR•

PUT IN AT THE BOAT LAUNCH at the end of Main Street, a somewhat nondescript spot smack-dab between two restaurant-bars. (If parking is an issue, just leave your vehicle on the street nearby or at the 400 State Trail parking lot off Commercial Street.) The setting here is pretty but a little disorienting at first, for on the other side of the right bank is a lake, created by a former dam in downtown La Valle. The dam, like all the previous dams on the Baraboo River, has been removed, though some concrete blocks and rocks remain, causing the rapid.

Take the channel on the right, as the one on the left is shallow and erratically rocky. There are two drops in the right channel, the first one bigger. The rapid itself is not technically demanding, but it's not one to take for granted either. A small wave train continues for 25 yards below the second drop. On the right, you can catch an eddy that recirculates to the rapid, if you wish to run it a second or third time.

For the next mile, the Baraboo flows in mostly broad strokes, with just a few meanders through an undeveloped floodplain. The river width will vary between 45 and 65 feet, the bottom mostly sandy (though the banks often are muddy). The setting here is intimate and quiet. The tree line on the right will thin out and give way to a pretty view of an open meadow and rolling Driftless hills in the background. A straightaway leads to the WI 33 bridge. An occasional obstacle will require maneuvering around, but there should be no logjams or blockages to portage on this trip.

After a pleasant meander around another meadow, the bank on the right will rise, and before you will loom a sandstone outcrop about 30 feet high and running along the water for a few hundred feet. Soon another outcrop will appear on the right, this one more modest and receded from the bank. All of the outcrops on this trip will be adorned with hemlock and pine. A rusty metal bridge resting on foundations of huge rock slabs appears next. On the downstream side, a small island splits the river in two channels; choose the left one, as the right is often clogged with deadfall. (This is one of the many bygone bridges of the 400 State Trail, which connects Reedsburg and Elroy along a former railroad track. Time was when a passenger train from Chicago to Minneapolis took just more than 6.5 hours to complete the distance, or

400 minutes, from whence the repurposed state trail received its name.) The prettiest bluff yet looms into view as the river bends to the right.

After a gentle horseshoe-shaped meander, you'll see a creek entering from the left as well as a wayside boat launch. If you wish, you can call it quits here, but you'll be forfeiting a fun exploration. Assuming you're still on the water, turn into the mouth of the feeder stream, called Big Creek (although it's pretty narrow and shallow). There is a current, but paddling upstream on the creek is not much of a workout. You'll paddle through a culvert to the other side and then up as far as you can to a rapid, where you will take out on the left or right. Immediately upstream of the rapid is a huge artificial waterfall 40–50 feet tall. It's actually the dam that creates the sprawling Lake Redstone that lies on the other side of the berm. There are hiking trails to the left and right of the dam that lead to the top.

Feeling venturesome? Schlep your boat up and over the berm, down to the rocky shore directly below, or to the left where there is a beach, and launch into the lake, where there's a no-wake ordinance. An abundance of sandstone striations—nooks and crannies, slits and crevices, tapered spires and billowy pillows—awaits your discovery. True, there are several private residences along the way, but this portion of the lake is like a little taste of the Dells on the Wisconsin River (thankfully, minus the Duck tour boats; see Wisconsin River A, page 292). I wouldn't go out of the way just to paddle Lake Redstone by itself, but tacking it on as a fun adjunct to the rapids, splendid isolation, and awesome sandstone bluffs along the Baraboo River from La Valle makes for a fun and varied day trip.

•THE•FUDGE•

ADDITIONAL TRIPS From the take-out at the Big Creek confluence down to Reedsburg are 8 miles of monotonous paddling, plus two portages at logjams. The river runs here through low-lying wetlands with little topography. The take-out in Reedsburg is a little difficult to locate as well. Unfortunately, the section from Reedsburg to Rock Springs cannot be recommended either, due to significant deadfall. It's definitely pretty, but more work than it's worth.

CAMPING **Wonewoc Legion Park** (North Road/CR G; 608-464-3114) and **Chaparral Campground** (316 Dreamland Drive, Wonewoc; 608-464-3200)

RENTALS **Beyond Boundaries** (113 Center St., Wonewoc; 608-464-7433) and **Chaparral Campground** (see above)

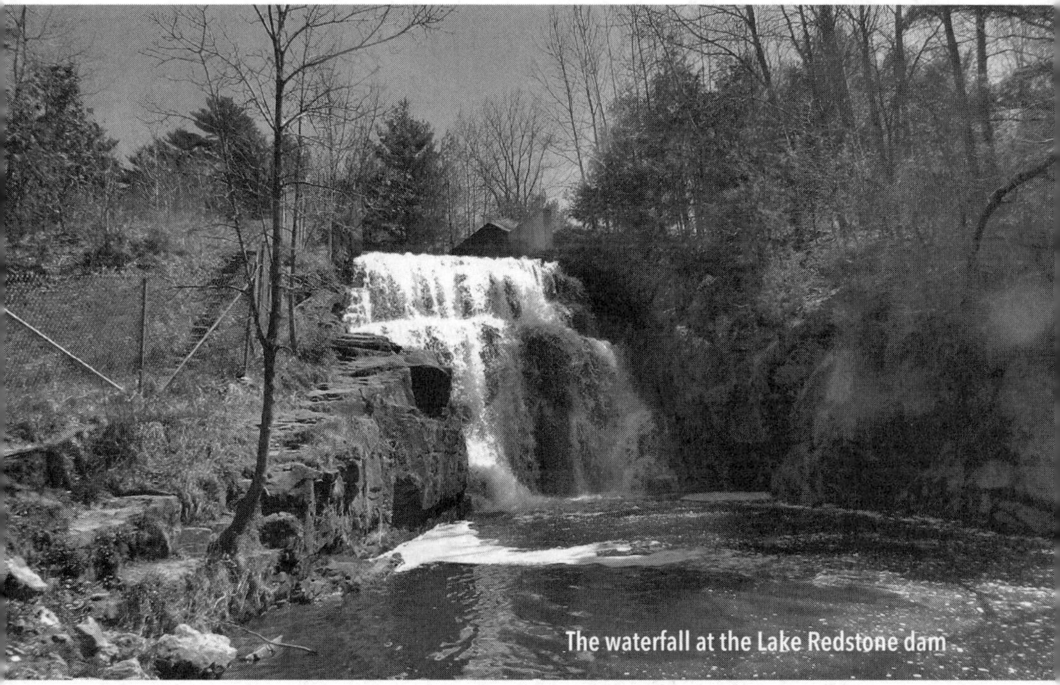

The waterfall at the Lake Redstone dam

Food for Thought At some point you'll have to return to the put-in, where you probably noticed that there are bars and restaurants on either side of the boat launch: **The River Mill** (305 W. Main St., La Valle; 608-985-7723) and **Fishy's Bar and Grill** (100 Commercial St., La Valle; 608-985-7710).

In Reedsburg, there's the **Corner Pub** (100 E. Main St.; 608-524-8989), which makes its own beer and sometimes hosts live Wurlitzer music. For great Italian food, treat yourself to a feast at **Calabria Pizza and Pasta** (251 E. Main St.; 608-524-7888). And for some of the absolute best craft beer selections you'll find anywhere in Wisconsin, stop by **Viking Liquor** (1625 E. Main St.; 608-524-3880). All in all, Reedsburg is a really cute town worth poking around in.

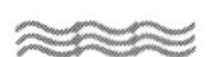

46 Baraboo River C: ROCK SPRINGS TO NORTH FREEDOM

•THE•FACTS•

Put-in/take-out Parking area for Ableman's Gorge at WI 136 bridge in Rock Springs/ North Freedom Park

Distance/time 8 mi/Allow for 4 hrs

Gradient/water level 1.5 fpm/The Baraboo should always have enough water for paddling, but it will be unsafe when the visual gage on the WI 136 bridge reads 13' or higher.

Water type Quietwater

Canoe or kayak Kayak preferable; canoes would have to portage around deadfall more frequently.

Skill level Beginner

Time of year to paddle Early spring or late fall

Landscape Quartzite gorge, Baraboo Range, hardwoods, pastures

---

OVERVIEW A stream steeped in history, this trip is a geologist's dream, as the river cuts through the pink quartzite cliffs of the Upper Narrows of the Baraboo Range and underneath ancient railroad bridges. There are logjam issues here, however. Wildlife includes minks; red, blonde, and black squirrels; muskrats; bald eagles; great blue herons; hawks; and turkeys.

SHUTTLE 5.3 miles. From the take-out, turn left onto Walnut Street, then right onto CR I. Turn left onto WI 136 and follow it into Rock Springs. After you cross the bridge, turn right to stay on WI 136. Drive through the beautiful Upper Narrows; then, before you cross the bridge, turn left into the parking area for Ableman's Gorge—or stay on WI 136 to the next bridge.

TAKE-OUT N43° 27.404' W89° 51.793' **PUT-IN** N43° 29.434' W89° 55.087'

•THE•FLAVOR•

IT'S NOT OFTEN THAT I RECOMMEND PADDLING UPSTREAM, but it's worth it on this trip at the very beginning; the gradient is so minimal that it's hardly a workout. In so doing, you paddle west along the north-facing slope of Ableman's Gorge, one half of

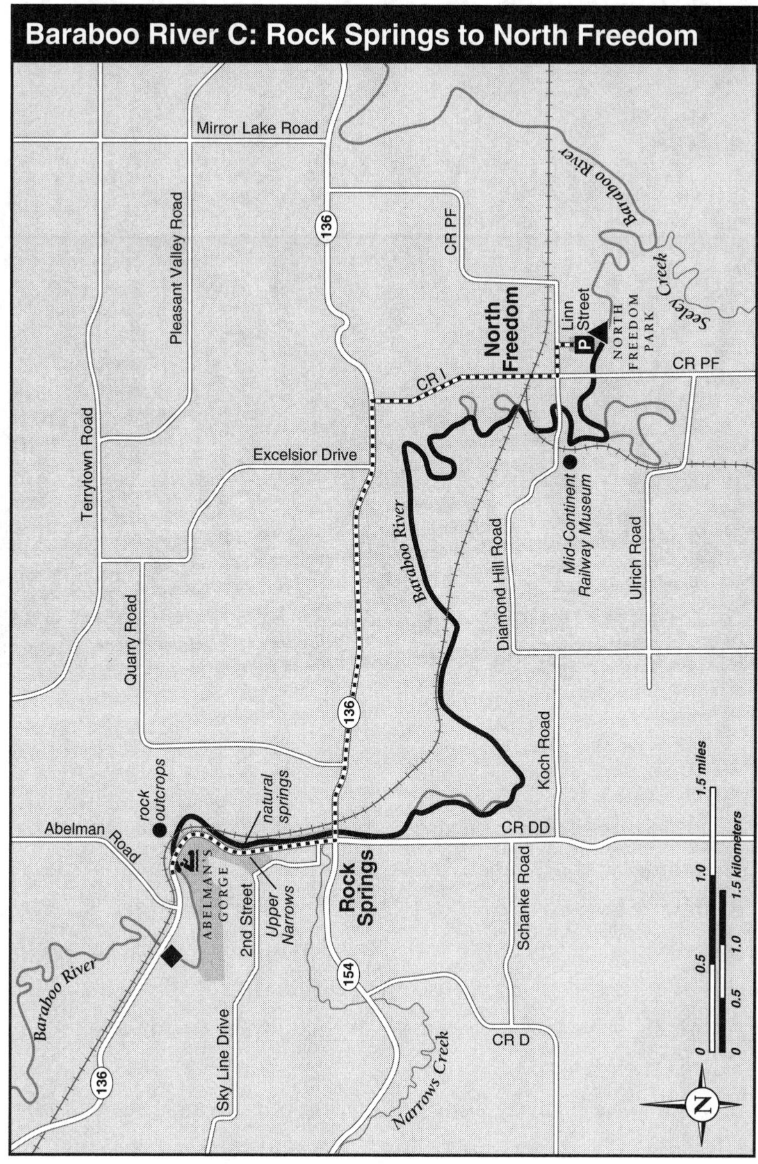

the magnificent cliff the river cut through to create a gorge many hundreds of millions of years ago, thus constituting what is called the Upper Narrows of the Baraboo Range. (It's called "Upper" because this trip corresponds to the western terminus of the Baraboo Range, an ancient mountain chain that today resembles an oval that's 30 miles wide and 10 miles long. The Lower Narrows lie 10 miles downstream from the city of Baraboo, along WI 33.)

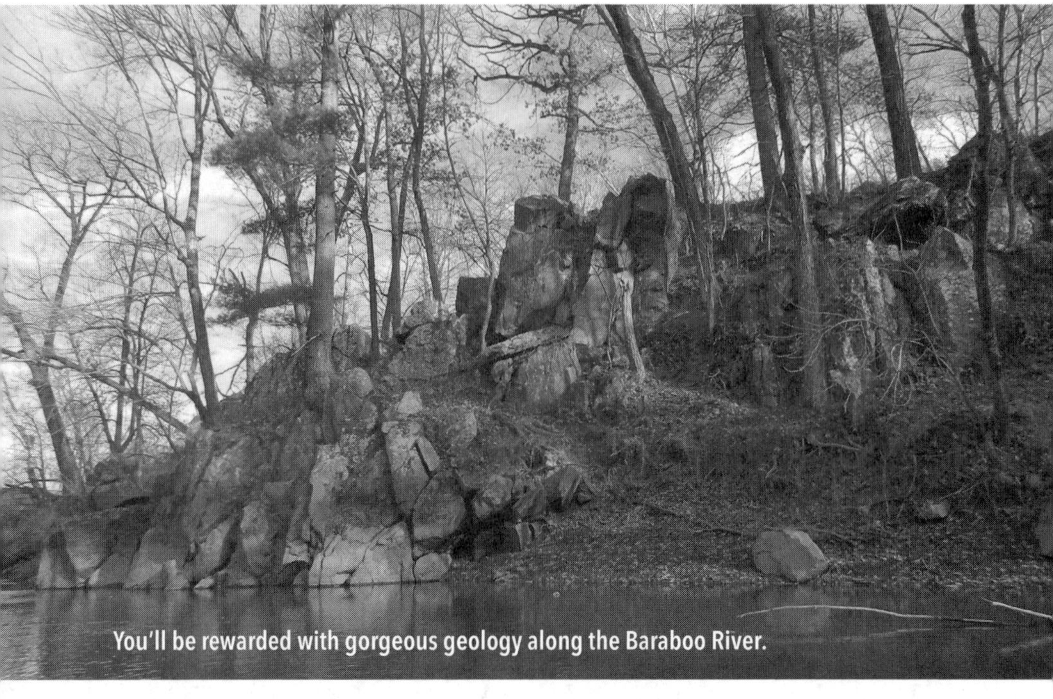
You'll be rewarded with gorgeous geology along the Baraboo River.

Ableman's Gorge, a protected state natural area, offers some fine hiking. It's one of three such gorges in the Baraboo Range; the other two are in Devil's Lake State Park (page 258) and the Lower Narrows (see "Additional Trips"). On the water, this slope has an otherworldly feel where hemlock, birch, and pine trees are juxtaposed with a loose jumble of quartzite boulders ensconced within the cliff. Once the river bends to the right (north), you've seen the best of Ableman; turn around and let yourself go with the flow of the current.

Approaching the highway bridge where you put in, you'll see the other half of the Upper Narrows rising above the railroad grade with an attractive outcropping. You will pass the first of many handsome old railroad bridges. Another outcrop comes up on the left as the river bends to the right. The hill on the left soon becomes studded with talus, weathered rock debris in huge heaps. The next and arguably most magnificent outcrop looms above the river on the right as you pass under another railroad bridge. This is the south- and east-facing slope of Ableman's Gorge and the showiest section of geology on this trip. Rising 200 feet above the river for about a mile, the rock formations here are world renowned.

Long story short: This is a buried mountain that has been exhumed by erosion, together with the serendipitous assistance of a quarry. Nowhere else in the Midwest are the forces of metamorphic geology better displayed. Indeed, it was at Ableman's Gorge where Professor Charles Van Hise of the University of Wisconsin–Madison pioneered the field of structural geology, using the gorge as an outdoor laboratory. To this day, researchers and students alike seek out Ableman's Gorge as a kind of mecca. The only thing less than wonderful about this effect is that the road runs parallel to the river, so the sights and sounds of traffic are present. The view and overall feeling from the river are nonetheless exhilarating.

All that romance aside, deadfall obstructions and logjam pileups are problematic on the Baraboo River, and this trip is no exception. Conditions change all the time, and the river is prone to spectacular flooding, which flushes out old pileups while scattering and depositing newer ones downstream. You should expect to have to portage at least a few times. Clever maneuvering, a handsaw, and the willingness both to duck under and scrape over obstructions will diminish some of the portages.

After Ableman's Gorge, things settle down a bit. The river is atypically straight and wide, making obstructions here unlikely. On your right, you'll see a natural springs pouring out of a pipe—the town isn't called Rock Springs for nothing. It's accessible via a pull-in from WI 138 (there is no direct access from the river); you'll often see cars here with folks filling up jugs. Shortly after the springs, also on the right, Narrows Creek empties into the Baraboo River. You'll pass under the road bridge in town, where a hand-painted gage on a pier tells you how high (or low) the river is. The Baraboo on this trip should always have enough water for paddling, but it's best to keep off it while it's high.

After the bridge, again on the right, is a small park with a wooden stairwell that can be used as a put-in or take-out. The river continues straight and south for a short while. You'll see and hear a huge farm co-op on the left, followed by an unfortunate logjam that's been there forever. On the left bank is a visible portage path; while the bank itself is steep, it takes you around the logjam and then down to a flat, accessible area where reentry is easy.

As the river heads east, a ridge in the distance will come into focus. The landscape becomes wild and beautiful again. Moss-patched limestone outcrops line the right side at water's edge, past which the river will run along an attractive slope; for half a mile, all you will see are pockets of boulders embedded in the hill and towers of pines. The river will bend to the right and once again run parallel to the railroad grade, then bend to the left before passing under the next railroad bridge. On your right is a lovely little hill with gorgeous quartzite outcrops.

The next section of river is flatter but still quite pretty. It's wider than upstream, so deadfall is less of an issue. A gentle incline will be found just beyond the left bank. In a pleasant straightaway, there is a prairie feel on the left, where an abandoned car and some old farm equipment are grandfathered into the landscape. After this tranquil stretch, the river turns sharply to the right and meanders for the next mile; here you will likely run into some obstruction issues. There is a decidedly nonpublic area on the left with a tire swing, picnic tables, fire pit, and floating pier—and a NO TRESPASSING sign. Another logjam follows. Again, not all of these obstructions require automatic portaging; many can be negotiated with pluck and determination.

You'll pass under another railroad bridge supported by limestone pilings. On the right bank is a brief, unusually open stretch of pasture, with an occasional lone tree set in solitude. Walls of woods enclose on each side of the river shortly after this, followed by another railroad bridge. The river abruptly turns to the left, then to the right, as it passes under a road bridge signaling the town of North Freedom.

The current gently takes you westward below the bridge. Before turning left, you'll see a red building and several old-time trains ahead. This is the engine house of the Mid-Continent Railway Museum (see "The Fudge"); after this, the river bends to the left, then again to the right as it heads east into town. You'll pass under one more bridge at County Road PF. A farm atop a hill on the right is the last pleasant sight to take in before you find the take-out on the left at North Freedom Park, which has water and restrooms.

•THE•FUDGE•

ADDITIONAL TRIPS If you're feeling wanderlust and geological curiosity—and why wouldn't you, especially in Sauk County?—combine this trip with the **Lower Narrows of the Baraboo Range** way downstream. It's a short and easy 3.5-mile addendum about 8 miles east of the city of Baraboo. To get the full effect of this once-mighty mountain range, put in at Luebke Landing on CR W and take out at the intersection of WI 33 and CR U.

The Lower Narrows are arguably less dramatic than the Upper Narrows, and WI 33 cuts through the gorge, but it's still pretty. *Spoiler alert:* The sound of cars and trucks on the highway will be constant. Also, the take-out off WI 33 is very muddy and requires a schlep of about 50 yards from the river to the parking area at the state historical marker. It's definitely worth it, though, considering how old and special the Baraboo Range is.

CAMPING **Devil's Lake State Park** (S5975 Park Road, about 3 miles south of Baraboo; 608-356-8301) and **Mirror Lake State Park** (E10320 Fern Dell Road, about 10 miles northwest of Baraboo; 608-254-2333)

RENTALS **Wisconsin Canoe Company** (608-432-5058, thebestcanoecompanyever.com) and **Beyond Boundaries** (113 Center St., Wonewoc; 608-464-7433)

FOOD FOR THOUGHT Specializing in spectacularly large pancakes, the **Railroad Inn Cafe** (104 E. Walnut St., North Freedom; 608-522-4485) is the perfect place for breaking fast before a rugged day on the river.

SHOUT-OUTS If railroads interest you, check out the offerings of the outdoor **Mid-Continent Railway Museum** (E8948 Museum Road, North Freedom; 800-930-1385, midcontinent.org).

Even if you don't go for an extended hike, I strongly encourage you to walk up to the base of **Ableman's Gorge.** On WI 138, there is a pull-out for the natural springs mentioned earlier; chances are you will see cars parked there and folks filling jugs with the clear, clean water, which I also recommend. Across the road, a short walking trail leads to the base of the Ableman. It's one of those moments when you'll forget that this is the relatively flat Midwest. With a little imagination, enfolding yourself in the rocky panorama of the gorge makes you reflect upon the fact that the Baraboo Range used to be a mountainous terrain on the order of Yosemite.

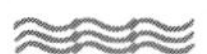

47 Baraboo River D: BARABOO RAPIDS

•THE•FACTS•

Put-in US 12 south of Gander Mountain parking lot or Haskins Park

Take-out Glenville Landing at WI 113 bridge. See "The Flavor" for an alternative take-out.

Distance/time 3.7 mi or 4.8 mi/Allow for 2 hrs

Gradient/water level 11 fpm through downtown, then 2 fpm leading to the take-out/ Consult USGS gage 05405000. *See additional information below.*

Water type Class I rapids downtown, quietwater for the remainder of the trip

Canoe or kayak Either

Skill level Beginner

Time of year to paddle Anytime, as long as the water isn't low

Landscape Downtown Baraboo, followed by tree-canopied plains with the Baraboo Hills in the background

---

OVERVIEW This is a trip of contrasts: an urban beginning and a rural ending, Class I rapids and gentle meanders. Wildlife includes great blue herons, ducks, geese, turtles, muskrats, and bald eagles. The river here is a travelogue of history, both human and geologic.

WATER-LEVEL ADVISORY The Baraboo River is 120 miles long but drops just 150 feet from beginning to end. That's a paltry 1.25 fpm. However, one-third of this drop—11 fpm—occurs along the 3-mile section in downtown Baraboo, which is the focus of this trip. As such, this is the only trip in the book that can be designated as a whitewater paddle at the right levels.

When you check the USGS gage, keep in mind that the light rapids downtown can be run from as low as 400 cfs to as high as 1,300 cfs. Below 400 cfs, the river is too shallow, whereas all the rapids wash out above 1,300 cfs. For the casual paddler, 400–600 cfs is perfect. For whitewater enthusiasts, the Baraboo is hardly challenging, but a minimum of 800 cfs is required to form big waves and play spots.

CAR SHUTTLE **4.1 miles.** From the take-out, turn right onto WI 113 and follow it into town. At the Broadway/WI 123 intersection, turn right. Go north half a mile and turn left onto Eighth Avenue/WI 33. Then you have a choice to make:

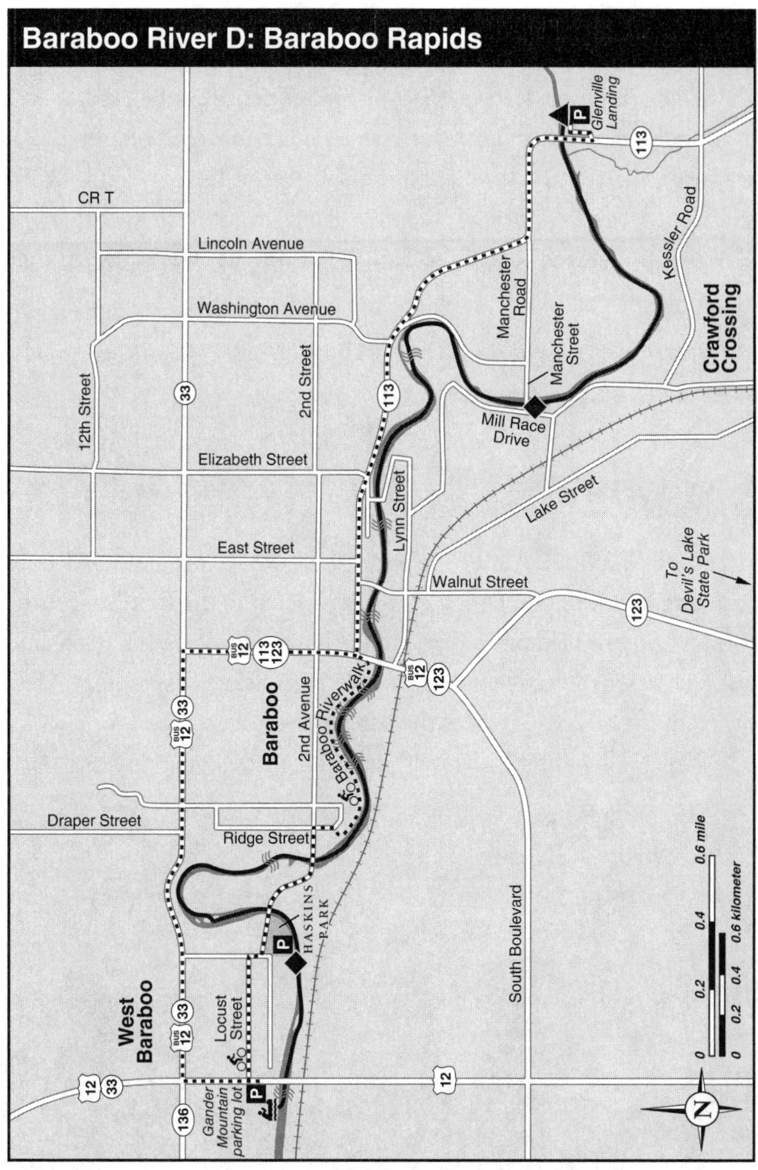

If you want to run the rapid described in the profile, turn left off of WI 33 onto West Pine Street/US 12, then right into the Gander Mountain parking lot. Park in the southeast corner of the lot and look for the path down the bluff to the water.

To skip the rapid, you can put in at **Haskins Park.** Instead of turning right into the Gander Mountain parking lot, turn left onto Locust Street, then right on Willow Street to Haskins Park. Put in just past the parking lot.

BIKE SHUTTLE **3.2 miles.** Past the intersection of Ash Street and WI 11, cross the road and access the path on the left for a portion of the Ice Age Trail, which runs parallel to the river. (This trail is designated as Wisconsin's only State Scenic Trail, as well as 1 of only 11 National Scenic Trails; however, a state-trail pass is *not* required.) Follow the yellow marker tags. After the trail leads you onto Second Avenue, stay on the street and cross the Attridge Park bridge, then a second bridge at Shaw Street. Turn left onto Willow Street to put in at Haskins Park, or turn right on Willow and then left on Locust to put in at Gander Mountain.

TAKE-OUT W89° 42.839' **PUT-INS** N43° 28.249' W89° 46.225' (Gander Mountain), N43° 28.195' W89° 45.693' (Haskins Park)

•THE•FLAVOR•

PUT IN AT THE US 12 BRIDGE. How? The public is allowed to park and walk down to the river via the Gander Mountain parking lot. Drive down to the southeast corner of the lot and park. A few trampled paths descend the hill to the water. It's steep, but not too precipitous. Put in wherever seems safest and most accessible; you may need to walk west, away from the bridge, to where the bank is the least steep.

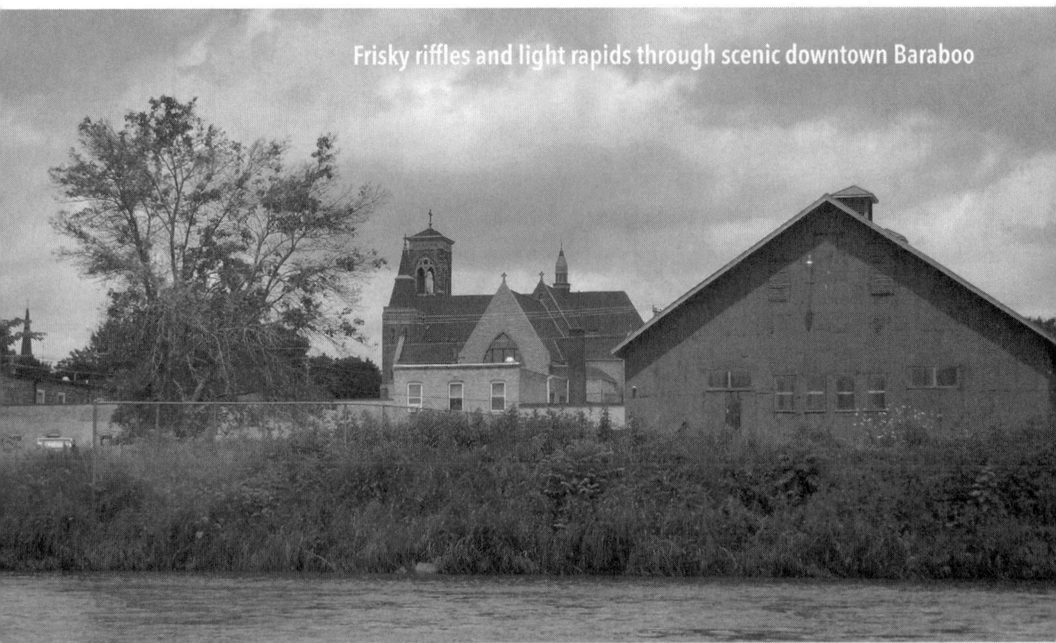

Frisky riffles and light rapids through scenic downtown Baraboo

Immediately on river right lies a rapid just upstream of the bridge that is one of the best anywhere on the Baraboo. Just watch out for fishing line! There are no additional rapids between US 12 and Haskins Park, but this first rapid is definitely worth running and surfing. But if that sounds like too much of a hassle or too intimidating, for simplicity's sake, put in instead at Haskins Park, only half a mile downstream. The park has all the amenities: picnic tables, bathrooms, water, and plenty of parking. There's even an easy lead-in to the water from which to launch your boat.

A tiny rock island precedes the first bridge, after which the river bends to the left (north) then immediately bends back to the south in a rather unusual loop. Riffles ruffle the surface, and the Ice Age Trail can be seen on the left, parallel to the river. A lively rapid lies just downstream from the attractive footbridge in Attridge Park. As with all the rapids on this trip, in normal conditions this rates a Class I. While smack-dab in downtown Baraboo, the river retains a natural-setting feel. Even when it's just riffly, always keep a watchful eye out for submerged boulders: They're scattered everywhere in the streambed, and bumping into one, while somewhat inevitable, can be a jolting enough surprise to catch you off-guard and cause you to lose your balance. In the unlikely event that you do fall in, don't panic—just stand up. The river is usually quite shallow.

Between the Second Avenue and Broadway Street bridges are two baseball fields on your left. The best rapid lies in between the Broadway Street and Ash Street bridges. Stay to the left—you'll see a brick building on the left bank by a set of power lines. Two tiny islands braid the river into three channels; you want the left one, as the other two are impassable. This rapid is hardly dangerous, but don't take it for granted either. Don't be surprised either if a clap of water falls on your lap!

After Ash Street, you'll see first some attractive buildings and a church on the left, followed by the Circus Museum on both banks. Baraboo was home to the Ringling Brothers, and circus traditions are observed to this day. Expect to see and hear elephants, tents, trains, calliope music, clowns, and whirligigs. You can even improvise a detour, get out, and buy some ice cream. Riffles persist in this section, but the gradient begins to slacken some at this point. Don't let your guard down just yet, though. After a parking lot on the left, the river will curve to the right; a large island splits the stream into two channels. Both are runnable, but the right channel is more fun. In the right channel, a rapid with a small hole at its base offers an opportunity for play.

The remainder of the trip is slower but also less developed. The landscape is flatter than it is upstream, with the exception of occasional views of the Baraboo Hills in the background. Expect to spook a great blue heron here, maybe a bald eagle, too. The river meanders lazily east and south past the bridge at Manchester Street—if you've come just for the rapids, those are done, so you can take out here on the right, downstream of the bridge (**N43° 27.600' W89° 43.811'**).

Continuing on to the designated take-out, you'll see isolated sandbars and mudflats here and there in the next mile. A cream-colored brick building on the left announces the last bridge at WI 113. The take-out is just downstream of the bridge, on the right. Mind the mud! There are no facilities here, but parking is plentiful and river access is excellent.

•THE•FUDGE•

ADDITIONAL TRIPS You can add 3.4 miles to this trip by putting in upstream at the **Giese Park** wayside by Hatchery Road, which has room for a few vehicles plus a rather eccentric outhouse almost as old as the Baraboo Range itself. It's a pretty stretch featuring a few modest bluffs and outcrops, though houses are numerous approaching US 12 and roads are nearby as well. Additionally, you can take out downstream of WI 113 at **Luebke Landing** on County Road W, but this segment is muddier, flatter, and prone to downfall.

CAMPING **Devil's Lake State Park** (S5975 Park Road, about 3 miles south of Baraboo; 608-356-8301); **Durward's Glen,** for cabins and private rooms (W11876 McLeisch Road, about 10 miles southeast of Baraboo; 608-356-8113); and **Wheeler's Campground** (E11329 WI 159, about 3.5 miles south of Baraboo; 608-356-4877)

RENTALS **Wisconsin Canoe Company** (608-432-5058, thebestcanoecompanyever.com)

FOOD FOR THOUGHT For great food and probably the best malted milkshake you'll ever have, make your way to the **Little Village Cafe** (146 Fourth Ave., Baraboo; 608-356-2800).

SHOUT-OUTS While you're in Baraboo, spend some time downtown around the square, a thriving, locally owned scene. Where else will you find the **International Clown Hall of Fame** (102 Fourth St.; 608-355-0321)? For the more cerebrally minded, **The Village Booksmith** (526 Oak St.; 608-355-1001) is a bibliophile's dream come true.

It's worth noting that at one time there were as many as 11 dams along the 120 miles of the Baraboo River. Today there are none—making the Baraboo one of the longest free-running rivers in America.

48 Black Earth Creek: OLSON ROAD TO LIONS PARK

•THE•FACTS•

Put-in/take-out Olson Road/Lions Park

Distance/time 3.7 mi/Allow for 2 hrs

Gradient/water level 8 fpm/80 cfs at USGS gage 05406500 is perfect. At lower levels, you'll scrape, but too much higher and the creek becomes turbid.

Water type Constant riffles, several small rapids, one Class II rapid (in high water)

Canoe or kayak Kayak

Skill level Experienced

Time of year to paddle Lush in summer, better views of bluffs in early spring/late autumn

Landscape Rolling hills of a glacial valley, residential, hardwoods

---

OVERVIEW A spectacular short trip through a glacial valley with constant riffles, a modest rapids, a hilly landscape, and a short run through town, this stretch on the renowned Black Earth Creek will have you coming back for more. Wildlife includes beavers, muskrats, wood ducks, great blue herons, sandhill cranes, blue-winged teals, snapping turtles, trout, and red-tailed hawks.

CAR SHUTTLE **2.7 miles.** From the take-out, head out of Lions Park, then turn left (east) onto Hudson Street. Turn right onto Brodhead Street, then left onto US 14. Turn right onto CR KP, then left onto Olson Road.

BIKE SHUTTLE **3.1 miles.** In 2013–14, the village of Mazomanie opened the **Wolf Run Trail,** a 2-mile bike/pedestrian trail, thanks to the Wolfs, a prominent local family who donated the land for the project. This trail is part of a larger project called the **Good Neighbor Trail,** which will eventually connect Mazomanie to the Madison suburb of Middleton. Head east on Hudson Street as above, but then turn left onto Crescent Street to access the Wolf Run Trail. Cross the creek over the footbridge, then proceed underneath US 14 and outward to Wisconsin Heights High School. At the trailhead behind the school, cross the railroad tracks and proceed on Olson Road.

TAKE-OUT N43° 10.799' W89° 48.290'

PUT-IN N43° 09.367' W89° 46.579'

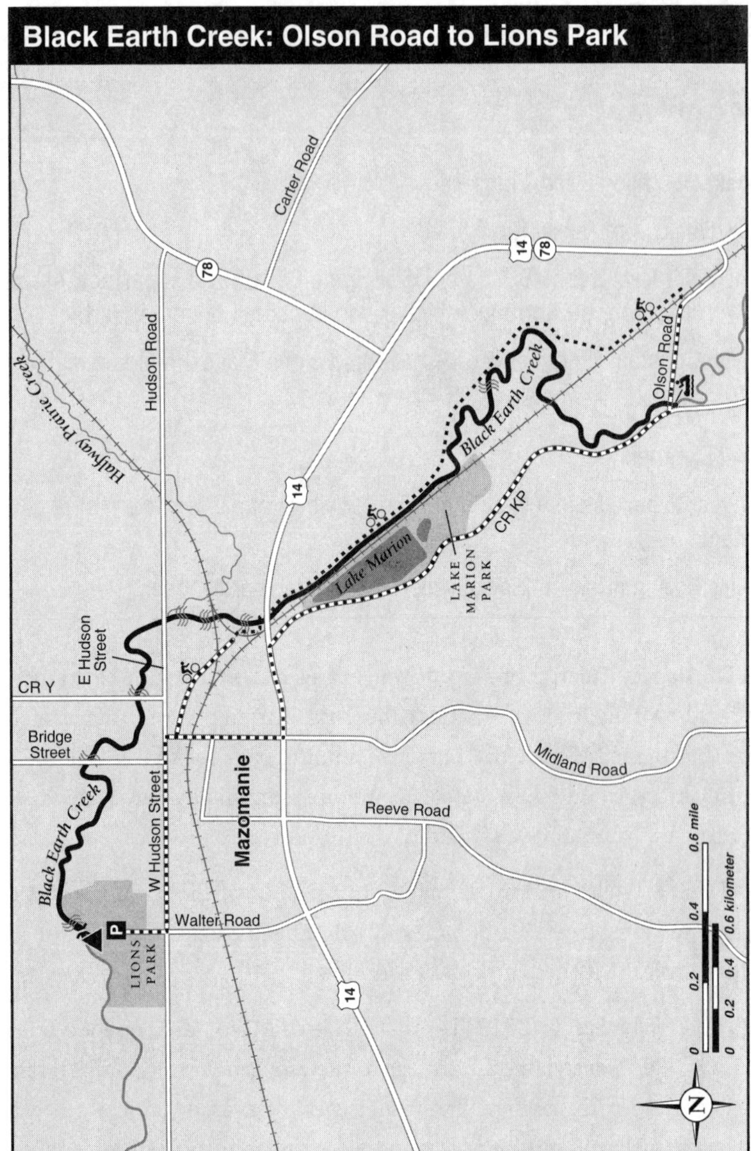

•THE•FLAVOR•

PUT IN AT OLSON ROAD ON THE UPSTREAM SIDE of the bridge, river right. For the first mile, the stream is gentle but not sluggish. The water should be clear, and the odds of spying trout are excellent, as Black Earth Creek is a renowned Class I trout stream with many vested interests, private and public, seeking to protect its watershed and make it more accessible to paddler and angler alike. The creek is only 30 feet wide for this entire trip. Views of the beautiful landscape abound with hills, for Mazomanie is situated at the frontier of the Driftless Area. Some 13,000 years ago, give or take, a glacier as nearby as Middleton receded, and the meltwater carved through the valley. (Today, the bedrock in the towns of Cross Plains and Black Earth lies some 200 feet deep, due to the glacial sand and gravel.)

A few meanders take you past a greenhouse on the left just before the first of several railroad bridges. After more meanders, the creek will bend to the left as you approach two sets of rapids, the first a Class II in high water, the second a Class I. The first has reputable gusto and is good fun; the second, also fun, is easy and nothing to worry about. The first rapid can be easily portaged on either bank, if need be, but running it is irresistible. Catch the eddy on the left and paddle back into the rapid for some fun surfing. Or take out at either bank and run the rapid again; the banks are low, so getting in and out is easy. Be careful, though—the water is powerful here, and the bottom is at least 7 feet deep in the middle of the creek.

Now you're into a long straightaway, but don't worry: The scenery to the right is gorgeous, and the stream is nonstop riffles. A berm on the left separates the creek from Lake Marion, an artificial pond that is a relic from the bygone railroad days that first put Mazomanie on the map. Locals have strategically placed small boulders to create mini-drops from here all the way to the US 14 bridge. The purpose of these drops is to help oxidize the water for trout habitat, but it serendipitously makes for nonstop paddling fun. On your right, you'll see a red barn and silo, part of the property owned by the Wolf family, who have generously donated much land along the creek for public use and advocacy.

The US 14 bridge comes into view, notably huge for such a small creek. Thrilling riffles are continuous. After the bridge, the views of hilly landscape give way to secluded, intimate hardwoods. A footbridge spans the creek past a red pavilion on the left, followed by two railroad bridges, the first easy, the second a little tricky. Approach the first bridge carefully, as debris tends to collect here between the pylons. Portage along the left bank if necessary. Below the bridge, the creek swiftly passes high banks on both sides that abut the backyards of several houses in Mazomanie. That said, there's still a hardwoods feel to the scenery, plus the current is so much fun you won't really care. You'll pass by large concrete slabs, as well as the former foundations of an extinct mill. There's even a motorized zip line in the backyard of one house.

Evocatively named Halfway Prairie Creek comes in on the right; this is the same little stream that drains pretty Indian Lake at the county park off WI 19 to the northeast.

Another fun Class I rapid lies at the State Street bridge; choose the left channel. More riffles follow past some low-hanging but not dangerous trees, leading to yet another small rapid. The creek will bend to the left and then make a quick turn to the right, after which you'll see the pedestrian bridge at Lions Park. Below the bridge is one more fun Class I rapid. The take-out is a bit inconspicuous, but it's on the downstream side of the bridge, on river right. Run the rapid first, then turn back around to the bridge. Walk across the footbridge to the parking area, 400 feet to the south.

•THE•FUDGE•

ADDITIONAL TRIPS Below Lions Park, the creek changes character. Volunteers do a great job clearing out potentially dangerous strainers, sweepers, and logjams, but the creek is narrow and meandering, thus making it prone to obstructions. From Lions Park to Blynn Street lie 5 riffly miles, but these impediments can be tricky and turn a great day into regret. At the time of this writing, the Lions Park–Blynn Street section had been cleaned up and cleared out, but because the creek becomes agrarian and eventually runs parallel to US 14, that section has not been included in this official trip. That said, it's still a fun and pretty addendum with oak savannas, riffles, and more hilly vistas. There's one intimidating-looking cattle gate below a bridge, but don't worry: It pushes forward (downstream), so it won't obstruct your progress.

Upstream, some paddlers put in behind **The Shoe Box** shoe store (1314 Canal St., Black Earth), 2.7 miles above Olson Road. There is some deadfall to avoid, the surroundings are predominantly agricultural, and the sound of US 14 is never far away, but it's otherwise pleasant.

The section from Cross Plains to Black Earth is definitely not recommended due to narrowness, shallow conditions, and the number of frustrating downed trees, dangerous cattle gates, and low-clearance bridges. Above Cross Plains, the creek is fit only for fly-fishing.

CAMPING **Blue Mound State Park** (4350 Mounds Park Road, Blue Mounds; 608-437-5711)

RENTALS **Rutabaga Paddlesports** (220 W. Broadway, Madison; 608-223-9300) and **Wisconsin River Outings** (7554 US 12, Sauk City; 608-375-5300)

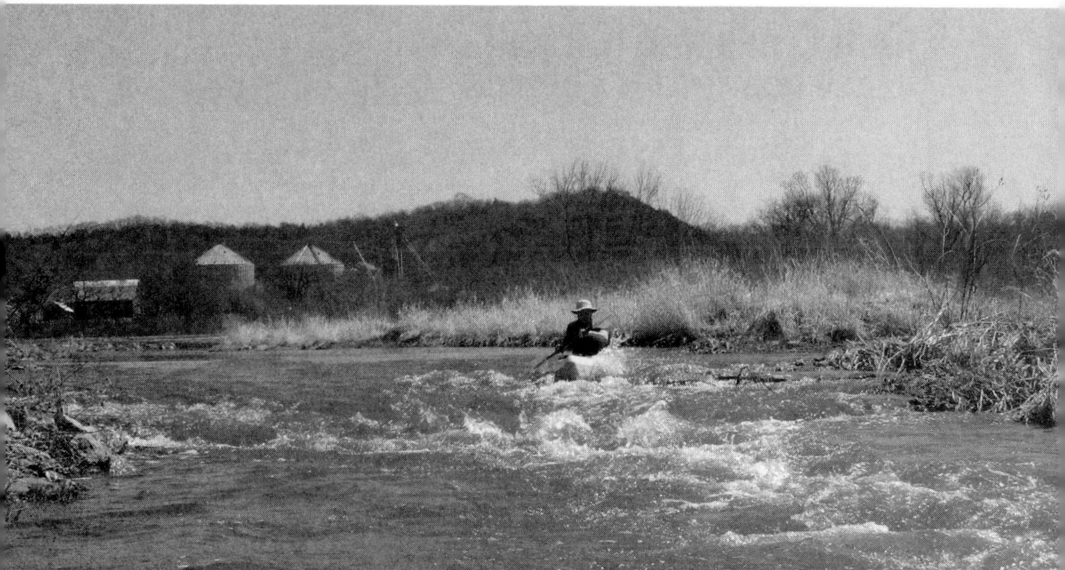

A splashy Class I-II drop on thrilling Black Earth Creek

FOOD FOR THOUGHT For upscale, locally sourced cuisine in a gorgeous restored building, stop in at **The Old Feed Mill** (114 Cramer St., Mazomanie; 608-795-4909).

SHOUT-OUTS **Mazomanie** is a real gem of a town, with as many as 34 buildings downtown listed on the National Register of Historic Places. Considerable praise must be given to the Wolf family for their dedication to making the creek and its surroundings more available to the public (see wolfruntrail.net for more info).

Thanks also to **Capitol Water Trails** (capitolwatertrails.org) and the **Black Earth Creek Watershed Association** (becwa.org) for their tireless work to clean up our streams while working with landowners to promote safer access to the water and educate the community about preserving our natural treasures. As recently as the early 2000s, Black Earth Creek was an unsightly mess of agricultural runoff and logjams. Today, it is an outstanding creek for paddling, thanks to the sweat equity and outreach of private visionaries and public groups.

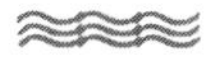

49 Dell Creek and Mirror Lake:
DELLWOOD AND LAKE DELTON IN SAUK COUNTY

•THE•FACTS•

Put-in/take-out WI 23/Timme's Mill County Park. See "The Flavor" for an alternative put-in.

Distance/time 3.2 mi/Allow for 2 hrs

Gradient/water level There is no gage, but there's always enough water in the lake itself. The marsh area just downstream from WI 23 does run low in dry spells.

Water type Flatwater with lake paddling

Canoe or kayak Either

Skill level Beginner

Time of year to paddle Spring, early summer, autumn (for beautiful foliage)

Landscape Grassland savanna, marsh, sandstone outcrop canyon, state-park lake with minimal development

---

OVERVIEW This pretty trip on both a small creek and a skinny lake allows for a variety of put-in/take-out options amidst an array of landscape settings, from grassland savanna to marsh to canyon to lake, nearly all of it on public land. Residing wildlife are bald eagles, swans, sandhill cranes, turkey vultures, great blue herons, egrets, owls, deer, ducks and geese, coots, turtles, pileated woodpeckers, and blue jays.

CAR SHUTTLE **6 miles.** From the take-out parking area adjacent to the Dell Creek/ Mirror Lake dam, drive north on Burritt Avenue and turn left (west) onto Xanadu Road; then turn left (south) onto WI 23. The put-in will be on the left before you cross the bridge, on the downstream side of Dell Creek.

BIKE SHUTTLE **4.7 miles.** From the take-out parking area, head south on Burritt Avenue, which becomes Ishnala Road; then turn right (west) on Fern Dell Road. Merge onto Mirror Lake Road as it doglegs south; shortly after you cross Harrison Creek, veer right onto Turtle Road and then make another right onto WI 23. The put-in will be on the right, on the north side of the bridge.

Note: To park at the main put-in above or the alternative put-in mentioned in "The Flavor," you must buy a Wisconsin State Parks vehicle-admission sticker ($8 per day or $28 per year).

TAKE-OUT N43° 35.058' W89° 47.839' **PUT-IN** N43° 33.554' W89° 50.523'

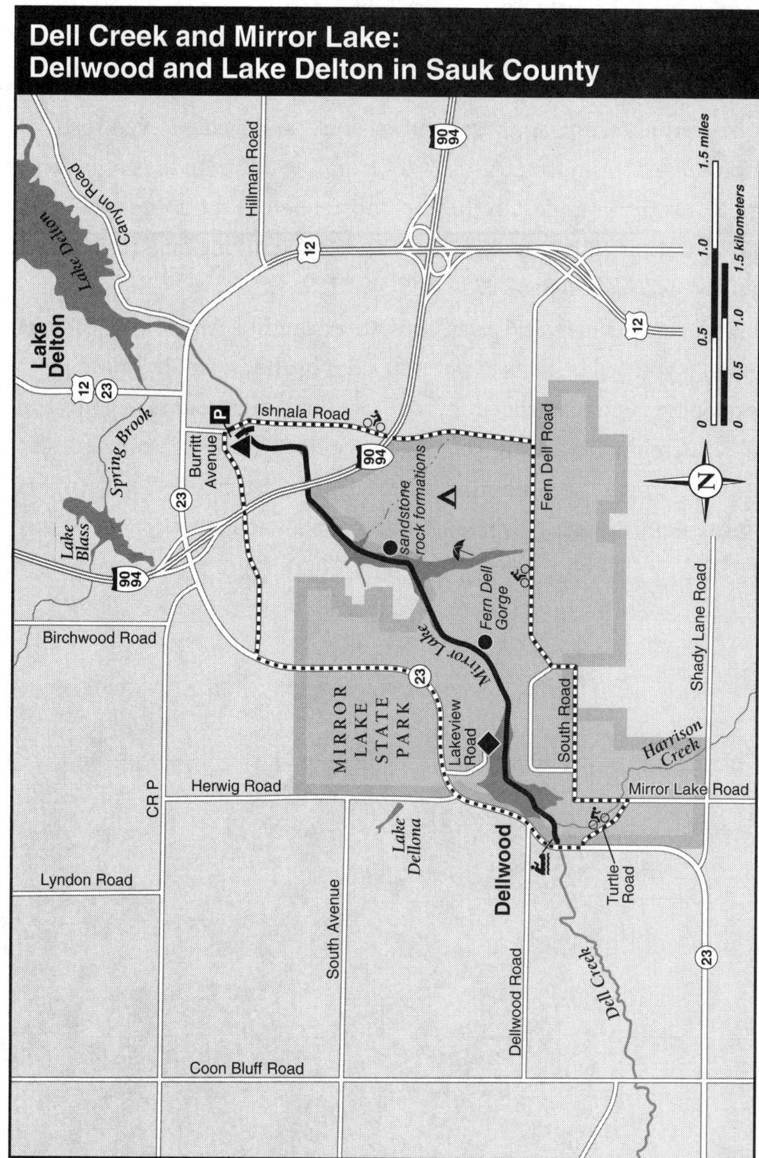

•THE•FLAVOR•

PUT IN AT WI 23 ON THE DOWNSTREAM SIDE of the bridge, on river left. There's no designated parking area here, but it's all public land, and there's plenty of room to park a vehicle or two off the road. Access to the creek is easy and clean. You can paddle upstream for a mile or so to get the full benefit of Dell Creek itself before the lake effect. It's quite pretty and almost entirely undeveloped.

Turning back downstream, almost immediately after WI 23, the creek begins to widen into a marsh. Mirror Lake is an impoundment comprising 137 acres and is roughly 4 miles long. Wild rice, originally hand-planted, provides habitat for sandhill cranes, blue herons, geese, and wood ducks. The marsh widens even further but constricts soon thereafter. In fact, the distance from the put-in to the gorge section in the state park is less than 1 mile. On the left, shortly before the gorge begins, is an alternative put-in option with easy access and an actual parking area for several vehicles, just off Lakeview Road (**N43° 33.880' W89° 49.825'**).

Now the marsh tapers and gives way to the beautiful canyon area leading into Mirror Lake. Here, you will be flanked on both sides of the stream by stunning sandstone outcrops popping out of the woodsy hills 50 feet high. Take your time going through the gorge; it's positively splendid. On your right atop a hill nestled in the lush woods is the Seth Peterson Cottage, the last building in Wisconsin that Frank Lloyd Wright designed and the first (of only a few anywhere) that the public can rent overnight.

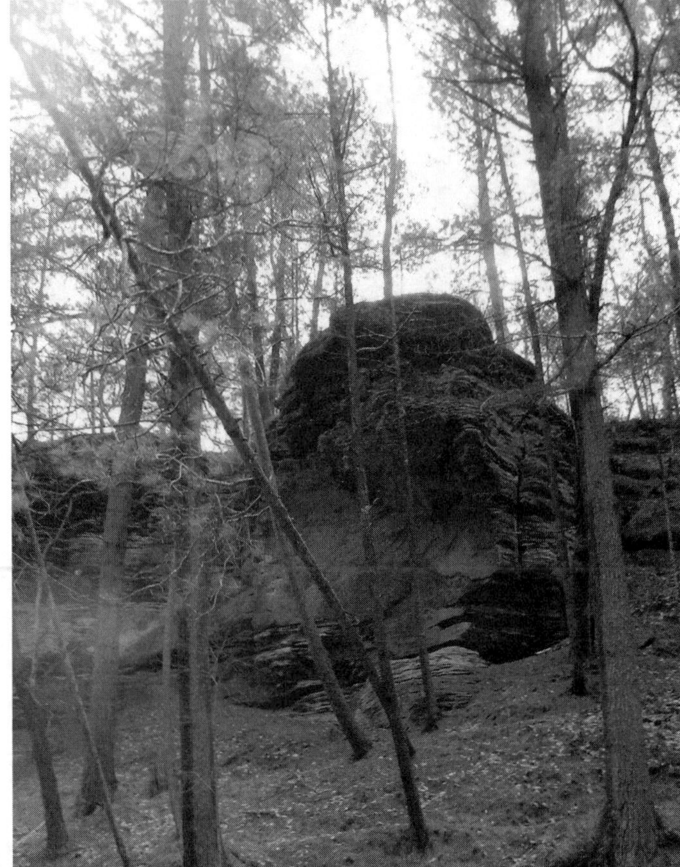

The gorge in Mirror Lake features spectacular rock outcrops.

Beyond this, also on the right, is the Fern Dell Gorge State Natural Area, where you can hike through the ravine. The lake section of the state park begins in earnest shortly after this. Mirror Lake is skinny and irregularly shaped, so the full-blown effects of wind are mitigated. On your left, you'll see buildings. The western shore of Mirror Lake once was a popular resort area for the wealthy and influential Ringling Brothers and friends. From the late 1800s to the early 1930s, there were pavilions and hotels, bathhouses and boat rentals, but most fell into disrepair after the Great Depression. In 1966, the state bought most of the land on the west end of the lake and created the park. Today, 70% of the shoreline is public land.

Where the gorge and lake proper meet forms a kind of T-bone; you can turn left (north), right (south), or paddle straight ahead to the other shoreline (east). If you turn right, you will head to the beach, concession stand, and restrooms. Some gentle hills line the right bank, but this southern "horn" section is modest and unadorned—and bustling in summer. There are two inlets on the left, but they don't lead to anywhere terribly interesting. Instead, paddle straight ahead to the eastern shoreline of the skinny lake, where the prettiest bluffs and rock outcrops are found on the right-hand side, similar to those found on the Wisconsin River in the nearby Dells. (Incidentally, the word *dell* comes from the French *dalles*, meaning "narrows," but it always refers to rock formations rising above streams; hence the names Dell Creek, Lake Delton, Wisconsin Dells, and so on.) These Cambrian sandstone cliffs are magnificent in their ridged and rippling beauty. They line the lake here, so you can paddle right up to them and feel the gritty sandstone rubbed between your fingers.

Moving on northward now, you'll see on your right the famed Ishnala Supper Club. The cabin originated as a trading post in 1826 but was turned into a swanky restaurant in 1953. Pine trees still grow through the floor and ceiling. (*Ishnala* is said to come from the Ho-Chunk [Winnebago] for "by itself alone"; before being purchased by settlers and turned into a trading post, the grounds had long been a ceremonial place.) It's pricey to have a cocktail here, much less dine, but it's worth checking out. Immediately before Ishnala is another ravine on the right that you can paddle into. There's a natural spring here, and past it is a hiking trail that takes you through a small but beautiful rock canyon. (Past Ishnala, there used to be a cabin indecorously called "Hags Crag," after two old schoolteachers who lived there on a rock overlooking the lake.)

The lake begins to narrow again as it approaches the monolithic twin bridges of I-90. Resembling a futuristic vision from Epcot, the bridges tower above you 100 feet high and are buttressed into striking sandstone cliffs. Shortly after the bridges is an atypical sharp bend to the left. On the right-hand side is a mini-ravine. Even as late as April (depending on the winter), there sometimes is a north-facing frozen ooze of ice and snow seeping out of the rock, the smallest glacier you ever saw. A spring pours out of the holler in the steep hillside and through a cleft between the sandstone. It's worth getting out of your boat to explore.

A little more than half a mile later, you'll hear the dam (really more of a spillway) at Ishnala Road and see a dizzying horizon line along with a sign telling you where to take out. There's a convenient concrete pad for easy access on the left. This spot is popular with the fishing public, and there's a parking area that accommodates several vehicles. This is the primary take-out option, unless you wish to paddle farther downstream.

Either way, check out the Grotto, a mini-cave with a blizzard of lurid graffiti. Back in the day, it was a make-do saloon aptly called "The Hole in the Wall," one of the first three taverns in the Dells area. There was no running water or plumbing as late as 1967. Today it still smells of urine and is probably resurrected on the sly as a BYOB hangout for bored teens. It makes for fascinating history, though.

The dam has a history, too: It was first operated as a gristmill for self-rising pancake flour in the 1860s. Farmers would bring their grain to be stone-ground at the mill and then seek shelter from the heat within the cool recesses of the cave, where they'd have a cold one (or several).

•THE•FUDGE•

ADDITIONAL TRIPS A 3.2-mile paddle may not be worth an hour's drive for some (for others, it's perfect), but rest assured that one can tack on additional miles to make a full day of paddling. One can portage around the Dell Creek/Mirror Lake dam and continue downstream, where Dell Creek feels more like a creek again. A metal staircase descends to a safe spot away from the dam, at the bottom of which you can reenter the water. Just below the dam on the left is a gorgeous sandstone bluff; unfortunately, there's also a house right there. From here to the beginning of Lake Delton is less than a mile of mostly modest houses and cabins. As such, roads encroach, and deadfall begins to be a nuisance. By the dam, you've seen the very best that Dell Creek and Mirror Lake have to offer.

If you do continue on, the best take-out is immediately after the Adams Street bridge (just after the US 12 bridge), where there is a public boat launch on your right before Lake Delton begins to sprawl. Paddle a quarter mile past the boat launch, then turn left (west) around a peninsula and into the mouth of **Spring Brook.** Here, you can paddle upstream as far as conditions allow, and you will be rewarded with more stunning sandstone outcrops and less development.

At 1.5 miles, there is another dam around which you will need to portage; above it is Blass Lake, across or around which you can paddle to the other side, where Spring Brook continues. The total additional mileage here is up to you and how far upstream you can or want to paddle. Just remember that it's a there-and-back trip—*no public take-out options are available.* Water levels are shallow, and deadfall is problematic. Nevertheless, it's a beautiful oasis escape of red sandstone, lush green ferns, and copper-clear water in a mini-gorge environment surrounded by the tornadic tourism of the Dells.

Alternatively, you can add 2 miles by putting in upstream on Dell Creek at Coon Bluff Road, upstream side on river left. Park along the road. Here, the creek is a narrow stream that's totally different than it is downstream. The current is surprisingly good and the water clarity excellent. The creek meanders quite a bit through a savanna with zero development. This section comprises the lower **Dell Creek Wildlife Area,** a lowland public-access area with a North Woods feel. It's a very pretty area, and together with the variety of environs below the highway, you get a best-of-all-worlds smorgasbord of creek and lake. The bad news? The creek is extremely narrow, and you have numerous low-hanging branches and "tree debris" to contend with for 1.5 miles of this 2-mile segment. *Do not attempt this in a canoe!*

CAMPING AND RENTALS **Mirror Lake State Park** (E10320 Fern Dell Road, about 10 miles northwest of Baraboo; 608-254-2333). For rentals only, try **River's Edge Resort** (20 River's Edge Road, off CR A, Wisconsin Dells; 608-254-6494).

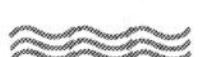

50 Devil's Lake State Park: BARABOO IN SAUK COUNTY

•THE•FACTS•

Put-in/take-out Lake Road, just west of the park's south-shore entrance and beach

Distance/time 3 mi round-trip/Allow for 2 hrs

Gradient/water level N/A

Water type Flatwater

Canoe or kayak Either

Skill level Beginner

Time of year to paddle Anytime, but the park is very congested on summer weekends

Landscape Glacier-formed gorge composed of quartzite bluffs

OVERVIEW A beautiful clear-water lake towered by a 500-foot-tall quartzite gorge in the heart of the Baraboo Range, the scenery alone on this trip beckons, as does its history, for here you will find the aftermath of ancient oceans, volcanoes, and glaciers. Combine this paddle with a dozen different hiking options—and the chance to spot turkey vultures, great blue herons, deer, and songbirds—for a magnificent day outdoors.

Note: You must buy a Wisconsin State Parks vehicle-admission sticker to enter the park ($8 per day or $28 per year).

SHUTTLE N/A **PUT-IN/TAKE-OUT** N43° 24.758' W89° 44.257'

•THE•FLAVOR•

DEVIL'S LAKE LIES IN THE HEART OF THE STATE PARK named after it. Drive to the park's south entrance, on Lake Road; register at the ranger station if your vehicle doesn't have a state-park sticker, and pick up a map. Make a U-turn and head back on Lake Road, going west. The boat launch, 1 mile west of the ranger station, has ample parking and a restroom.

Very little in the Midwest captures the imagination as does the geology in Devil's Lake State Park. The bluffs surrounding the lake are part of the Baraboo Range, an ancient mountain chain more than a billion years old, making them some of the oldest rocks on the planet.

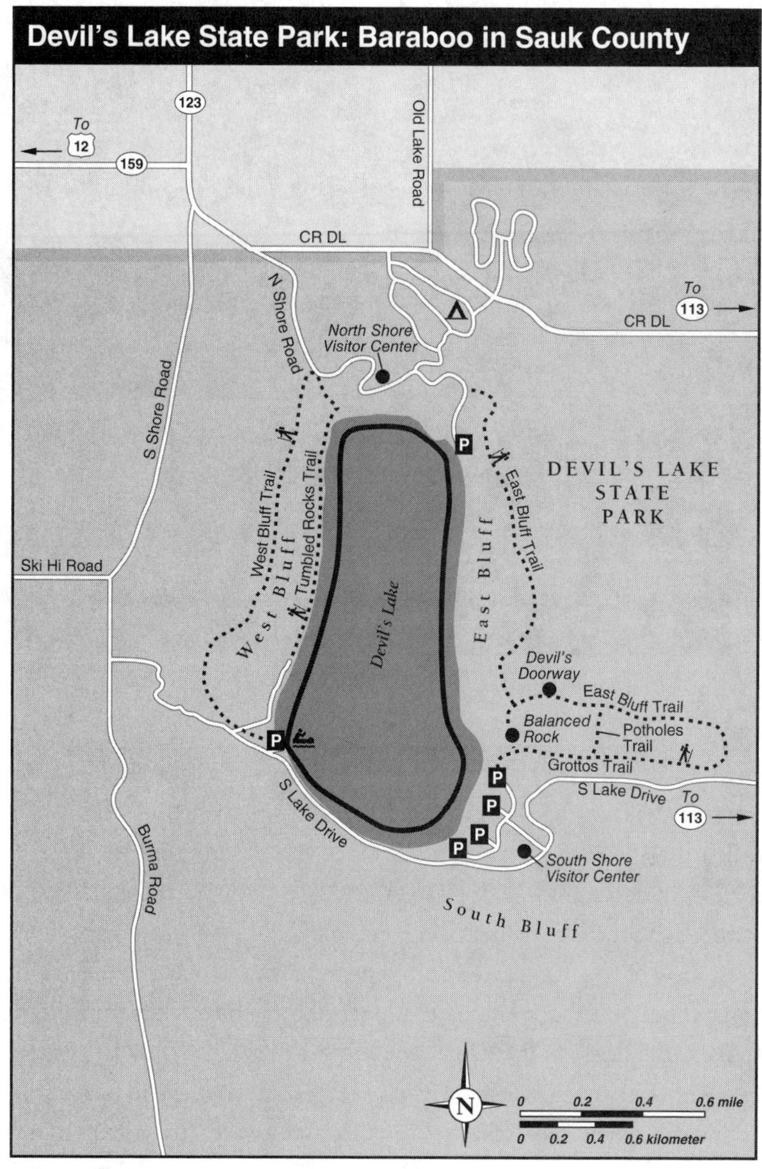

In addition to offering stunning scenery, Devil's Lake is an excellent place to practice rolling and wet entries—there is no current, the water is clean, and the shoreline is shallow. It won't take you long to paddle around the lake, so I recommend dividing your time in the park between your boat and a pair of hiking boots. The hiking trails are excellent, allowing you to experience the gorgeous geology from different perspectives; many of these are part of the Ice Age Trail, a thousand-mile-long

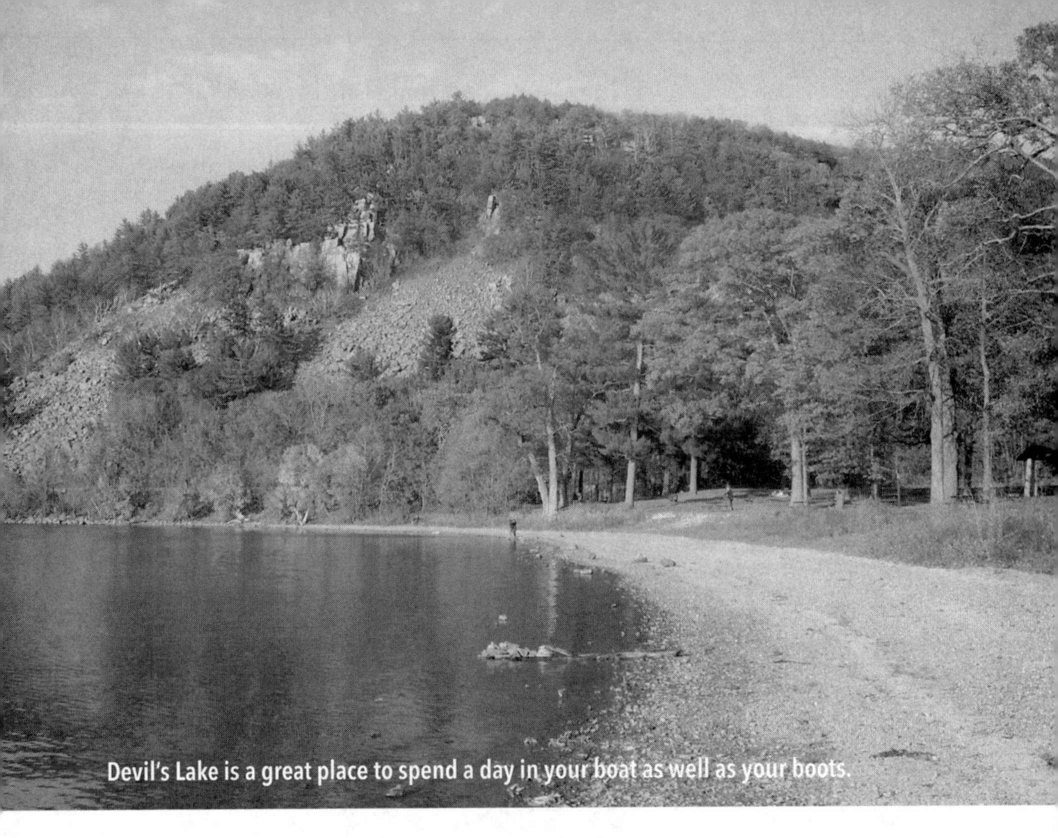
Devil's Lake is a great place to spend a day in your boat as well as your boots.

trail from St. Croix Falls to the Door County Peninsula, via Janesville, that traces the demarcation of the last glacial advance.

While on the water, you can paddle clockwise or counterclockwise, of course. The lake varies in depth from 40 to 50 feet, with a circumference of just over 3 miles. Scattered throughout the park, including on the beaches, are erratics and kettle ponds that house a slew of frogs and rare salamanders. From the put-in, the East Bluff towers 500 feet above you and contains the most photogenic rock features in the park, including Balanced Rock, Devil's Doorway, and the potholes.

If you know where to look and you patiently train your eye to take in the minutest detail, you can actually see Balanced Rock from the water (though it's more impressive close up on a hike). Crudely resembling an inverted trapezoid, Balanced Rock is a huge but slender boulder perched on a flat ledge, improbably upright, defiant of gravity or wind. Devil's Doorway is composed of two similar but thicker monoliths, with boulders at their tops, leaning against one another and creating a kind of portal. The potholes are rounded depressions in smaller boulders created by swirling ice melt in cavities that formed when the glaciers began receding. Also high up on the East Bluff is a pygmy forest of stunted hickory and ash trees.

The South Bluff, also called Devil's Nose, is a huge swath of public land between US 12 and WI 113, the majority of it mesic forest. Two highlights of South Bluff are a beautiful small gorge called Pine Glen, and Messenger Creek, a spring-fed stream in a valley hundreds of millions of years old. You can't paddle the creek, but its mouth is immediately north of the put-in, and from it, you can hike into the gorge, following the path of the streambed. Two other excellent hikes to consider while in the park are the East Bluff Trail and Parfrey's Glen.

Fun lore to ponder: The Ho-Chunk named Devil's Lake *Tawacunchukdah,* or "sacred lake"; the story is that the bluffs are the result of a battle between thunderbirds and water spirits. Today, one can still see a 150-foot bird mound on the southeastern shore, representing the upper world, as well as bear and panther mounds on the northern shore, representing the lower world.

•THE•FUDGE•

CAMPING There are three park campgrounds on the north shore of the lake (608-356-8301).

RENTALS Canoes and kayaks may be rented at either of the park's beaches (608-356-8301).

SHOUT-OUTS If you're coming from the south, I recommend with my whole heart this fun-filled itinerary: Cross the Wisconsin River on the free ferry north of Lodi. Stop at **Parfrey's Glen** for a short hike into the gorge, then go to the park and paddle Devil's Lake for an hour or two. Head up the bluffs for a spirited hike, but save room for daylight. Stop by **The Barn Restaurant and Bar** (S5566 WI 123, just south of Baraboo; 608-356-2161) for great bar food and an incredible variety of craft beers.

Take US 12 south to **Dr. Evermor's Foreverton** art park (S7703 US 12, Sumpter; 608-219-7830) and immerse yourself in the spectacular steampunk wonder of scrap-metal masterpieces. A cross between the works of Dr. Seuss and Tim Burton, these fantastical sculptures are out of this world. Be sure to call before you go to make sure someone's there.

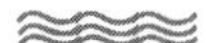

51 Lemonweir River:
MAUSTON DAM TO TWO RIVERS BOAT LANDING

•THE•FACTS•

Put-in/take-out Dam in Mauston off Roosevelt Street/Two Rivers Public Boat Landing at the Wisconsin River. See "The Flavor" for an additional access point.

Distance/time 20 mi/Allow for an overnight stay

Gradient/water level 1.2 fpm/Below 200 cfs will be slow and bottoming out; consult USGS gage 05403500.

Water type Quietwater

Canoe or kayak Either

Skill level Experienced

Time of year to paddle Spring and autumn

Landscape Sandbars, hardwood forests, floodplain bottoms, high bluffs

---

OVERVIEW This tranquil river trip with sandbar-camping options culminates in a maze of wild bottomlands. As pretty as it is peaceful, the Lemonweir is home to bald eagles, great blue herons, hawks, muskrats, raccoons, clams, songbirds, plovers, dragonflies, deer, warblers, scarlet tanagers, and ospreys.

SHUTTLE **13 miles.** From the take-out, head up the hill and turn right on Cliff House Road. At the stop sign, turn left onto 28th Avenue and turn immediately right onto 56th Street. At the stop sign, turn right on County Road HH. From here, you have a choice:

For the more direct route, stay on CR HH, cross the river, and then turn left on WI 82. Stay on WI 82 to Mauston; turn left on Roosevelt to below the dam.

For the more rural route (and better for bike shuttling), turn left on 54th Street from CR HH before crossing the river, then turn right on Townline Road. Turn left on 53rd Street, which will become CR N. Turn right onto 19th Avenue and cross the river; then turn left on WI 82 and take it to Mauston.

At the take-out, allow for a moment to familiarize yourself with the surroundings. The take-out is at a nook on the south shore of the Lemonweir River's confluence with the Wisconsin River, and it is easy to miss if you don't know where to look.

TAKE-OUT N43° 45.689' W89° 51.155' **PUT-IN** N43° 47.822' W90° 4.151'

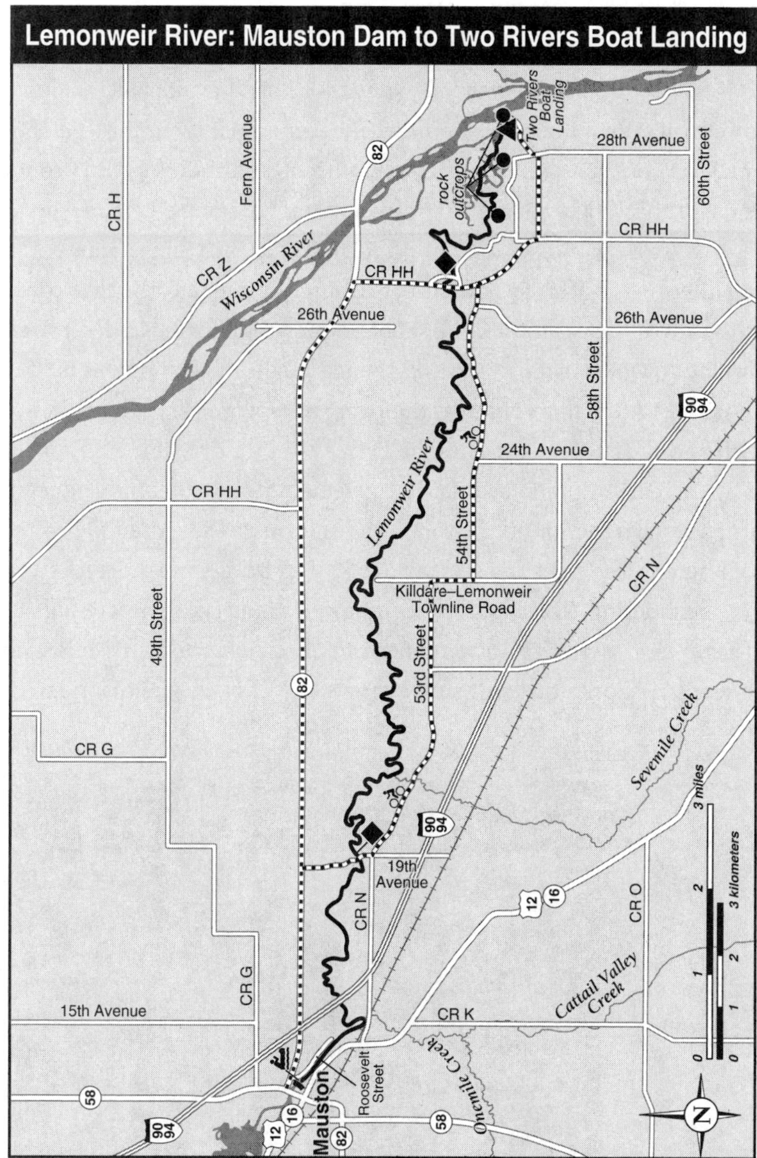

•THE•FLAVOR•

PUT IN BELOW THE DAM ON RIVER LEFT (north bank). There are no facilities, but the parking is quite adequate. There are some riffles immediately downstream, the only ones of the long trip, so enjoy them! After a long straightaway the river will make a notable S-shaped loop as it heads east and passes beneath the interstate. After this, the

Lemonweir begins its classic meandering, and you will start to see the many oxbows and sloughs for which the river is famous—or infamous, depending on your take. You will begin to see its other chief characteristic as well: sand (sandbanks, sandbars, sand on the bottom); it's ubiquitous and exquisite. The Lemonweir is reminiscent of the lower Wisconsin River, but it is much narrower and more meandering. This combination enhances its intimacy, but this intimacy can bewilder you, as the Lemonweir does have a wild feel to it. Just follow the current and you'll stay in the main channel.

After a short straightaway downstream from the interstate, the river comes to a T; you want to turn left (east) toward the set of power lines. (There is a deceptive temptation to turn right, which takes you to a dead-end slough. The Lemonweir is full of these 50–50 decisions.) After this dilemma, the river will flow in easy straightaways before bending left and right as it approaches the 19th Avenue bridge, at the 4.5 mile mark for this trip. This access is a pretty spot and a convenient place to get out and stretch your legs. There's a small reservoir off the southern bank where there used to be a mill.

From here to the next access near the CR HH bridge is a 12-mile stretch with significant meandering. This is classic Lemonweir country. There are logs to dodge now and again, but there should be no need to portage since the river is wide. Since there are few landmarks but so many oxbows, it's easy to feel disoriented on the

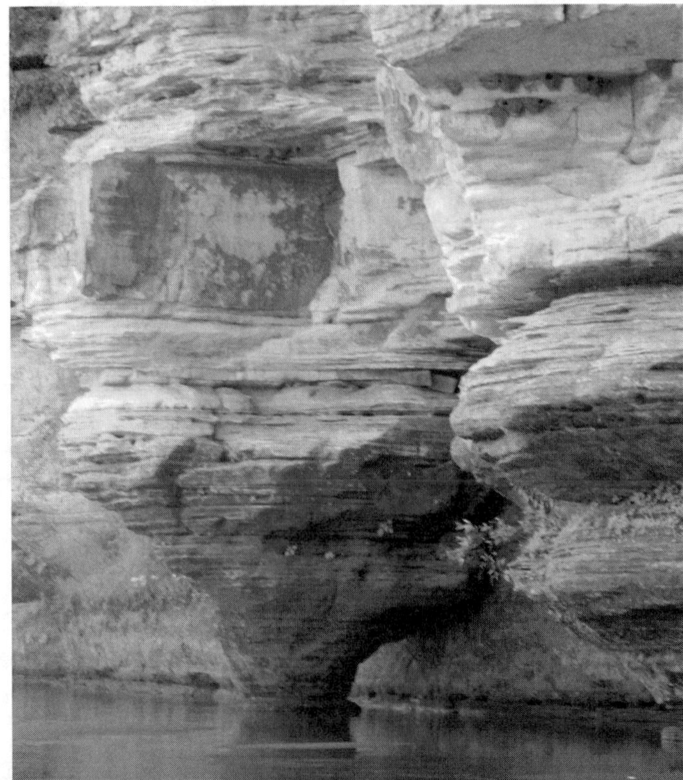

Incredible sandstone cliffs lie at the mouth of the Lemonweir at the Wisconsin River.

water, which in turn makes it difficult to gage how far you should practically paddle for an overnight trip. Call it the "Lemonweird." Just keep in mind that on this river, 2 miles per hour is a fair rate of travel. (Or if you have GPS, you can take all the fun out of not knowing where you are!)

Occasionally you will see houses (mostly cabins), but only briefly. For the most part, there simply is no development on either bank. Rather, the paddling experience is one of being adrift in a world of sandbars, oxbows, and sloughs. (This mosaic of backwaters also is why you absolutely do not want to paddle this trip after a recent rain: Mosquitoes will maraud you mercilessly. In fact, depending on when you paddle this mini expedition, you might encounter lots of dragonflies. Harmless to humans, they snack on mosquitoes—all hail the dragonfly!)

CR HH will appear and is immediately followed by a snowmobile bridge downstream, where there's access on the left (**N43° 46.263' W89° 53.174'**). There are no facilities, but it is a great put-in/take-out spot just the same. Depending on your schedule for the following day of this overnight trip, you may want to find a sandbar to camp on near CR HH and save the last segment of the river to the take-out (3.3 miles) for the morning. You'll want to allow 2 hours to explore these floodplain bottomlands, since they're pretty but can also be confusing. Along with the oxbows and sandbars, the two salient features in these final miles are wooded islands and outcrops.

The mouth of the Lemonweir resembles a labyrinth of islands, sloughs, swales, and oxbow lakes; together, these comprise the Lemonweir Bottomland Hardwood Forest State Natural Area, an old-growth floodplain forest that is especially fun to explore in spring.

To find the bluffs and rock outcrops, as well as the most reliable way not to get lost, follow the right shoreline as best as possible. The beautiful sandstone outcrops are on the south shore of the river, plus there's one more just downstream from the take-out (technically on the Wisconsin River). The first outcrop is almost 2 miles downstream from CR HH, preceded by a grassy floodplain. Tucked back a bit, it's nonetheless 50 feet high and is almost double that with the pine trees crowning its top.

The main channel will swing to the left and then the right. Through the braided islands, you'll begin to see glimpses of the Wisconsin River and hills in the background. The next bluff is recessed back in a bay near the take-out. Where you actually end up at the delta depends on water levels and your own reckoning. The easiest way to find the take-out is to look for a large and absolutely lovely bluff on the Wisconsin River's west shore. The base of the bluff is dyed algae green, evidence of how high this huge river can rise, the rest a rippling white and beige.

Here you have two choices: spot the bluff and make a U-turn to the right and paddle upstream to the take-out *or* paddle up to the bluff itself. I highly recommend seeing the bluff, because its formation really is one of the prettiest anywhere in the Dells. It lines the river for a thousand feet, its palette of colors magnificent: green, cream, and sunburned red. Sculpted by wind and waves for thousands of years, the sandstone textures bulge and undulate or are whittled down to tapered spires and fissured lines. There's even a petrograph near the base of the bluff just a bit downstream that depicts a deer being hunted by humans. This bluff begins the famous Dells, so whether the rock art is authentic or forged as a hoax is debatable; either way, it's still pretty cool.

Be careful as you turn around and paddle upstream to the take-out, since the current along the bluff is rather strong. You'll make a counterclockwise hook to the left. Once you're out of the main channel of the Wisconsin River, there's no current, so it's an easy glide to the take-out only 500 feet away. Located at the bottom of a hill, the take-out is excellent and has plenty of parking and even bathrooms.

•THE•FUDGE•

ADDITIONAL TRIPS I personally don't recommend the Lemonweir upstream of Mauston, although there's a lot of river there. It's not as pretty, plus there are dams and a hell-awful lot of deadfall obstructions. There's also the 7-mile jaunt down the **Wisconsin River** between the Two Rivers Public Boat Landing and the first public take-out on the right at River Bay Campground and Marina, just past huge Louis Bluff. This is a fun trip in its own right with many sandstone cliffs and pretty sandbar islands, but you do have to paddle through a bit of lake-like water.

CAMPING Primitive camping is permitted for free on sandbars.

RENTALS **Country Cruisin' Kayaks & Canoes** in Mauston (608-548-4280, facebook.com/countrycruisinkayakscanoes)

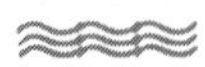

52 Neenah Creek A:
CHAUNCEY STREET TO COUNTY ROAD A

•THE•FACTS•

Put-in/take-out Chauncey Street (County Road I)/CR A

Distance/time 6 mi/Allow for 3 hrs

Gradient/water level 2 fpm/Levels should always be adequate.

Water type Quietwater with three rapids below bridges

Canoe or kayak Kayak

Skill level Experienced

Time of year to paddle Anytime, though it's especially pretty in autumn

Landscape Gentle hills with tall banks, pine and oak trees, open meadows, and marsh with oxbows

---

OVERVIEW This trip in a remote landscape with three thrilling rapids along clear water and sandy bottoms packs a lot of punch in a little distance. You'll see sandhill cranes, swans, geese, ducks, beaver, snakes, fish, killdeer, and muskrats.

SHUTTLE 4 miles. From the take-out, head north on CR A. Bear left and stay on CR A at the intersection with CR D. Turn left on Chauncey Street (a.k.a. CR I). The put-in is at the bridge.

TAKE-OUT N43° 43.954' W89° 33.679' **PUT-IN** N43° 46.774' W89° 34.583'

•THE•FLAVOR•

PUT IN AT CHAUNCEY STREET (a.k.a. CR I) upstream, on river right, if you want to run the Class II rapid below the bridge. If the water is shallow, the rapid might be too rocky to run. It's an adrenaline blast though. If you prefer to skip the rapid, head downstream to the makeshift steps leading to the water. Either way, the first thing you will notice is how spectacularly clear the water is. In fact, it's so translucent that your eyes need to adjust, because at first it seems like the sandy bottom is only an inch below you and that you're about to scrape the bottom and get stuck. Together with tall banks, tree canopy, and a narrow width of only 20–25 feet, the creek has all the feel of a beautiful, intimate stream—which it is.

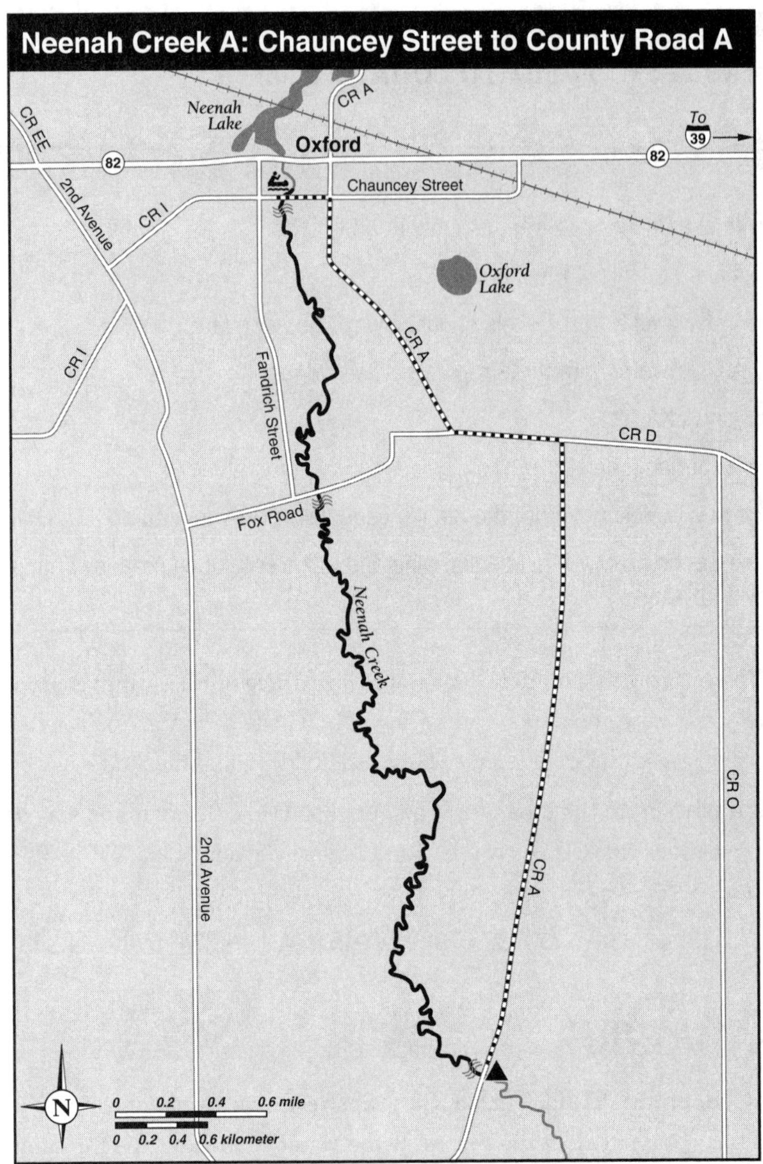

There are no large hills here, but the landscape does gently rise in places, usually with meadows, some accentuated with pine trees, others with handsome oaks. The first 2 miles of this trip are exceptionally pretty in autumn as colors begin to blush or burst. Also, along the shore you'll often see small- to medium-sized rocks; when surrounded by a carpet of fallen leaves on a crisp autumn day, the feeling is pristine. Soon the creek runs through a random culvert you'll need to duck under (or portage around if the clearance is too low), where there's a fun riffle on the downstream side. After this, you'll see and hear a miniature waterfall/gurgling spring on the left. Surrounded by moss-strewn rocks, the spring percolates from below, enhancing the wonder and wildness of this trip.

Shortly after the spring, you will encounter obstacles in the creek. All in all, you will probably need to portage three to four times during this trip, but these are easy, since the creek is sandy and shallow, and the banks around the deadfall are low. Some deadfall can be negotiated by ducking under or riding over downed trees, or by carefully pulling yourself through low-hanging limbs, without having to get out of your boat. You will see evidence of recent and ancient sawed-off branches and trunks. If you have the time and inclination, help a fellow paddler out by sawing off such obstructions or pulling them out of the creek altogether. Many hands (and handsaws) make light work.

Six-foot-tall clay banks will line the creek leading up to the Fox Road bridge, where below lies another fun rapid. This one is less intense than the one at the put-in, but it has a steep ledge. It's a lot of fun and not technically challenging, but it can easily be portaged, too. Take care to note the mud dauber nests lining the ceiling of the bridge; they resemble organ pipes. The current will slacken some below the bridge. For a short while, the surroundings take on a forested feel as the creek zigzags in earnest. Again, you may encounter an occasional obstruction.

Soon the landscape flattens out and the horizon widens, so obstructions will be a thing of the past. The bad news is the creek will start to meander like it's going out of business. If there's anything to appreciate about such oxbow slaloms, it's that they are the growing pains of baby streams; the more "crooked" a stream is, the more it meanders, the younger it is. Neenah Creek is still a toddler in geological time.

The water remains crystal clear, and you'll likely pass over clams and snails. Here and there, you'll see duck blinds and, farther away, a silo or two. While meandering around one tight bend, you'll see on your right a visually disorienting canal that is 2 feet higher than the creek, penned in by an earthen dam. A few gentle curves later you'll pass under a footbridge. A brief 0.5 mile with a bit more meandering leads you to the CR A bridge. As before, there is a small rapid below the bridge, this one the easiest of all three. Take out on river left.

•THE•FUDGE•

ADDITIONAL TRIPS Upstream of Chauncey Street is dull lake paddling created by the dam in Oxford. There is a beautiful trout stream section of the creek before the lake, but it's very narrow, shallow, and clogged with frustrating obstructions. Leave this part of the creek to the anglers.

Downstream from CR A, the creek meanders torturously back and forth. It's only 4 miles until the next bridge at CR P—or 2 miles as the crow flies—but it's a daunting 4 miles since it feels like you're never making progress. As such, it isn't recommended.

CAMPING Coon's Deep Lake Campground (348 Fish Lane, Oxford; 608-586-5644)

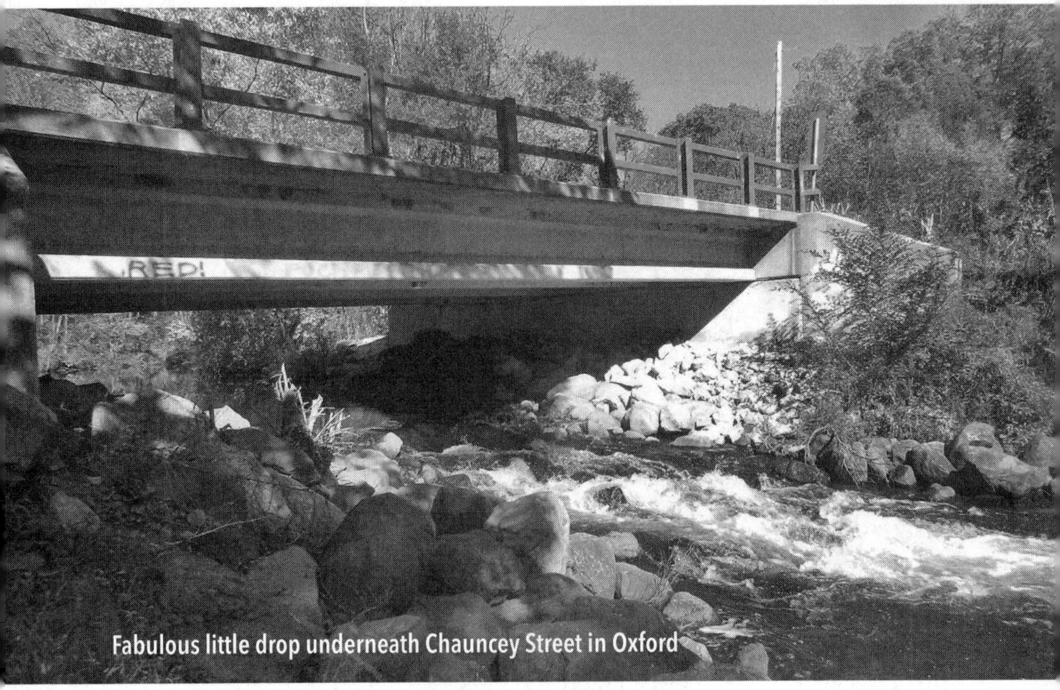

Fabulous little drop underneath Chauncey Street in Oxford

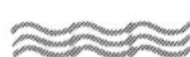

53 Neenah Creek B: COUNTY ROAD P TO MUSKRAT ROAD

•THE•FACTS•

Put-in/take-out CR P/Stevens Court or Muskrat Road (see note below)

Distance/time 9.3 mi/Allow for 5 hrs

Gradient/water level 3 fpm/There should always be enough water.

Water type Quietwater

Canoe or kayak Kayak preferable

Skill level Beginner

Time of year to paddle Anytime

Landscape Meadows, oak savanna, hardwood forest, marsh

OVERVIEW This is a supremely pleasant trip on a narrow stream with crystal-clear water and good current revealing a multitude of landscape environments with virtually no development along the way. Chances are good that you'll see bald eagles, sandhill cranes, wild geese, teals, turkeys, coots, water snakes, frogs, deer, ducks, beavers, muskrats, great blue and green herons, hawks, and owls.

SHUTTLE **5.6 miles.** From the take-out, head north on Stevens Court, then turn left on Grouse Drive. After a few doglegs, turn right on Miller Avenue. Stay straight on Miller as it merges with CR O. At the WI 23 intersection, stay straight and follow WI 23 north. Take CR O to the left where WI 23 splits to the right. Turn left on CR P to the bridge.

Note: Finding the take-out bridge is a bit bewildering, as there is no consensus on the actual name of the road that leads there—probably because the bridge lies right on the Marquette–Columbia County line. Coming in from the north, from Grouse Drive (Marquette County side), the street sign says Stevens Court. Coming in from the south, the road is unnamed in DeLorme's *Wisconsin Atlas & Gazetteer* before it forks at Corning Road and Muskrat Road, just south of the creek (Columbia County side). Google Maps labels Stevens Court as Fifth Court, which is certainly inaccurate. This much every resource agrees on: The road leading to the put-in is a quarter mile east of Fourth Drive at Grouse Drive.)

TAKE-OUT N43° 38.461' W89° 31.301' **PUT-IN** N43° 42.070' W89° 33.116'

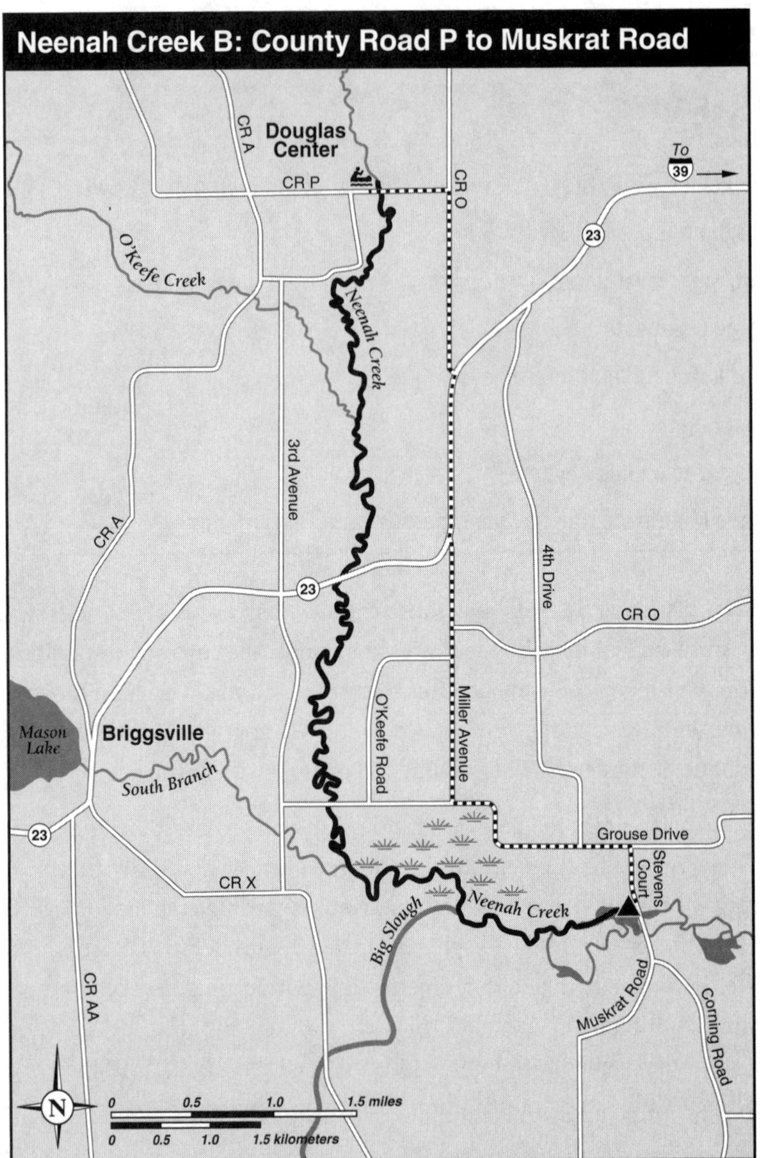

•THE•FLAVOR•

PUT IN ON THE UPSTREAM SIDE of the bridge at CR P, on river right. A makeshift footpath leads to the creek from the road. The setting here already is quite pretty, a lush meadow with handsome oaks. On the creek, you'll remark how utterly clear the water is: sandy with occasional water plants warbling in the steady current. The first mile is especially pretty. Stands of pine alternate with clumps of oaks, and where the banks are not flat, they flank the stream 10–20 feet high. There are moments of wild abandon where a menagerie of trees, both living and decorously decayed, envelops the environs. The creek is about 25 feet wide.

Soon, the creek widens a bit and the tree-lined peripheries dissolve; marshy meadowlands open before you. The foreground will be flat, but gentle hills peak above the tallgrass in the backdrop. The creek will meander intermittently, then relax to easy straightaways. On your right, O'Keefe Creek will quietly enter. But for a kinky wooden footbridge, there is zero development here until the bridge at WI 23. In fact, you will see far more duck blinds than barns. You'll come upon that poor footbridge on your right where the creek sharply bends left. Here, the creek leaves the marsh and flows past tall clay banks that you can see slowly eroding and tincturing the water just below the surface, a pretty cool effect. Trees enclose both banks once more.

The WI 23 bridge has a surprisingly low clearance, so be careful passing under it. For point of reference, you have paddled a little more than 3 miles at this point; you have nearly 6 more to go. After a few sharp turns, you'll pass under a footbridge. A woodsy section claims the creek's character next, where tall, tapered maples explode in autumn color. Take your time enjoying this, for between WI 23 and Grouse Drive, the creek meanders considerably. In a very short stretch, you will end up facing each cardinal direction at least twice.

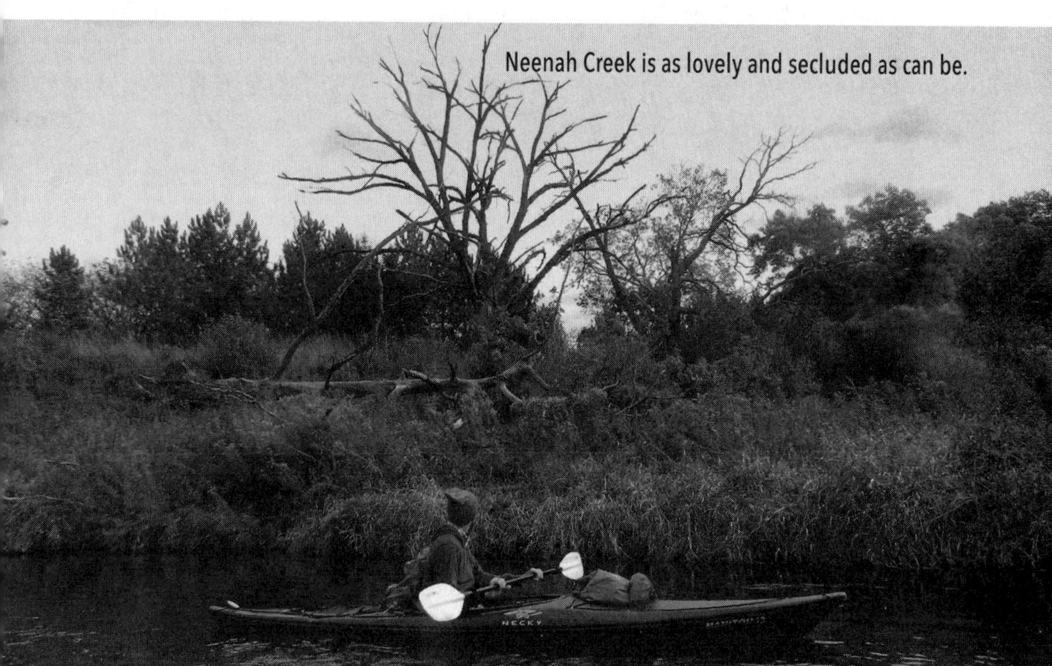

Neenah Creek is as lovely and secluded as can be.

At Grouse Drive, there are two short culverts to paddle through; there's a fun, rustic feel to it. The landscape here is a pleasant mix of marshy tallgrass with stands of tamaracks, oaks, and maples. Soon you will see the relatively huge mouth of the south branch of Neenah Creek on the right, after which point the main stream will double in width. There will be a few more zigzags, but they will be less angular than upstream.

At a gradual bend to the left, you will see the morass of Big Slough on your right with houses lining its shore off in the distance. From here, there's only a mile and change of paddling left before the take-out. It's a secluded section with a North Woods feel to it, so take your time. Be on the lookout for bald eagles and sandhill cranes. Be on the lookout, too, for hunters, as this final section is a licensed shooting preserve. The bridge at Stevens Court/Muskrat Road will appear before you with its wooden and poured concrete pilings. Take out on the upstream side on river left.

•THE•FUDGE•

ADDITIONAL TRIPS I don't recommend using WI 23 as a put-in due to the high volume of traffic. Alternatively, **Big Slough** is not without its own charms and can be paddled for a good 10 miles, but it's not as pretty as Neenah Creek. The same can be said about the south branch of Neenah Creek from Mason Lake to Big Slough, where it's slow, wide, and less attractive.

CAMPING **Coon's Deep Lake Campground** (348 Fish Lane, Oxford; 608-586-5644)

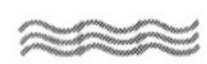

54 Neenah Creek C:
MUSKRAT ROAD TO COUNTY ROAD CX

•THE•FACTS•

Put-in/take-out Stevens Court or Muskrat Road (see note below)/County Road CX

Distance/time 4.8 mi/Allow for 2.5 hrs

Gradient/water level 1 fpm/There should always be enough water.

Water type Quietwater

Canoe or kayak Either

Skill level Beginner

Time of year to paddle Anytime

Landscape Meadowlands with low rolling hills

OVERVIEW The most scenic and least obstructed segment of delightful Neenah Creek, this little sojourn is a great wildlife area hiding in plain sight with virtually no development. The creek meanders here and there, and the water is clear. Add to this a fun rope swing perfect for cooling off on hot summer days, and this trip is a real gem. Short in its own right, it has two additional take-out options to make a longer day on the water (see "Additional Trips"). Expect to see bald eagles, sandhill cranes, wild geese, teals, water snakes, frogs, deer, ducks, beavers, muskrats, great blue and green herons, hawks, and owls.

SHUTTLE **4 miles.** From the take-out, go north on CR CX, then turn left onto Grouse Drive. Turn left onto Stevens Court to the bridge.

Note: Finding the take-out bridge is a bit bewildering, as there is no consensus on the actual name of the road that leads there—probably because the bridge lies right on the Marquette–Columbia County line. Coming in from the north, from Grouse Drive (Marquette County side), the street sign says Stevens Court. Coming in from the south, the road is unnamed in DeLorme's *Wisconsin Atlas & Gazetteer* before it forks at Corning Road and Muskrat Road, just south of the creek (Columbia County side). Google Maps labels Stevens Court as Fifth Court, which is certainly inaccurate. This much every resource agrees on: The road leading to the put-in is a quarter mile east of Fourth Drive at Grouse Drive.)

TAKE-OUT N43° 38.676' W89° 28.093' **PUT-IN** N43° 38.461' W89° 31.301'

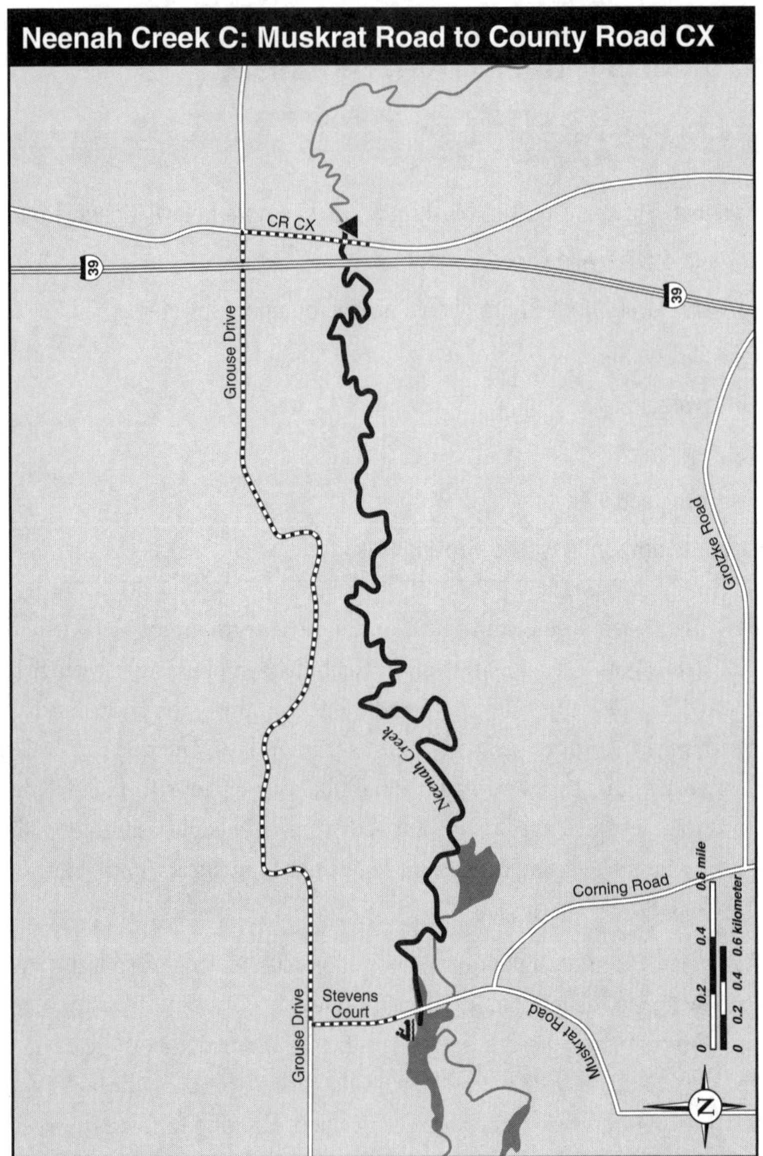

•THE•FLAVOR•

PUT IN AT THE UPSTREAM SIDE OF THE BRIDGE, on river left. It's not an official launch, but it's flat and dry. The creek is narrow yet wide enough to comfortably paddle a canoe. Despite the negligible gradient, there's still a decent current. Unlike the segments upstream, where the water is clear and the bottom all sand, here it's more convoluted. That said, something this trip has that you won't find upstream is a backdrop of lovely rolling hills, mostly on your right (to the south). You're in drumlins country, and while these are less dramatic than those seen on the nearby Fox River, the setting here is nonetheless quite appealing.

There will be some tree limbs to dodge and duck under, but you shouldn't have to portage around anything on this trip. The dead or dying trees in the stream enhance the natural setting. From the put-in to the interstate, there is just wonderfully nothing out here but the natural landscape in all its abandoned beauty. The feeling of solitude saturates the surroundings. As such, the wildlife on this trip is quite remarkable.

As you begin to hear the whirring din of the interstate, you'll come upon a sharp right-hand bend in the creek where, on the far right side, above an accessible log, someone thoughtfully placed a rope swing. I cannot tell you just how much fun this is, and I hope I don't need to explain why. Due to the position of the logs and an eddy on the inside bend, you can securely lodge your boat without worry. What's more, because the log is in the stream, you don't even have to think twice about whether you're trespassing on private property. So reach high, hold down hard, and have at it—just don't forget to let go!

The creek meanders a bit before heading straight under the interstate bridge. Immediately downstream from the interstate is a second bridge at CR CX, where an excellent access for taking out is on the downstream side on river right.

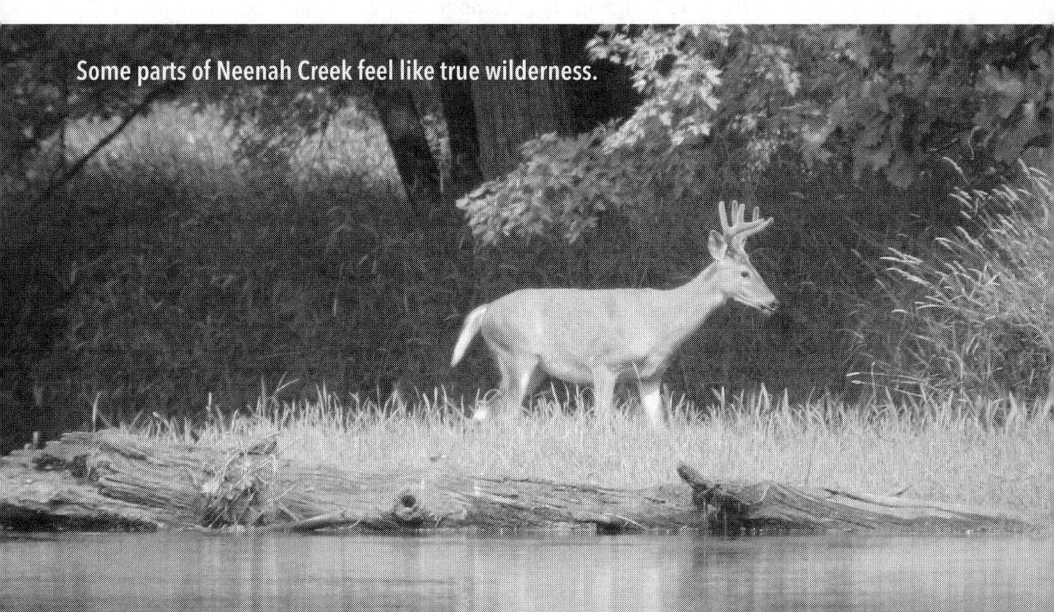

Some parts of Neenah Creek feel like true wilderness.

•THE•FUDGE•

ADDITIONAL TRIPS Instead of taking out at CR CX, you can continue down to the next bridge on CR CM for an additional 3.7 miles, or you can paddle into the Fox River and take out at the first bridge downstream of the confluence, also on CR CM, for a 10-mile trip. The section between CR CX and CR CM is not as pretty as upstream. For one, it's developed; for another, there's a lot more deadfall in the creek, some of which can be frustrating (especially in a canoe). It's more of a marsh, and the water clarity is muddier. Lastly, the take-out at CR CM is rather imperfect. There's only a short zigzag to the Fox River if you seek the experience of merging from a tributary to a bigger river.

The corresponding Fox River segment is nondescript, so you'd want to do it only for the novelty of paddling two streams on one trip. Again, the take-out for this—the bridge on CR CM half a mile east of the previous CR CM bridge over Neenah Creek—is imperfect but doable.

Incidentally, at this bridge on the Fox there used to be a settlement of unemployed but hopeful potters who had emigrated from England. A man by the name of Thomas Twiggs operated a store and blacksmith shop and set up a livery service called Emancipation Ferry to transport the newly arrived to and from the river. Alas, the settlement was not long for this world. Exhaustion and starvation, in part brought about by a lack of reliable supplies, led to its demise, as well as the tragic moniker of Desolation Ferry.

CAMPING AND RENTALS **Indian Trails Campground** is situated on a small lake (that incidentally does connect to the Fox River upstream of this trip) in Pardeeville, a few miles east of Portage (W6445 Haynes Road; 608-429-3244).

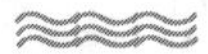

55 Pine River A:
PIER NATURAL BRIDGE PARK TO COUNTY ROAD AA

•THE•FACTS•

Put-in/take-out Pier Natural Bridge Park/CR AA

Distance/time 10.3 mi/Allow for 4.5 hrs

Gradient/water level 1.5 fpm/There is no gage, but water levels are usually good. Call Pine River Paddle and Tube (608-475-2199) for updated conditions, or check their Facebook page.

Water type Quietwater

Canoe or kayak Kayak preferable—only experienced paddlers should try canoeing this.

Skill level Experienced

Time of year to paddle Late spring, summer, or autumn

Landscape Driftless hills, several beautiful sandstone rock outcrops lining the river

---

OVERVIEW Paddle through a rock tunnel that's part of a natural bridge on your way through the rolling landscape of beautiful Richland County. This trip on the upstream Pine is pure Driftless Area, as you slowly meander around several sandstone bluffs and pastureland on a stream only 20–30 feet wide. Deadfall can sometimes be a problem, so it's best to call ahead for condition updates. Wildlife includes sandhill cranes, great blue herons, kingfishers, wood ducks, muskrats, beavers, butterflies, turtles, songbirds, trout, cows, bulls, sheep, and alpacas.

SHUTTLE 6 miles. From the take-out, head out northwest on CR AA to WI 80, then turn right on WI 80 and head north. Turn left into Pier Natural Bridge Park and head down to the northernmost point of the parking lot to the river.

TAKE-OUT N43° 22.383' W90° 23.046' **PUT-IN** N43° 26.851' W90° 21.863'

•THE•FLAVOR•

PUT IN AS CLOSE AS POSSIBLE to the rock bridge that is the centerpiece of this unique county park, located essentially off the far edge of the parking lot. Technically,

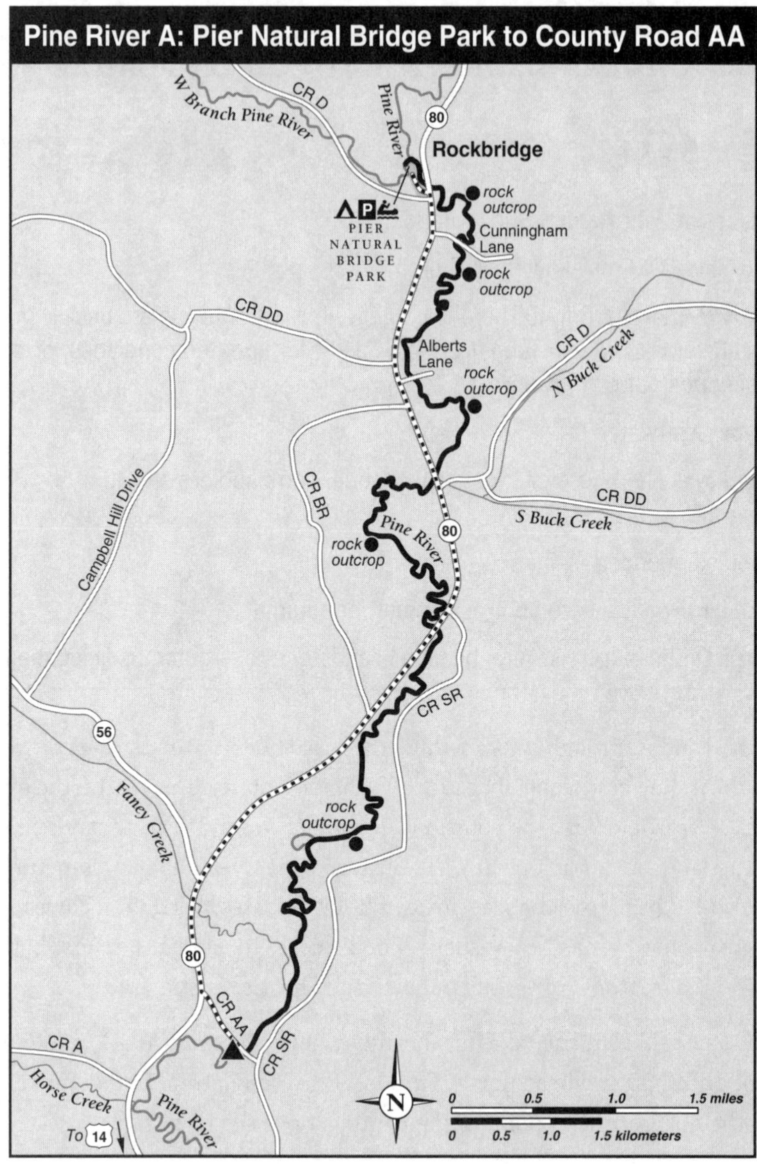

this is the West Branch of the Pine River, but you'll be on it for only 20 yards or so before it converges with the main stream. Paddle upstream through the rock and out to the other side. The natural bridge here rises 40 feet high and is more than 20 feet wide and 1,100 feet long. There's a ladder that gives you access for hiking around, as well as a tunnel that allows you to walk through the other side, where there is a mowed area allowing for up to six campsites.

After merging with the main stream, you'll still see the front side of the rock wall on your right before crossing the WI 80 bridge. Below WI 80, the river begins its characteristic meandering. Soon you'll see some lovely sandstone formations strewn with summer moss on the left. They're the first of many more to come, these tiny by comparison to those downstream. The next bridge, at Cunningham Lane, has a low clearance; in high water, you may need to portage around it. Shortly afterward are more outcrops on the left. The river will continue to meander before an atypical straightaway that leads you to the next (and fortunately last) low-clearance bridge.

From here, the Pine heads east to another series of sandstone rock walls. The deepest pools of water lie below the rock walls (many of which line the river). The upper Pine is often shale-hued to clear, a signature feature not only of Driftless streams, but trout-friendly waters, too. Pyramid-shaped bluffs in the near distance punctuate the pastoral landscape. Sometimes called (either with euphemism or exaggeration) the Ocooch Mountains, the Driftless hills may well be at their most rugged and New England–esque in Richland County.

Below the next WI 80 bridge, the Pine meanders again, and its course, together with its narrowness and the potential for downed trees, makes kayaking much preferable to canoeing (unless you're a skilled canoeist). The doodling of the river will reward you with the most glorious rock feature so far (other than the natural bridge): a 60-foot-high sandstone bluff on the right. Its grandeur is striking. You can sidle up to it and touch it (if you do, you're literally in contact with the past couple hundred million years). After this, the seemingly indecisive Pine makes another line for WI 80. Short banks give you a view of Steamboat Rock, in the near distance beyond the bridge.

The final leg of this trip, from the last bridge at WI 80 to the take-out, includes more straightaways than upstream but is more prone to obstructions. It's for this section in particular you want to inquire about conditions ahead of time. Pine River Paddle and Tube in Rockbridge does a fine job of clearing out obstructions, but the feel of a river changes daily. All in all, impressive rock outcrops remain; a particularly nice one lies 2 miles downstream from WI 80.

There are three straightaways here: The first is directly below WI 80, the next is between tight meanders, and the last is a nice long coast all the way to the take-out. The take-out is a floating dock generously provided by the parks department of Richland Center in conjunction with local Boy Scouts. The first of five along the Pine River within the city, these structures are supremely convenient and most appreciated. This one is on the downstream side of CR AA, on the right.

•THE•FUDGE•

ADDITIONAL TRIPS There are several put-in options upstream of Rockbridge, where outcrops are spectacular, but river access is more difficult and obstructions are problematic.

CAMPING Pier Natural Bridge Park in Rockbridge (WI 80 North; 608-647-4673)

RENTALS Pine River Paddle and Tube in Rockbridge (608-475-2199, facebook.com/pineriverpaddleandtubellc)

FOOD FOR THOUGHT For a fine variety of healthy local food, stop by the Pine River Food Co-Op (196 W. Court St., Richland Center; 608-647-7299).

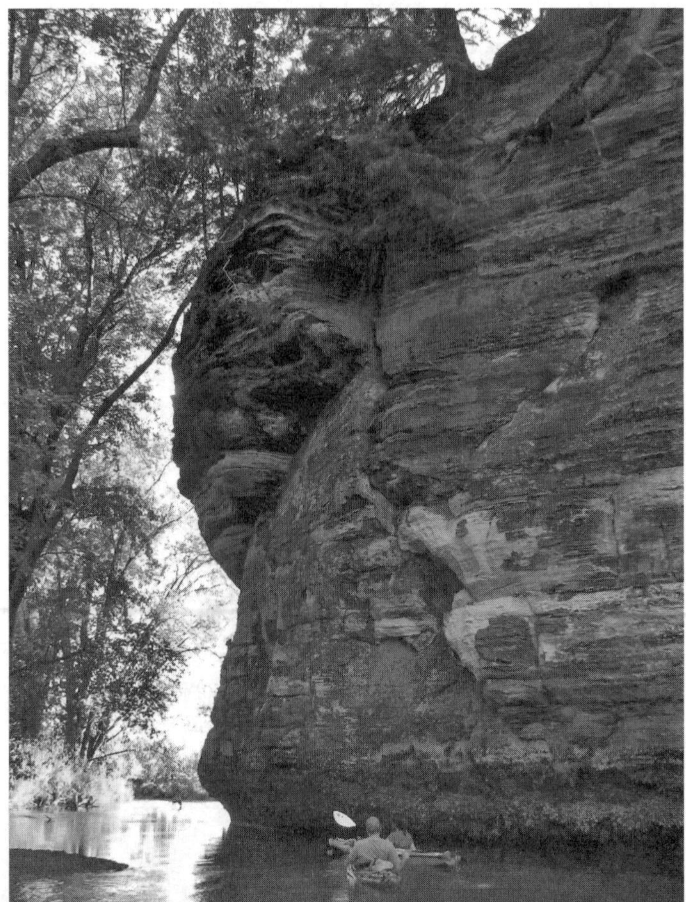

The upper Pine River has breathtaking sandstone cliffs and rock outcrops.

56 Pine River B: COUNTY ROAD AA TO BOHMANN DRIVE

•THE•FACTS•

Put in/take-out CR AA bridge/Bohmann Drive

Distance/time 8.1 mi/Allow for 3.5 hrs

Gradient/water level 4 fpm/There is no gage, but adequate water is rarely a problem; too much water, however, makes it a better fit for paddlers with some experience. Call Pine River Paddle and Tube (608-475-2199) for information on current conditions (no pun intended).

Water type Quietwater with one Class II rapid that can be easily portaged

Canoe or kayak Kayak preferred

Skill level Experienced

Time of year to paddle Anytime

Landscape Driftless hills, bottomlands, light urban, rural countryside

---

OVERVIEW A fun, varied trip with a thrilling Class II rapid and several unique accesses designed just for kayakers, this middle section of the Pine is sure to satisfy all sorts of paddling taste buds. Turkey vultures, sandhill cranes, wood ducks, muskrats, and snapping turtles add to the delight.

CAR SHUTTLE **4.7 miles.** From the take-out, head north on Bohmann Drive, then turn left at the traffic light onto US 14. At the next traffic light, turn right onto WI 80 (Main Street) into downtown. Turn right onto Industrial Drive after 2 miles. Turn left onto CR AA, then bear left, staying on CR AA where CR SR splits. The put-in at the bridge is just ahead.

BIKE SHUTTLE **5.1 miles.** Head north on Bohmann, then turn left onto the Pine River Trail before US 14. Follow the trail to Krouskop Park, then turn left onto WI 80 (Main Street). Turn right onto Industrial Drive and follow as above.

TAKE-OUT N43° 18.890' W90° 22.702' **PUT-IN** N43° 22.388' W90° 23.042'

•THE•FLAVOR•

PUT IN ON THE DOWNSTREAM SIDE, river right, of the CR AA bridge. Immediately, you'll see a floating dock anchored to the bank with a grooved channel designed for kayaks to slip into and out of the water. It is truly the perfect way to launch a boat.

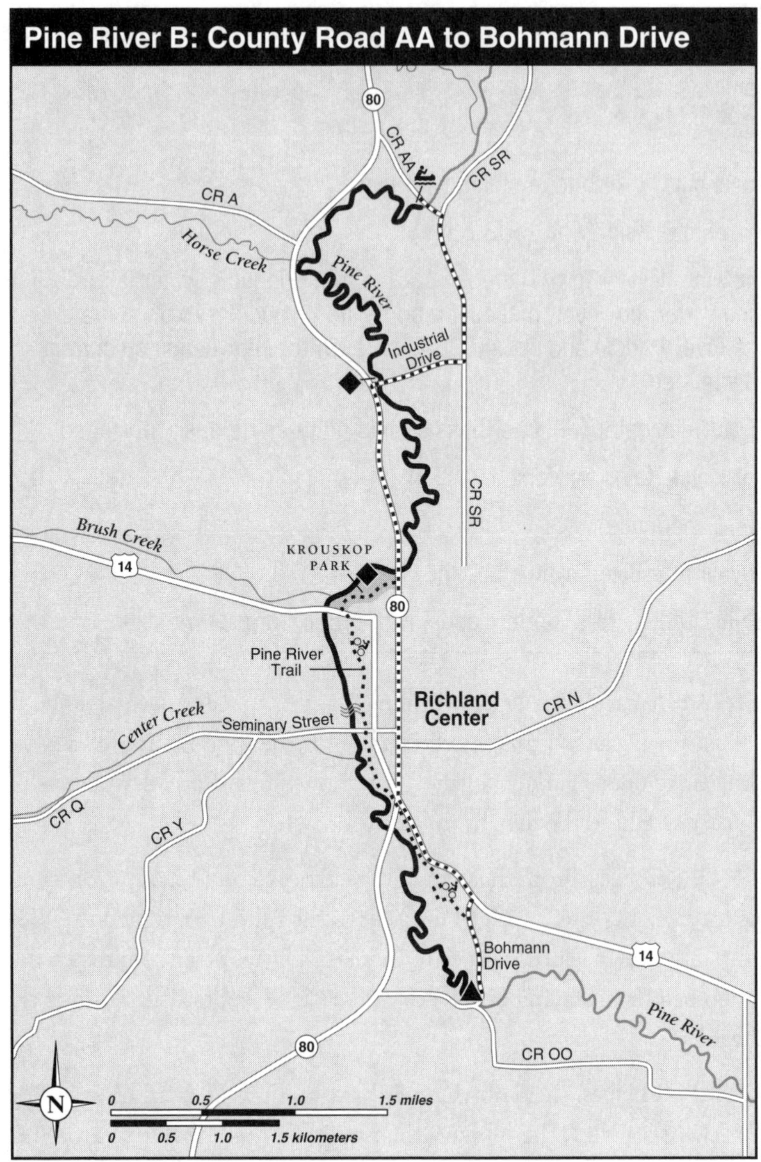

The current is brisk but not pushy unless the river is high, in which case you will need to have excellent boat control for the occasional strainers and hairpin turns midway into the trip. The river here is representative of what to expect throughout: 40 feet wide with a sandy bottom and a clear/slate-gray hue. Even though this trip is only a hair over 8 miles, it can be broken into four distinct sections. In this first section, after a small island splits the channel in two, you'll be rewarded with the first of many beautiful views of the so-called Ocooch Mountains (Driftless hills). These uplands are everywhere in Richland County, like white-capped waves on an inland sea undulating one after another for as far as the eye can behold.

After briefly running parallel to WI 80, you'll pass some large buildings, and the Pine will meander quite a bit to the east and become more secluded. This second section is quite woodsy, and there are some obstructions here, but you shouldn't have to portage. (The local outfitter does a commendable job keeping the river clear of dangerous snags and impediments; plus, this section of the river is used during an annual race in July, adding to its cleanup.) There should always be a path to weave through the downed trees and floating logs that you'll likely encounter, but due to the steady current and surprising depth of some of the pools, you'll want to be mindful, and beginners in particular should wear their PFDs. The gradient also gradually picks up, so you want to have good boat control.

The bridge at Industrial Drive will signal the halfway point of the wooded section, and the next floating dock will appear on the right downstream from the bridge. The landscape does begin to gradually open up as you head into town, with outstanding views of the huge hills (or "mountains," if you wish) on the right.

Now the Pine curves toward the next bridge at WI 80 in the trip's third section. A small island splits the channel again; far left or right both work, each with a very gentle riffle. A pedestrian bridge, part of Krouskop Park, one of the two Pine River Trail terminuses, comes into view. The third floating dock will be on the left, a great place to rest or to use the bathroom. For better or worse, it's worth noting that the river runs just to the west of downtown, not through it, so don't expect to see much of an urban scene.

Before bending to the left at the US 14 bridge, you'll see a phalanx of flags on your right. On a windy day, the sound of their crisp snapping is quite acoustic. Below the bridge, the river runs unusually straight for about 1 mile. On your right, you'll see a few houses, while all of the land on the left is a pleasant city park. In the middle of everything is a unique wooden suspension bridge for pedestrians. Surprisingly long, it straddles what used to be a pond. Shortly downstream comes the exhilarating exclamation mark of this trip: a Class II rapid where there used to be a dam. For those wary of getting wet, whether splashed or capsizing, there's good news: The fourth floating dock is cleverly located upstream of the rapid on the right.

The rapid is safe and just good, clean fun. It consists of two drops. If you have a spray skirt, it's wise to wear it for this, especially on a spring or autumn day. There's

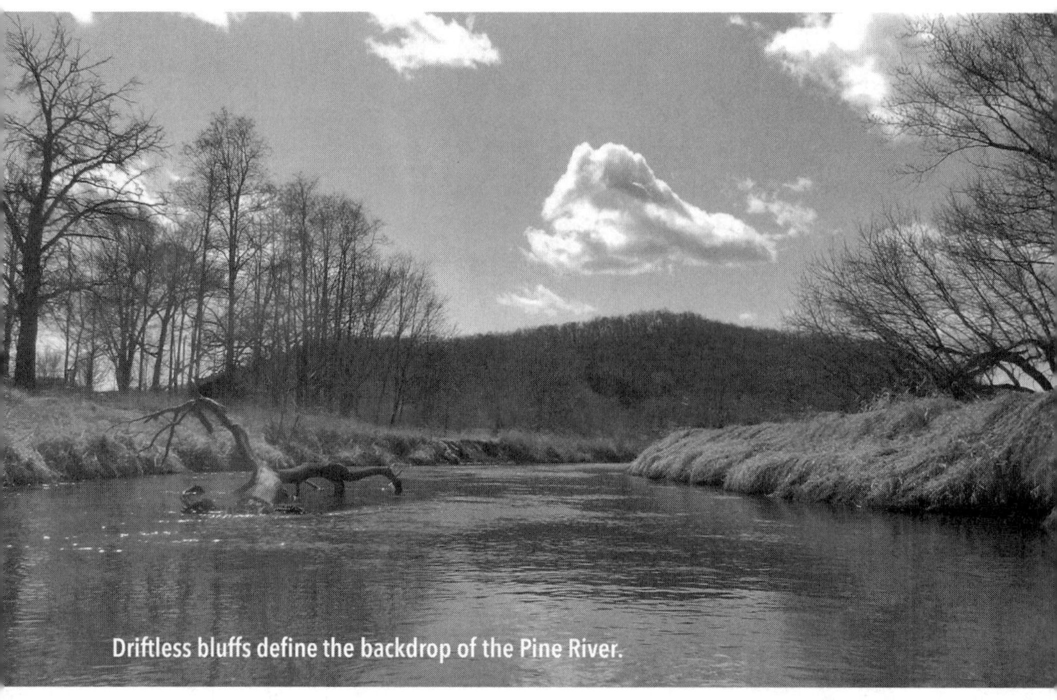

Driftless bluffs define the backdrop of the Pine River.

only one boulder to watch for, on the left at the bottom of the rapids, but staying clear of it is no problem. Catch the eddy on the right to paddle back into the rapid for some super-fun surfing. Still better, the bank on the right is so low that getting out using the convenient dock makes running and rerunning the rapid supremely easy. Either way, take a moment to look upstream of the rapid; the view of the Driftless hills with the spilling whitewater is quite a sight.

After the next bridge at Seminary Street, the river begins to meander again in a densely wooded area. This last section features small islands, a limestone retaining wall on the left, and a brief, modest limestone outcrop on the right. Things will thin out again soon, and you'll see a huge processing plant on the left, plus a rock quarry off in the backdrop. You'll pass under WI 80 one last time, after which there will be a mix of condos on the left and farmland on the right. More beautiful hills come back into view. Another red pedestrian bridge appears, followed by a humongous logjam that you'll paddle past. Too soon, the bridge at Bohmann Drive appears, the fifth floating dock on the left. You can paddle right up its slight incline like a seal.

•THE•FUDGE•

ADDITIONAL TRIPS Continuing past Bohmann Drive is not recommended because it's flat, the views of the hills are subdued, and most of the landscape is distracted by large farms on the right and US 14 off to the left.

CAMPING **Pier Natural Bridge Park** in Rockbridge (WI 80 North; 608-647-4673) and **Alana Springs Campground,** west of downtown Richland Center (22628 Covered Bridge Drive; 608-647-2600)

RENTALS **Pine River Paddle and Tube** in Rockbridge (608-475-2199, facebook.com/pineriverpaddleandtubellc)

FOOD FOR THOUGHT For a fine variety of healthy local food, stop by the **Pine River Food Co-Op** (196 W. Court St., Richland Center; 608-647-7299).

SHOUT-OUTS Thanks to the **Richland Center Parks and Grounds Department** and **Troop 81's Eagle Scout Project** for providing the awesome floating docks along the Pine River.

One of Frank Lloyd Wright's buildings, the **A. D. German Warehouse,** at 300 S. Church St. in Richland Center, is there for the exploration—it's a 4-story red-brick-and-concrete temple to storing such wares as tobacco, coffee, flour, and sugar (wrightinwisconsin.org).

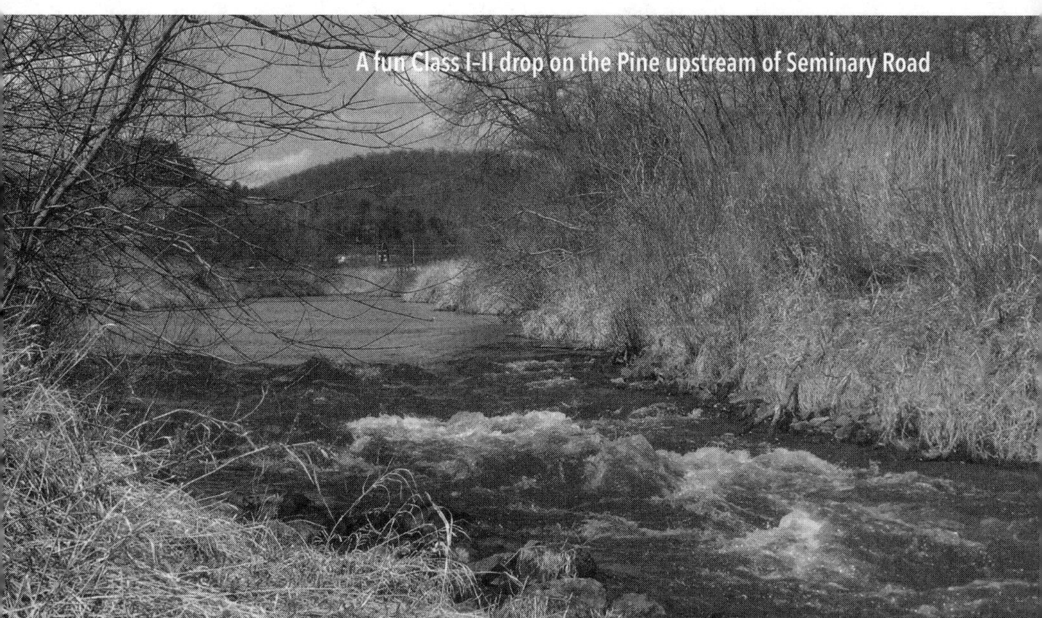

A fun Class I-II drop on the Pine upstream of Seminary Road

57 Pine River C:

TWIN BLUFFS DRIVE TO WISCONSIN RIVER

•THE•FACTS•

Put-in/take-out Wayside Park off of Twin Bluffs Drive/Buena Vista Boat Landing at Wisconsin River

Distance/time 8.8 mi/Allow for 3.5 hrs

Gradient/water level 2 fpm/There is no gage, but there should always be enough water for this trip. If the water is very high, though, it can be very dangerous, so call Pine River Paddle and Tube (608-475-2199) to check conditions before you go.

Water type Quietwater

Canoe or kayak Either, but canoes will struggle to clear low bridges during high water.

Skill level Experienced

Time of year to paddle Anytime

Landscape A pretty mix of hardwood forests and farm pastures surrounded by endless miles of Driftless hills and bluffs

---

OVERVIEW This stretch of the Pine River's final leg before it empties into the Wisconsin River meanders through a mix of bottomlands, pastures, and towering bluffs. Combine this paddle trip with a pedal shuttle along one of the prettiest bike trails in the state for a magnificent day outdoors. Along the way, you're likely to encounter such wildlife as muskrats, woodpeckers, frogs, turtles, hawks, cows, blue-winged teals, and bald eagles.

CAR SHUTTLE **6.5 miles.** From the take-out, head west on WI 60 to CR TB to Twin Bluffs Drive for the scenic route with exquisite views of the valley. Follow Oak Street after leaving the boat landing, then turn left onto Fulton Street. Turn left onto WI 60, then right onto CR TB after crossing the bridge. Follow CR TB up, down, and around the bluffs until it comes into the tiny hamlet of Twin Bluffs and the county road becomes Twin Bluffs Drive. Cross the bike trail, and the wayside landing will be on the right.

BIKE SHUTTLE **5 miles.** Follow Oak Street after leaving the boat landing, then turn left onto Fulton Street. Catty-corner to the intersection of Fulton and WI 60 is an

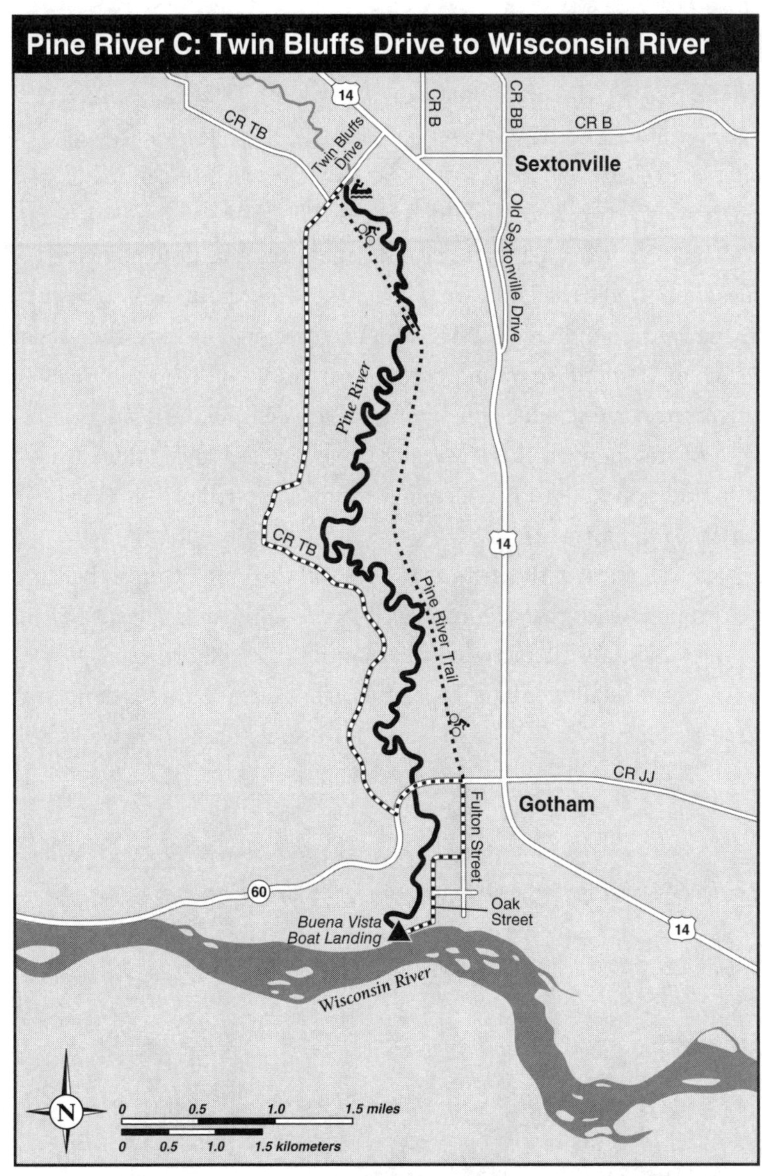

inconspicuous entry point to the Pine River Trail, a 14.3-mile crushed-limestone path along what was once a railroad, connecting Richland Center, Twin Bluffs, Gotham, and Lone Rock (no state-trail sticker is needed for access). Take the trail all the way to Twin Bluffs Drive, then turn right to wayside park at the river.

TAKE-OUT N43° 12.568' W90° 18.270' **PUT-IN** N43° 16.565' W90° 18.642'

•THE•FLAVOR•

PUT IN AT THE QUAINT WAYSIDE PARK along Twin Bluffs Drive (a.k.a. County Road TB). There are no facilities, but there is plenty of room to leave a few vehicles, and the access to the water is excellent. What the river looks like here will be essentially consistent for the remainder of the trip: a meandering stream about 50 feet wide with a mix of sand and mud along the bottom, high-grass banks, and occasional deadfall in the water.

Unless you paddle the Pine after a severe storm, expect there to be enough passage to maneuver around fallen trees without portaging. Despite the modest gradient, the current is good. Accordingly, you don't want to be on this river when the water is high; the current will be pushy, and negotiating all the deadfall will be tricky to the point of treacherous; plus, there are three low-clearance bridges that could be an issue. In addition, due to the meandering nature of the river, weird eddies and small whirlpools will form in high water that can be challenging.

The salient feature of this trip, as in most on the Pine River, is the surrounding landscape through which the river courses. You are in the magnificent Driftless Area, so bluffs, steep hills, and attractive ridges abound. But this trip is slightly more distinctive, due to the duality of landscapes the river meanders around: floodplain bottoms and sweeping meadows nooked beneath towering bluffs. You won't be bored.

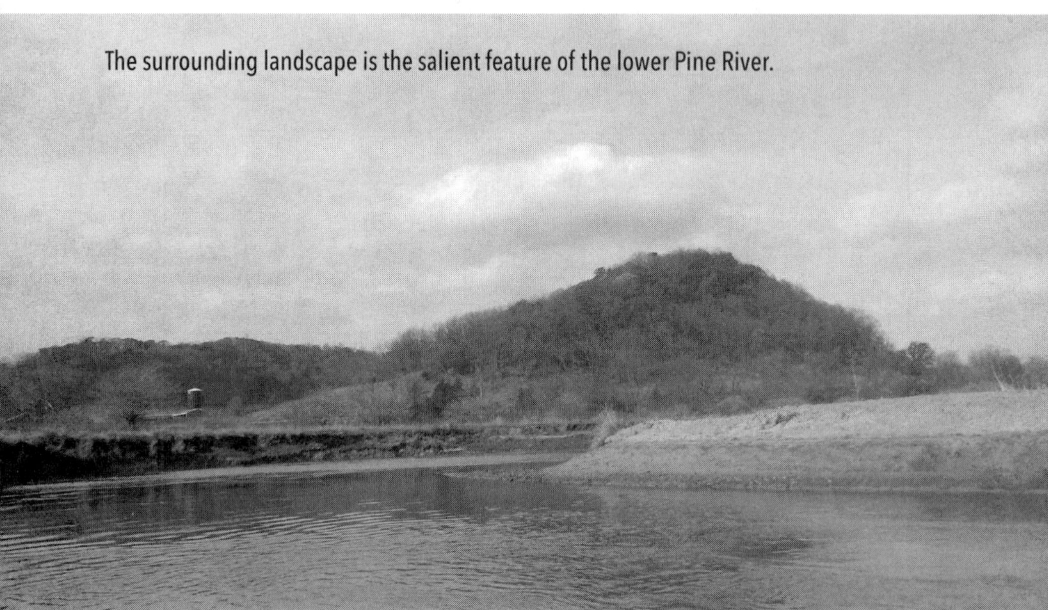
The surrounding landscape is the salient feature of the lower Pine River.

Within the first hundred yards after the put-in, you'll be rewarded with panoramic views of the pretty hills to the west and north. Just a mile down is one of many bridges along the Pine River Trail. Deadfall tends to collect at the pilings of the bridge on the river right, but there should be open clearance on the left side. A hardwood-bottomlands feel follows below the bridge, with occasional glimpses of pastures and bluffs through occasional breaks in the trees. Don't be surprised to see cattle. As always, yield to creatures many hundreds of pounds heavier than you!

Here and downstream, you'll appreciate how much the Pine meanders, sometimes as sharply as 180-degree turns doubling back on themselves; oxbow sloughs will be intermittent. The woods will clear and the rolling hills in the background will begin coming into sharper focus. There's a sandy bank some 15 feet high on your left, just past a fallen tree that hovers above you.

Perhaps the prettiest section on this trip begins as the banks shorten and grassy pastures extend to a continuous ridge a few hundred feet high. The first of three rusty antique farm bridges will appear, followed by a logjam with a clear passage on the far left side. For the next 2 miles, you'll keep coming back to the ridge due to the meanders. In the middle of the stream, two long-gone trees lean against one another rather like a tepee, and you can pass beneath them. Also in this section lies one hairpin turn with deadfall that's a little tricky to maneuver around; it's not complicated, but you should be mindful.

The first of only two houses on the trip will appear in front of you as the river bends sharply to the right; it's a thousand feet away and none too obtrusive. In short order, you then will paddle under the second dilapidated farm bridge followed by the only road bridge on the trip, at WI 60. The river does widen below the bridge, and there is an uncharacteristic but welcome straightaway that follows. Relax and soak it up; there's little deadfall to dodge, fewer oxbows, and a little more than a mile of river left before the take-out.

The third and final metal farm bridge will appear after a left bend. Another tall sandbank will appear on the left, below telephone wires. A straightaway flanked by a canopy of trees follows, and the soft rise of the left bank hints at the humongous Wisconsin River on the other side. The Pine will make one final series of bends around a small bluff—right, left, left—before leading immediately to the Wisconsin. The ancient-seeming remains of trees protruding from the water like piers from an abandoned dock are all that's left before the confluence. The take-out is on the left, at a concrete-lined launch. Or you could venture a bit into the Wisconsin, but keep in mind that the current will be significantly stronger and paddling upstream can be a workout.

•THE•FUDGE•

ADDITIONAL TRIPS You can put in farther upstream at an excellent access at CR OO and add 4.5 miles to this trip, but the scenery is none too spectacular.

CAMPING The only public campground in the area is at **Pier Natural Bridge Park** in Rockbridge (WI 80 North, 15 miles north of Twin Bluffs Drive; 608-647-4673) and **Alana Springs Campground,** west of downtown Richland Center and 10 miles northwest of Twin Bluffs Drive (22628 Covered Bridge Drive; 608-647-2600).

RENTALS **Pine River Paddle and Tube** in Rockbridge (608-475-2199, facebook .com/pineriverpaddleandtubellc)

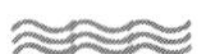

58 Wisconsin River A: UPPER AND LOWER DELLS

•THE•FACTS•

Put-in/take-out River Bay Resort and Campground public boat launch/public boat landing at Norway Drive

Distance/time 11.4 mi, 13.7 mi including a circumnavigation of Blackhawk Island/ Allow for 6–8 hrs

Gradient/water level 2 fpm/Always adequate, but when the river is high, dangerous rapids occur in the Narrows.

Water type Quietwater with strong current and occasionally dangerous waves (see Planning Advisory on page 294)

Canoe or kayak Kayak preferably, though the Lower Dells and Blackhawk Island are suitable for canoes.

Skill level Beginner

Time of year to paddle Spring or autumn; the river is very congested in the height and heat of summer.

Landscape Spectacular sandstone cliffs lining the river with occasional canyons, coves, rock islands, sandy beaches, and lots of pine trees

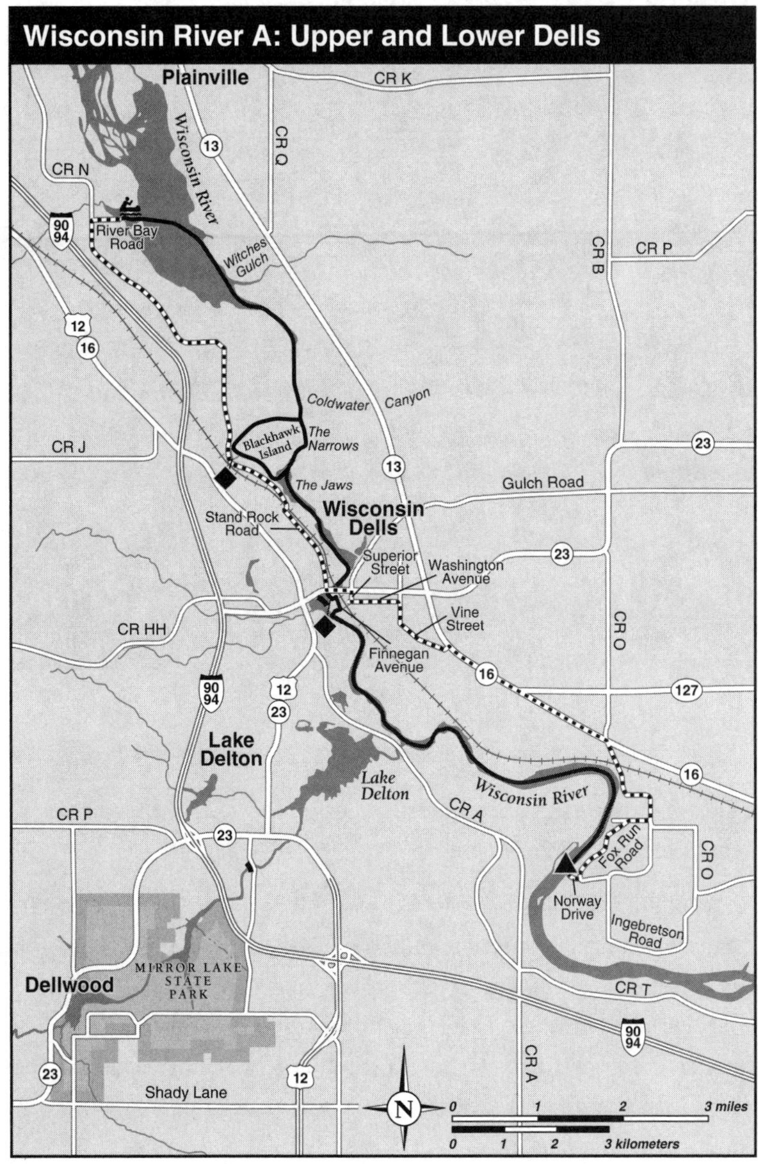

OVERVIEW A unique combination of both the Upper and Lower Dells sections of the Wisconsin River, this truly is one of the most scenically spectacular river trips anywhere in the Midwest. Coral-colored sandstone cliffs, coves, and canyons have been sculpted by wind and wave for millennia and are on display for miles on end. This trip is an absolute must-do for any paddler, veteran or novice. Bald eagles, deer,

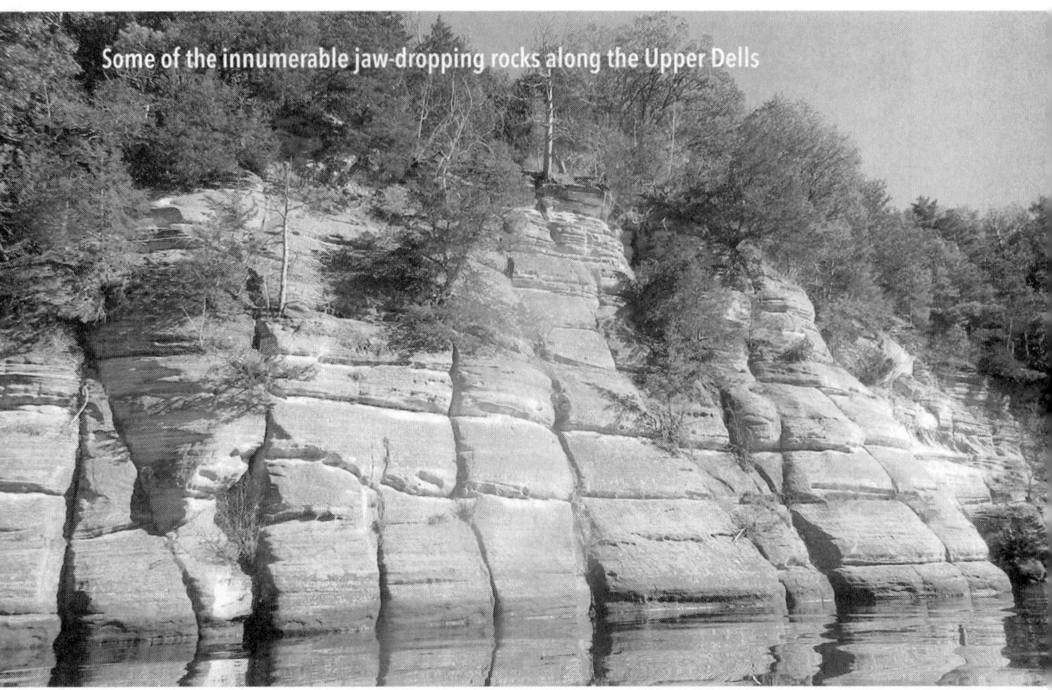
Some of the innumerable jaw-dropping rocks along the Upper Dells

and great blue herons are not uncommon, but given the volume of traffic on the river, don't expect to see too much wildlife.

PLANNING ADVISORY While this trip begins in a wide, lake-like swell created by the dam, the river quickly constricts only a mile or so from the put-in. The reason a section is called the Narrows is that the river tapers from 4,000 feet wide to 700 to 200 to 50 within 2.5 miles. That's a lot of water being funneled. Compounding matters further, there is little to no shoreline in this section. Instead, both sides of the river are lined with magnificent sandstone rock walls, resulting in a rollicking current as waves bounce off the walls.

A no-wake zone through this section of the river is in effect from mid-May to mid-October. If you paddle this trip before or after that window of time, approach the Narrows cautiously. Large tour boats run up and down the river here, not to mention private powerboats and the occasional Jet Ski, all of which create a sizable wake, which in turn bounces off the rock walls and sends waves from in front and behind. I have taken first-time kayakers down the Narrows, and no one has ever tipped or capsized; a little water in the boat is all but inevitable. Just remember that when a wave is coming your way, turn your boat into it so that the bow is perpendicular; canoes and kayaks get swamped when they're parallel to a wave.

The Narrows is one of the most thrilling sections on this already delightful trip, but ambivalent paddlers can circumvent the narrowest of the Narrows by turning into the right channel of Blackhawk Island and going counterclockwise around the huge island and back into the main section of the river downstream.

SHUTTLE 12 miles. From the take-out, turn left onto Fox Run Road, then bear right onto Erickson Drive. Turn left onto CR O, then left onto WI 16. You can take WI 16 and then turn left onto Broadway/WI 33 at the traffic light into downtown Wisconsin Dells, or, if you want to skip the long delay of pedestrians and mayhem, turn left onto Vine Street 2 miles from the intersection of CR O and WI 16, then left onto Washington Avenue. You'll next turn right onto Superior Street and then take a left onto WI 33/Broadway.

Cross the river on WI 33 and take your first right onto Stand Rock Road, then a right onto Fitzgerald Road/CR A, where the road comes to a T; pass under the railroad bridge. On the other side of the bridge the same road is called CR A, CR N, and 28th Avenue; it's a little confusing but basically intuitive in that the road runs parallel to the west shore of the river. You'll pass Blackhawk Island on the right. Stay on CR A/CR N/28th Avenue as it bears left (west and away from the river), then heads north again. Turn right onto River Bay Road. Look for signs for River Bay Campground and Boat Launch. You'll have to give up a $5 parking fee to put in here.

TAKE-OUT N43° 34.999' W89° 43.672' **PUT-IN** N43° 41.149' W89° 49.582'

•THE•FLAVOR•

THIS TRIP HAS TWO DISTINCT PARTS: the Upper Dells, or the portion above the dam in downtown Wisconsin Dells, and the Lower Dells, the portion below the dam. The dam requires portaging, which also suggests separation, and to an extent the upper and lower portions of the river do each have their own characters. But to regard the Dells as two separate trips is not only unnecessary, it prevents the imagination from experiencing the river the way it was before the dam. Therefore, the trip I've prescribed combines the two "sections" into one journey, allowing the paddler to taste what the first rafters encountered long ago.

That said, there are but two road bridges that cross the river in the 21-mile section between the Castle Rock dam and the dam in downtown Wisconsin Dells.

And public landings are few and far between. Consequently, the length of your trip depends on (a) where you choose to put in and (b) how much of the "lake" section you wish to endure. The lake section is roughly 2.5 miles long, and if the wind is from the south, the paddling is arduous. I recommend the River Bay Resort public boat landing, because it clips off most of the lake section. It does cost $5 per vehicle, and you do forfeit some scenic highlights, but you'll get the best of the Dells. Plus, it docks the *Princess K*, a paddleboat from a bygone age.

Once you are past the bay and into the main channel (which is enormously wide, at half a mile), look upstream for a moment, where you'll see Louis Bluff looming above the river. Back in the last ice age, this part of the state was covered by a humongous body of water called Glacial Lake Wisconsin, and Louis Bluff was an island, with only its crown above water. On a much smaller scale, you might see partially submerged tree stumps in the bay. This "shrunken forest" is the result of when the bay froze over, and local farmers sawed down the trees that stood above the ice for firewood. Make a beeline to the other side (the east bank) where towering palisades line the river in a gloriously undulating manner. These walls seem to ripple in the sunlight. This marks the beginning of the Upper Dells.

After the palisades, turn left into the slot canyon called Witches Gulch. Gorgeous crags of sandstone line both shores with tenacious pine trees improbably rooted in the rock. Eventually you'll see a walking plank on the left that belongs to one of the tour-boat companies. If you're feeling curious, you can paddle all the way down to what looks like a dead end, where two sandstone outcrops nearly kiss. If the water level is low enough, you can paddle underneath the walkway, through a cave-like fissure, and through to the other side—called Witches Cauldron. There isn't much to see on the other side, but the novelty is fun (unless you're claustrophobic). Just keep clear of the big boats.

Exit Witches Gulch with caution if the wind is out of the southwest, as the water can get choppy. The river begins to narrow in earnest here. There's very little shoreline development for the next few miles, as most of the land belongs to the state (though it does lease to the tour-boat companies). Approximately 1 mile after Witches Gulch on the left is Rood's Glen, another pretty slot canyon into which you can turn. The nice thing about Rood's Glen is that the tour boats don't go down here, so it's a pleasant oasis for paddlers. (In fact, I've never seen any motorboats down here.) As the name implies, it's a lovely glen and particularly becoming in spring. That said, the huge Chula Vista Resort looms in the foreground.

Exiting the glen, Steamboat Island is the next attraction in the main channel. It's visually deceptive in that it looks like another canyon detour due to the bend in the river. Paddle to the left of the island where a narrow channel permits. In spring, water seeping over the stratified rocks on the left bank marks a contrast to the attractive hemlocks atop the cliffs.

On the opposite bank soon after Steamboat Island is an inconspicuous cave through which you can just barely paddle. Again, it's a novelty experience at best. Look for stratified sheets of rocky shoreline about 7 feet high on the right bank on a diagonal angle. You'll eventually see the entrance to the "cave"; the exit is 15 feet or so downstream underneath a tree. One more side canyon can be slipped into on the left, at Coldwater Canyon, another gorgeous oasis of lush green and otherworldly ferns with sandstone. Here, the gangplank will be on your right. All the way at the end, you'll see an old brick building restored mostly for private functions.

(Some 700 feet downstream from the mouth of Coldwater Canyon is yet another side canyon on the left called Artist's Glen. Like Rood's Glen, it's quite lovely and is too narrow and shallow for motorboats, but by now you might have had enough of side canyons.)

Immediately past Coldwater Canyon is the head of Blackhawk Island. If you go right, you'll paddle around the island counterclockwise. The water here is slow but shallow; as a result, the big boats don't use this side channel. Blackhawk Island was

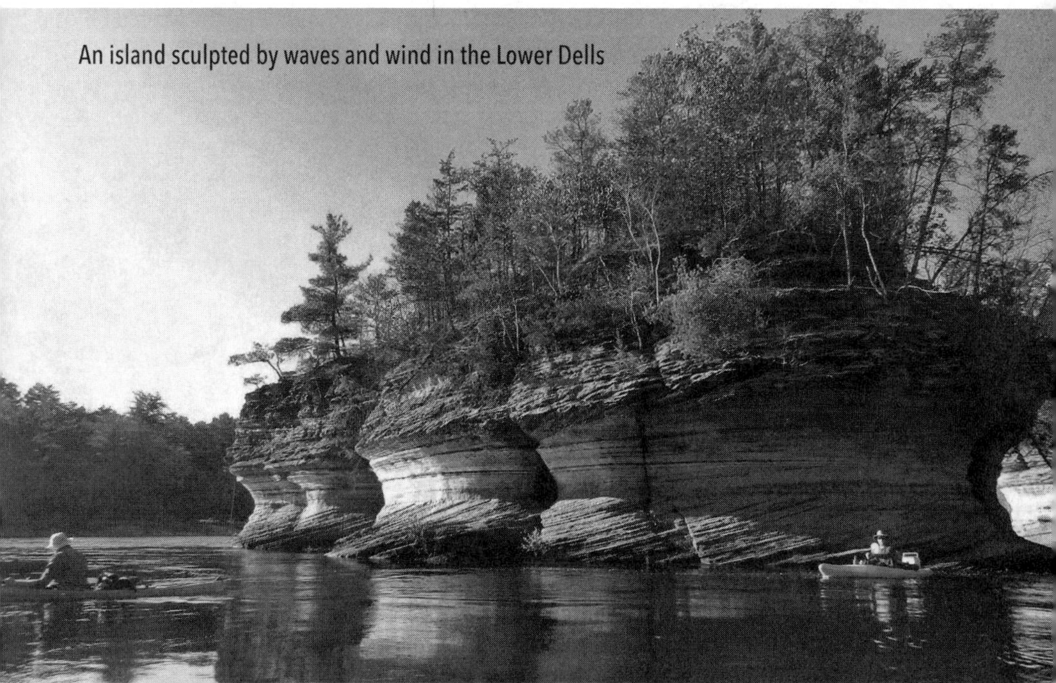

An island sculpted by waves and wind in the Lower Dells

originally part of the shoreline, but it was torn asunder during a cataclysmic flooding event in the last ice age, which scoured the riverbed and created much of the dramatic landscape that we see today. Today it's quite magnificent and offers many picnic spots. Even if you don't turn right into the side channel, the giant island is definitely worth paddling around.

If instead you go left, you'll enter the illustrious Narrows. With the exception of the headwaters of the Wisconsin River below Lac Vieux Desert, nowhere else in its 430 miles is the Wisconsin River so narrow as it is in this spot. Unlike up north, where it's a mix of marsh and forest, here high rocks line the skinny river, creating rollicking waves or, in high water, making weird whirlpools and dangerous eddies.

Historical photographs from the 1800s depict fearless (or foolish) lumbermen on makeshift rafts barreling down churning rapids. Many perished; most were phobic of the Dells. The Narrows can still be squirrelly, but nothing like it once was. Just the same, you do need to pay attention and respect the power of water *(see Planning Advisory, page 294, to learn more about how to manage this section of the trip).*

Where the river abruptly turns to the right—colloquially called Devil's Elbow; in the lumber days it was a formidable bend that dashed many a raft—look to the right on the east face of Blackhawk Island. (If you squint and the light is right, you might discern the worn inscription carved into the sandstone: LEROY GATES, DELLS AND RIVER PILOT, 1849–1858. A colorful character, Leroy Gates was a skilled pilot

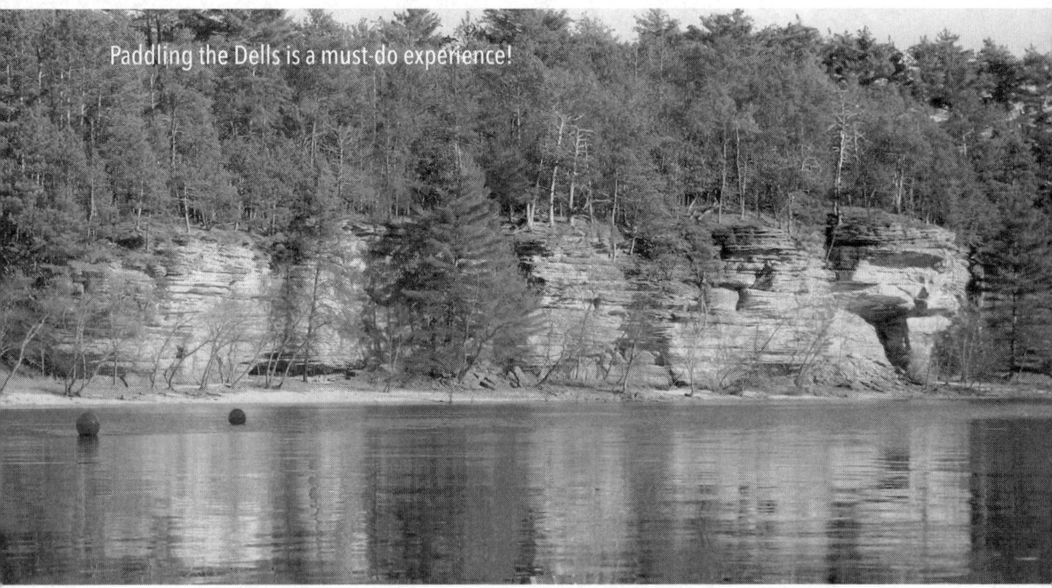
Paddling the Dells is a must-do experience!

guiding logging rafts through the rapids, so the inscription can be seen as the first act of vandalism in the name of vain posterity or simply the first act of commercial advertising in the Dells.)

After this, the river widens again. On the left is an especially pleasant beach that makes for a great place to picnic or just stretch your legs. On your right is the southeastern face of Blackhawk Island, which is stunning. Circumnavigate Blackhawk Island clockwise or continue downstream. On your left, a naturally chiseled rock can look like a face in profile. Two more geological landmarks remain in the Upper Dells: Chimney Rock and the Jaws. First comes Chimney Rock, on the left, a solitary spire more or less looking like a chimney. Just downstream are the more impressive Jaws, two sandstone promontories where the river again narrows; below these, the river is 120 feet deep.

Past the Jaws, the river swells to several hundred feet wide again, while the first signs of town can be seen on the left. The river swings to the right though, toward downtown. Follow it, and don't be lured into the bay. After Crandall's Bay, you'll pass under two bridges, the first of which is a double-decker railroad bridge. You'll also begin to see a whole lot of kitsch poking out here and there, whether miniature golf or touristy chintz. That such squalid commercialism and tackiness exist cheek-by-jowl with such extraordinary natural beauty is one of the oddities of Wisconsin Dells indeed, but not at all accidental.

After the second bridge, you'll see signs telling you to take out on the left-hand side, past which are orange buoys signaling the Kilbourn Dam. The take-out, undeveloped but adequate, leads you up a rough trail uphill. Once at the top, you have to portage through a parking lot to the trail leading to the put-in below the dam. The schlep is short, but the trail leading back down to the river, while quite pretty (unless littered), can be tricky for some, as it's steep and can be slippery. The descent is only 50 feet or so. It's absolutely worth the minor inconvenience, which you'll recognize immediately at the bottom, when you first take in the huge, beautiful sandy beach surrounded by undulating sandstone bluffs and root beer–hued water. Despite being so close to the dam and to downtown, the beach remains surprisingly secluded. Have a picnic here, go for a swim, hike along the rocky bluffs, or cast a line. You should savor this spot before putting back in.

Spoiler alert: The magnificent geology of the Dells does not go on forever. Below the dam, the spectacular rock features last for only another 2.5 miles (the take-out is 5.7 miles from here), so savor your time on the river.

Paddling upstream a smidge to see the dam is worth your while, but caution is critical: The current will be very strong. Moving on downstream, the river is wide, but the scenery remains spectacular, with another palisade of colossal sandstone bluffs lining the shoreline left and right. Soon you'll you see a private resort on the right and the mouth of Dell Creek. (Less than a half mile upstream of Dell Creek is Lake Delton, which drained into the Wisconsin River in 2008 during high-rain floods that breached the dam.) Just past this is the official USGS gage, which also notes the high-water mark on the river, which was back in 1938 when the river rose 17 feet. The best section of the Lower Dells comes next.

On the right is a large island with sinuously rippled sandstone layers called Sugar Bowl. To the right of Sugar Bowl is Grotto Rock, an equally yet uniquely gorgeous bit of geology where a fissure in the rock allows for canoes to pass inside and through, a thrilling experience. (There's a house on top of Grotto Rock, but once you're at the rock itself, the view is unspoiled.) After you pass through the cool cave, head over to the left shore to Lone Rock, an even larger island crowned with pine trees. The swirling lines of sandstone layers are just exquisite. Alas, the scenic splendor of the Dells ends here.

The good news is that the river remains lovely for the next 3 miles; wooded hills in the background still catch the eye. It will get wider and shallower, and large sandbar islands will begin in earnest. In fact, this marks the last phase of the Wisconsin River's basin; sandbars, rolling hills, and smooth water will frame the environment from here to its confluence at the Mississippi River, 130 miles downstream, a remarkable difference from its highland character 300 miles upstream.

After a sharp but long right-hand turn and one last woody hill on the left, the take-out will appear on the left rather modestly, so be sure to watch for it. It's an official boat launch, and taking out is a breeze. If you time your take-out just right, sunset here can be positively lovely.

•THE•FUDGE•

ADDITIONAL TRIPS You could put in upstream at the Two Rivers boat landing, one of the prettiest places to begin a trip anywhere in Wisconsin, but you will be adding 6 miles to this trip, which would make for a long day. And while 16-plus miles on the steady current of the Wisconsin River is not that crazy for a day of paddling, you do not want to rush through this trip; there are so many detours and diversions of jaw-dropping delight that demand your attention and reward dawdling.

CAMPING **Mirror Lake State Park** (E10320 Fern Dell Road, about 10 miles northwest of Baraboo; 608-254-2333) and **Rocky Arbor State Park** (WI 12/WI 16; 608-254-8001)

RENTALS **River's Edge Resort** (20 River's Edge Road, off CR A, Wisconsin Dells; 608-254-7707 or 608-254-6494), **Dells Watersports** (255 Wisconsin Dells Parkway S., Wisconsin Dells; 608-254-8702), and **Holiday Shores Watersports** (3901 River Road, Wisconsin Dells; 608-254-2878)

FOOD FOR THOUGHT There is no shortage of eateries in the Dells. The **Pizza Pub** (1455 Wisconsin Dells Parkway; 608-254-7877) and **Monk's Bar & Grill** (220 Broadway; 608-254-2955) are regular standbys. But for something entirely different, check out the **Cheeze Factory Restaurant** (521 Wisconsin Dells Parkway; 608-253-6065), a 100% vegan, non-GMO establishment. The food is incredible.

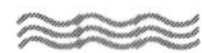

59 Wisconsin River B:
PRAIRIE DU SAC DAM TO SPRING GREEN

•THE•FACTS•

Put-in/take-out Below the dam in Prairie du Sac off Dam Road/WI 23 bridge in Spring Green. See "The Flavor" for two additional access points.

Distance/time 25.5 mi/Allow for 2 or even 3 days

Gradient/water level 2 fpm/Water is always plentiful, though in high water you will find fewer sandbars to camp on. Stay off the river during floods or thunderstorms. Consult USGS gage 05407000. Look for 4,500–10,000 cfs on the gage. Below 4,500 cfs, the river becomes shallow, but above 10,000 cfs, some of the sandbars will be under water.

Water type Quietwater

Canoe or kayak Either

Skill level Beginner

Time of year to paddle Anytime, though it will be busiest in summer

Landscape Wooded bluffs, sandbars, bottomlands, prairies

OVERVIEW The beginning of the end of the Wisconsin River, this overnight trip offers the best of the best on the river's final 92 miles before its confluence at the Mississippi River. You'll see beautiful wooded bluffs, endless sandbar islands, protected public land, oak barrens, swamps, prairies, 300-foot cliffs, cactus deserts, and a whole lot

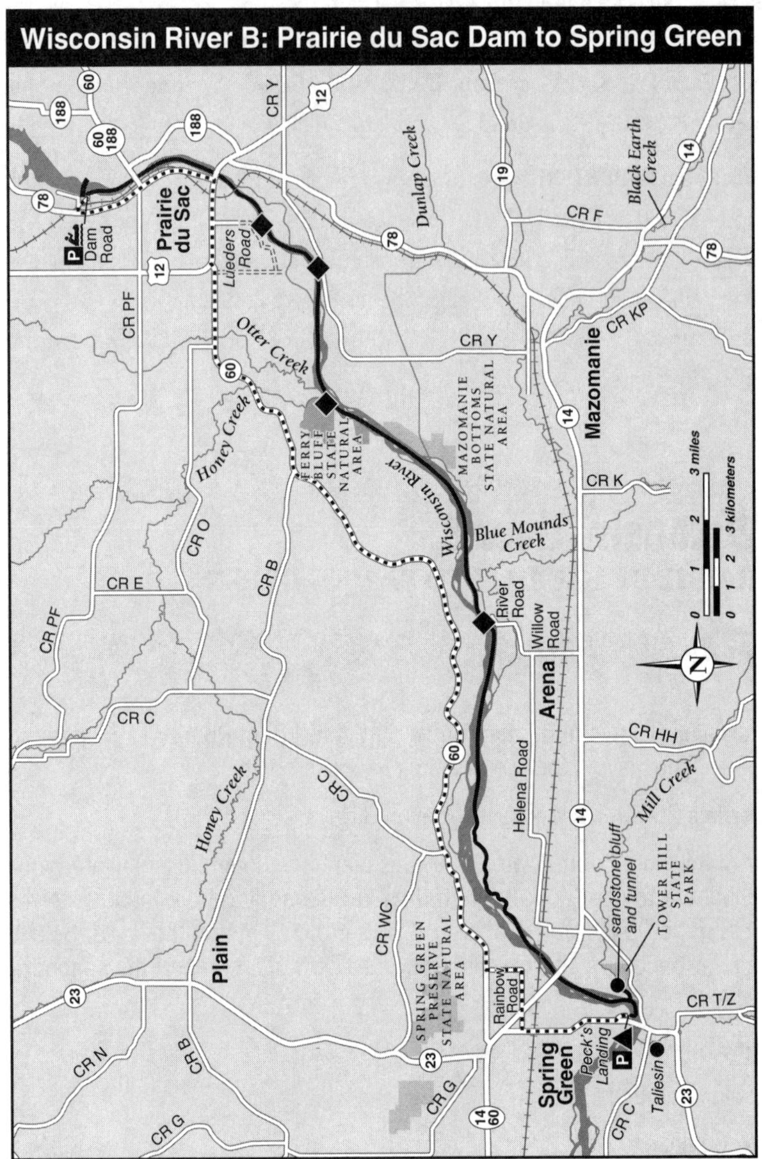

Wisconsin River B: Prairie du Sac Dam to Spring Green

of human history along the way—plus bald eagles, sandhill cranes, turkey vultures, turtles, woodpeckers, songbirds, clams, all sorts of fish and ducks, and deer.

SHUTTLE **27 miles.** From the take-out, turn right onto WI 23 and head north. After the railroads tracks. turn right onto Rainbow Road and head straight across US 14. Turn right onto WI 60, which you'll be on for most of the shuttle—a truly lovely drive. Turn right onto US 12. In town, turn left onto WI 78 into and past Prairie du Sac. Finally, turn right onto Dam Heights Road, then take a quick right onto Dam Road.

TAKE-OUT N43° 08.783' W90° 03.599' **PUT-IN** N43° 18.528' W89° 43.689'

•THE•FLAVOR•

PUT IN BELOW THE DAM, safely away from any discharge current. From this point forward, there are no more obstructions on the Wisconsin River, a notable exception to the rule on the "hardest working river in America" where a total of 26 dams dot the river's 430 miles. It's one of the longest, best-preserved free-flowing rivers anywhere in America.

The setting is beautiful from the get-go. The river is at its widest just below the dam, but the hilly bluffs will prevail for this entire trip. After the WI 60 bridge, there will be buildings on the right, but only briefly. Atop a hill on the left is the award-winning Wollersheim Winery, founded by a Hungarian immigrant in the 1840s (well worth a stop before or after this trip, but remember that glass is strictly prohibited on the river).

On the right is a public park named after native son and famed writer August Derleth, a literary lion whose colorful characters were often based on folks in Sauk City and along the river. There are small parcels of development on both sides of the river below the US 12 bridge, but again only briefly. Shortly downstream from US 12 is a railroad bridge where you want to stay as close to the right as you can; strong (and strange) whirlpools form here that can be dangerous. After this, you can relax and enjoy the wild and wonderful landscape that continues all the way to the take-out.

Half a mile down from the railroad bridge is an inconspicuous landing on the right off Lueders Road (**N43° 15.377' W89° 44.522'**). This is an excellent access that, if used, shaves off 4 miles of this trip. The entire left shore is undeveloped public land. After the mouth of Roxbury Creek on the left are the Mazomanie Oak Barrens. Beyond that, amidst two hills, is the site of the Battle of Wisconsin Heights, the penultimate scrimmage between Chief Black Hawk and the US Army in 1832. The landscape will be momentarily low, but sandbar islands braid the main channel. On your left will be a large boat launch off County Road Y (**N43° 14.338' W89° 45.517'**), another excellent access (there's a $5 fee).

On your left, you'll see a few cabins and then, on one of the small islands, is an eagle's nest that has been home to a single pair for several years. After the big river begins to bend to the left, you'll see a beautiful bluff looming 300 feet above the water. This is Ferry Bluff, a protected state natural area. Bald eagles nest here, which makes it off-limits to the public from November to April. But I positively insist that you explore this when it's open. A strenuous but rewarding trail takes you all the way to the top, where the view is unparalleled. The vista takes in the entire Wisconsin River valley, including Blue Mound, the highest point in southern Wisconsin, some 30 miles away. Turn into the mouth of Honey Creek on the right and paddle upstream 50 yards to a make-do landing on the left, above which is the trailhead.

Two more equally tall bluffs line the right shore after Ferry Bluff. As the river heads south, you'll pass countless sandbars, small islands, and beaches. (One of these beaches, on the left, the infamous clothing-optional "Mazo Beach," was closed by the state in the spring of 2016.) The next few miles are smooth sailing. The right shore remains bluff lined and lovely, while the left is home to the Mazomanie Bottoms, a floodplain forest with a Southern-swamp feel, accessible only in high water—rich in sloughs, ephemeral pools, draping vines, and migratory birds.

The river bends to the right and threads its way through more big islands. When choosing which to camp out on, make sure you find one that's at least a couple feet above the waterline. Rainfall from upriver or releases from the dam can raise the water in a matter of mere hours. I've twice been caught on the river camping during flash thunderstorms. The first time our party nearly lost a canoe because it hadn't been dragged high enough; the second time the water came within 2 feet of my tent. Just be smart and you'll have an unforgettable time. These sandbar islands are an absolute treasure and part of our heritage, but they do receive a lot of traffic, so please tread lightly and leave no trace.

For a short span, you'll see a few cabins on the left shore announcing the Arena boat launch (located slightly behind an island). On the right shore, a bluff named Sleeping Lion hovers above the river. Below the boat landing are two large islands on the left. If you hug the left channel, you can paddle up the mouth of Blue Mound Creek (which enters the river on the left), but it's interesting only as a novelty detour.

Wooded bluffs, sandbars, and small islands continue to call the shots, though this next segment toward Spring Green feels a little less wild than upstream. Behind the tree line on the left, where there used to be prairies, are miles and miles of agricultural fields. It's a huge operation that fortunately can't be seen from the river, but you might hear machinery. Behind all that is the site of Lake Louie Brewing Company in Arena, which makes great local ale. Two miles downstream is a huge long island with a narrow side channel to the far left that you can enter if the water is high enough. It will be slower and shallower, of course, but it's a fun excursion for variety.

As the river bends to the left in earnest, you'll enter a low-lying valley. Tall bluffs are still present on the right, but now they're in the background. Of particular interest is the sand prairie bluff at Spring Green Preserve, another state natural area protected by the good people at The Nature Conservancy. Nicknamed "Wisconsin's Desert," this bluff has a surface temperature that often exceeds 140°F and nurtures flora such as the prairie flameflower and prickly pear cactus, as well as three types of lizards, gophers, snakes, and wolf spiders. It's a few miles from the river, but absolutely worth checking out on a different occasion, perhaps during your shuttle.

After a few more long islands, you'll come upon a railroad bridge, the first structure spanning the river since the railroad bridge with the squirrelly current below Sauk City.

Half a mile downstream is the modern but mundane US 14 bridge. Keep to the left side of the river. Below the bridge and before the take-out, this mini-odyssey has 2 final miles steeped in rich history. The river heads directly south and seems to bounce off a bluff, ricocheting its course northwest in a horseshoe shape. As it bends to the right, look for the mouth of Mill Creek on the left; it's fairly wide and easy to spot. Paddle up the creek for half a mile (there's no current, so it's easy to do). You'll pass a few basic but pleasant campsites as well as a boat launch on your right, indicating that you are now inside the small but significant Tower Hill State Park.

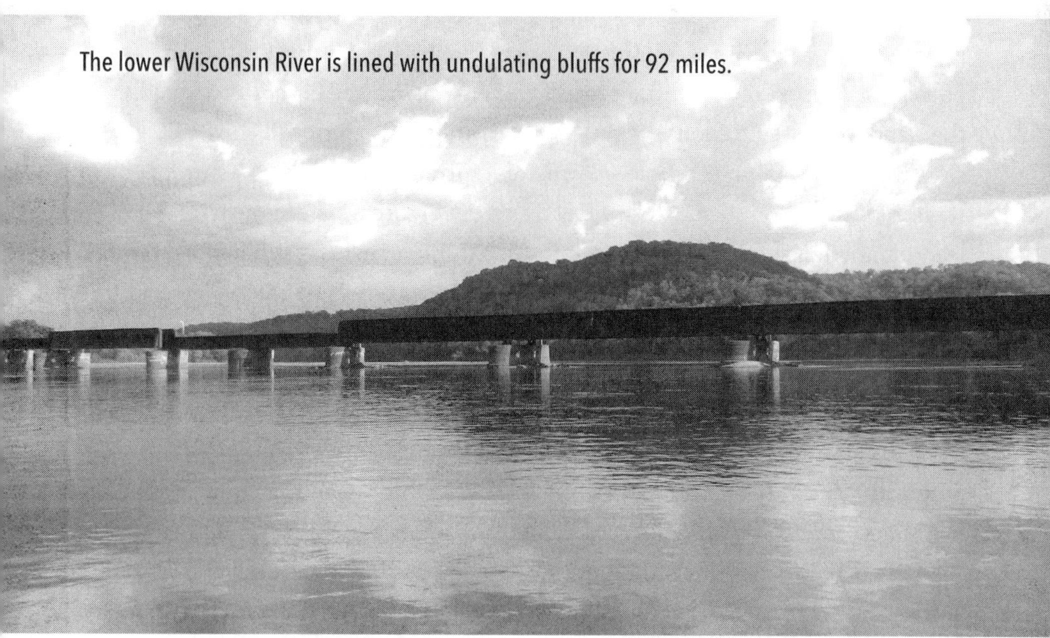

The lower Wisconsin River is lined with undulating bluffs for 92 miles.

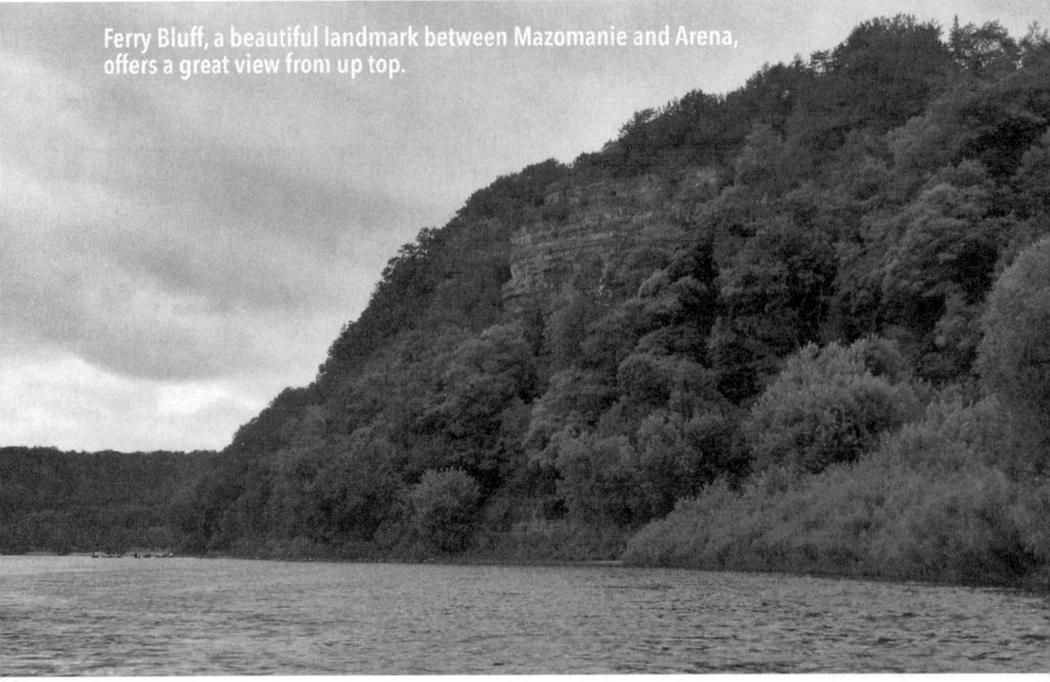
Ferry Bluff, a beautiful landmark between Mazomanie and Arena, offers a great view from up top.

Soon, on your right, will be a long wall of gorgeous sandstone 40 feet high, comparable to the Dells upstream. Immediately after it is a hand-dug tunnel that was part of the lead-shot manufacturing process of Wisconsin Shot Company. Directly above the hand-excavated tunnel is a 120-foot vertical shaft, above which is a 60-foot-tall shot tower atop the bluff. Lead was melted, mixed with arsenic, and dropped from the top of the tower, through the shaft, and down into a cistern of water below. The lead rounded in shape during the precipitous fall and cooled and hardened once submerged in water. Workers collected the shot and transferred it along railroad tracks out of the tunnel to be processed in buildings once present along the creek. A six-man crew could produce as many as 5,000 pounds of shot daily.

Leaving Mill Creek, the Wisconsin River bends to the right toward the wide bridge at WI 23. On the left is the Frank Lloyd Wright Visitor Center. There are more buildings designed by the brilliant architect per capita in Spring Green than anywhere else; he lived here for many years and was born and raised in nearby Richland Center. Just over the bridge, but indiscernible from the river, is the home Wright designed for himself: Taliesen, or "shining brow" in Welsh, an incredible work of art unto itself. Before you leave, take a moment at least to drive past the property, though paying for the tour is even better. Cross over to the right shore of the river; the take-out is on the right, just upstream of the bridge. This is a beautiful setting, perfect for a quick swim or picnic. A park is connected to the boat landing, and you'll find bathrooms and trash cans as well.

•THE•FUDGE•

ADDITIONAL TRIPS Upstream of the dam is the huge impoundment of **Lake Wisconsin,** where the wind is fierce and motorboats rule. A 7-mile trip begins at Dekorra and finishes in Whalen Bay, but there's a lot of shoreline development, the interstate highway bridge, and a few miles of lake paddling. There are some nice islands and outcrops, however.

CAMPING You may not camp along the shoreline, but all the sandbar islands are open to the public. Additionally, some pleasant campsites can be found along Mill Creek at **Tower Hill State Park** (5808 CR C, Spring Green; 608-588-2116).

RENTALS **Wisconsin Canoe Company** (608-432-5058, thebestcanoecompanyever.com), **Wisconsin Riverside Resort** (S13220 Shifflet Road, Spring Green; 608-588-2826), and **Wisconsin River Outings** (7554 US 12, Sauk City; 608-375-5300)

FOOD FOR THOUGHT Try **Blue Spoon Café** (550 Water St., Prairie du Sac; 608-643-0877); the **Woodshed Ale House** (101 Jackson St., Sauk City; 608-370-8200); or **Arena Cheese** (300 US 14, Arena; 608-753-2501), where fresh curds are made daily on premises. Consider as well **Spring Green General Store** (137 S. Albany St., Spring Green; 608-588-7070) and **Prem Meats** (E5028 US 14, Spring Green; 608-588-2164).

SHOUT-OUTS To get to **Spring Green Preserve** (springgreen.com/tower-hill-state-park) from Spring Green, take WI 23 north to Jones Road, turn right, and drive 0.75 mile. Turn left onto Angelo Lane to the parking area. Also consider a visit to the **Frank Lloyd Wright Visitor Center** (5607 CR C, Spring Green; 608-588-7090, taliesinpreservation.org).

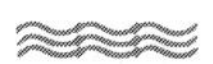

60 Wisconsin River C: LONE ROCK TO BLUE RIVER

•THE•FACTS•

Put-in/take-out Lone Rock boat landing at Otter Creek/County Road T on Coumbe Island in Blue River

Distance/time 21.7 mi/Allow for overnight trip

Gradient/water level 2 fpm/Water is always plentiful, though in high water you will find fewer sandbars to camp on. Stay off the river during floods or thunderstorms. Consult USGS gage 05407000. Look for 4,500–10,000 cfs on the gage. Below 4,500 cfs, the river becomes shallow, but above 10,000 cfs, some of the sandbars will be under water.

Water type Quietwater

Canoe or kayak Either

Skill level Beginner

Time of year to paddle Anytime

Landscape Wooded bluffs, sandbars, limestone rock outcrops, prairie savanna, pine barrens, sand dunes

---

OVERVIEW On this simply wonderful stretch of the Lower Wisconsin State Riverway, which is more isolated and less crowded than the previous trip, you will pass thrilling geological features, quaint towns, wonderful bluffs, and splendid sandbar islands. Look for bald eagles, sandhill cranes, turkey vultures, dragonflies, turtles, and various fish.

SHUTTLE **21.2 miles.** To find the take-out, travel north on CR T from Blue River and onto the bridge going across the river. The landing itself is on an island in the middle of the river (pretty cool, right?). As soon as you cross onto the island, you'll see a turnoff on your left to the boat landing. For the shuttle to the put-in from here, turn left onto CR T and follow it into town. Turn left onto WI 133 into Muscoda. (**Blue River Sand Barrens State Natural Area**, a microdesert with prickly pear cactus and roving sand dunes, is worth a quick look-see. Turn left onto Wightman Road from WI 133 at 2 miles from town.) Follow signs for WI 133 as the road doglegs right, then left. Follow WI 133 into and past Avoca. Stay straight where the road turns left to the big bridge. After a right-hand bend, you'll see the parking area and boat launch, on the left.

TAKE-OUT N43° 12.038' W90° 34.316' **PUT-IN** N43° 09.523' W90° 11.263'

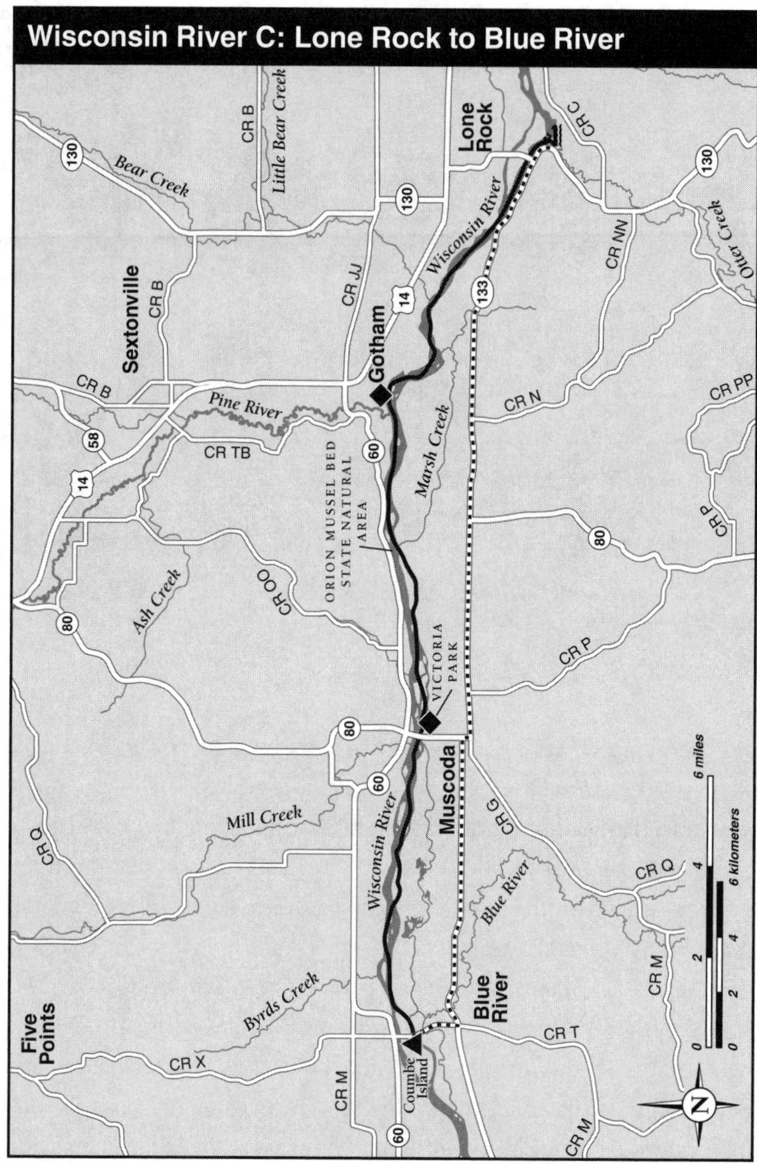

•THE•FLAVOR•

I CONTEND THAT THERE IS NOTHING, absolutely nothing, half as fun as canoe camping, particularly on the Lower Wisconsin River. Everything you need for food, shelter, clothing, and fun is in your boat, and you share it with a fellow sojourner. The river is magnificent. At sunrise, all the world's a soft hue of lavender-orange above the misty

The Lone Rock-to-Muscoda section has several beautiful rock outcrops.

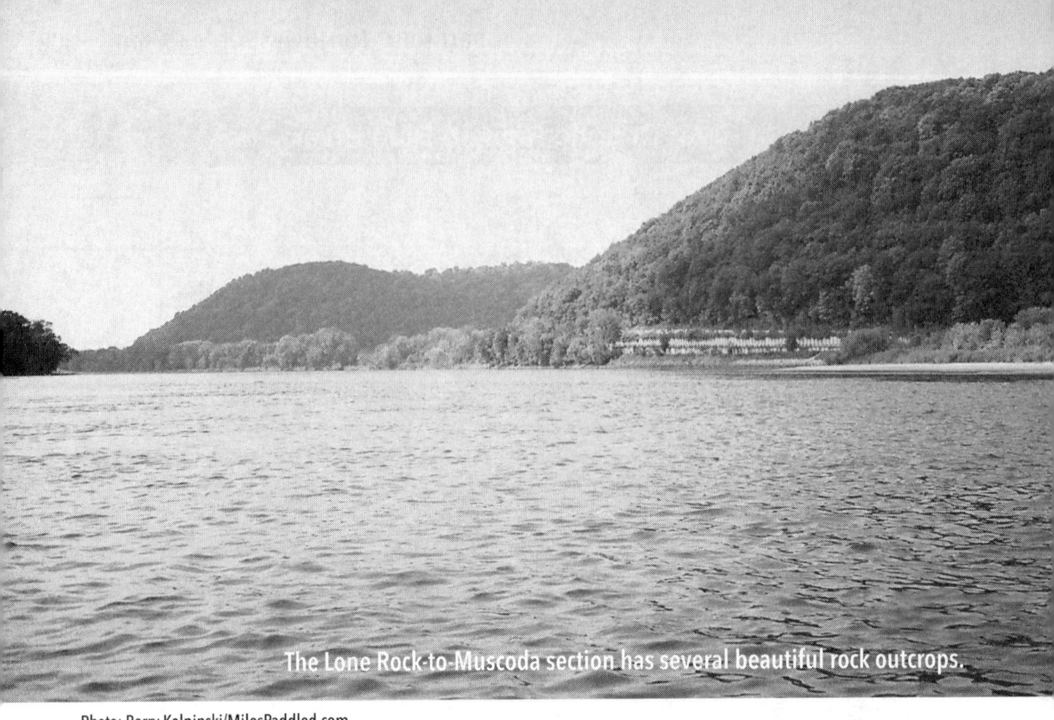

Photo: Barry Kalpinski/MilesPaddled.com

bluffs, and there's a rich stillness interrupted only by a pair of cranes bugling their trumpet cry. In a breathtaking but melancholy fog at dusk, or in a white-knuckles thunderstorm in the dead of night, or simply floating along on a lazy, hazy summer afternoon, it's just the most wonderful kind of paddling and camping I can think of. If you have never camped on the river, please do so, at least once, at least one night. But a weeklong journey is even better!

Put in at the boat landing at the mouth of Otter Creek off of WI 130 on the south bank of the river. There's plenty of parking. The river will appear surprisingly narrow here (that is, if you consider 500 feet to be narrow) due to that huge and aptly named Long Island, situated in the middle of the river. As you paddle around the gentle left bend, you'll be rewarded with marvelous views of exposed limestone. Such a rock wall is a rarity along the Lower Wisconsin in general, but on this trip, you'll see several. The antiquated bridge at WI 133 comes into view next, spanning no fewer than three separate channels of the river.

After the tip of Long Island, the river resumes its usual width of roughly 900 feet. Head on over to the right shore to take advantage of a fun side channel that passes along the southern boundary of Smith Slough and Sand Prairie, a protected state natural area that features an old oxbow lake, oak savannas, and sand dunes.

After returning to the main stream, you'll pass under a huge railroad bridge. Look for bald eagles in the trees. Incidentally, the coldest temperature ever recorded in Wisconsin was here in Lone Rock, at –53°F in January 1951. (The warmest recorded temperature, you ask? Also on the Wisconsin River, at the Dells, in July of 1936, when the mercury climbed to 114°F.)

After the mouth of Bear Creek on the right, the river takes a long S-curve first left, then right. Shortly thereafter, you'll pass some very pretty sand terraces on the right that signal the Gotham Jack Pine Barrens State Natural Area. Rich in such plant species as goat's rue and prairie coreopsis, this small oasis is a pretty tapestry of oxbow sloughs, sedge meadows, pine barrens, and dunes, today recovering from the overgrazing of yesteryear. The river will next make another big left turn. Look for the mouth of the Pine River on the right.

In the long straightaway that follows, the entire left shore will be dominated by the Avoca Prairie and Savanna State Natural Area. At 1,885 acres, Avoca is home to the single largest tallgrass prairie east of the Mississippi River and provides habitat for the endangered Blanding's turtle as well as the rare red-shouldered hawk and short-eared owl. Ephemeral wetland swales mix with sandy ridges and bur oaks in a landscape so unspoiled it appears pretty much as it did when Europeans first traveled down the river.

Rising more than 200 feet above the river, you'll see Bogus Bluff on the right, accentuated by a flash of exposed limestone, one of innumerable bluffs along the lower Wisconsin luring rumors of buried treasure or hideaways for fugitives and gangs. After this will be a more modest but still attractive sandstone wall on the right, much of it punctuated with swallows' nests. Soon you'll pass a quaint red cabin, also on the right, that reads OLD MAN RIVER. Stay to the right, where bluffs and WI 60 hug the shore. For about 3 miles now, the Orion Mussel Bed State Natural Area protects the particular habitat of rare species of mussel, invertebrates, and fish along the riverbed and shoreline here. Unlike the predominant sandy bottom of the Lower Wisconsin River, in this unique interval, the bottom is composed of rock and gravel substrate together with underwater sandstone ledges. (Look but don't take!)

Two quarter-mile-long islands appear in the middle and right before a much longer island on the left. Keep to the right shore. Where there are a few small islands past the long one, you'll see a boat landing on the right. Stop here for a moment to take a short walk (about a half mile there and back) to see some of the best-preserved effigy mounds anywhere in Wisconsin. Over a thousand years old, there are 15 total mounds depicting birds, bears, and lizards. To find them, walk north from the boat landing, west on Ginger Road, then continue west of Aigner Lane.

Back on the river, head toward the left and thread your way through a cluster of islands. Take a while to explore the back channels here. They provide shady relief on a hot day, plus there's a primitive privacy thanks to a lack of motorboat traffic here. On your left will be a large boat landing at Victoria Park in Muscoda (pronounced MUS-ka-day). From there to town, it's a 1-mile walk if you need supplies. Or, for something completely different, if you happen to be here on a weekend in mid-May, you can time your trip to coincide with the Morel Mushroom Festival, a festive celebration of edible fungus that's been going on for more than 30 years. If you've never sampled a morel and want neither to forage for them in the wild nor pay $30 a pound for them in a store, here's your opportunity, along with a small-town parade and beer tent to boot.

From Muscoda to the take-out are 7 easy miles along a straightaway, though this stretch is by no means boring. There is zero development along the left shore and hardly any on the right shore. Beautiful sandbars, lots of islands, and wooded bluffs undulate toward the distant horizon in a near-wilderness choreography. Sure, there are roads, bridges, and towns here and there, but they're more like the margins of a page in a book, there to structure the story, not detract from it. There are fewer highlights or salient features between Muscoda and Blue River compared to upstream; instead, here, you may wish simply to stop looking for or thinking about specific parts and rather soak in the whole in its impeccable simplicity. Depending on the water level, wind direction, and your own stamina, you may well reach the take-out in less than 2 hours.

To locate the take-out—you don't want to pass it by!—it's best to stay nearer the left shore. Although the river has been mostly straight since Muscoda, it does veer to the southwest (left) toward Blue River. If you can see the CR T bridge straddling a huge island, then you'll be all set. Follow the left channel to paddle along the southern edge of huge Coumbe Island. The landing is at the bridge on the island, on the down-stream side on the right.

•THE•FUDGE•

ADDITIONAL TRIPS You can add 7.1 miles by starting in Spring Green at the WI 23 landing, but it's a less attractive stretch of the river.

For a fun alternative, you can circumnavigate a fun side channel to the left of the take-out as long as the water is high enough. This slough adds 6 miles, and you can expect there to be little to no current. It makes

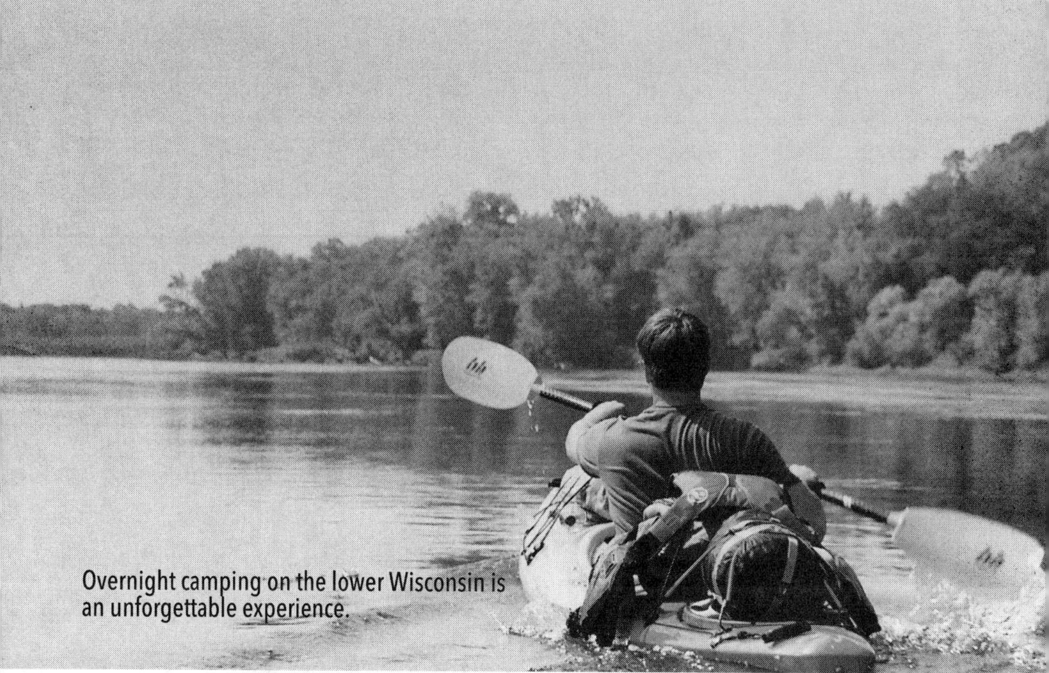
Overnight camping on the lower Wisconsin is an unforgettable experience.

Photo: Barry Kalpinski/MilesPaddled.com

for a unique adjunct trip all its own or added to this one if you're feeling ambitious. I recommend paddling it counterclockwise to avoid paddling upstream the main channel to the take-out.

While there are some 36 more miles of the Wisconsin River before its confluence with the Mississippi River, they lie beyond the circumferential jurisdiction of this book, alas.

CAMPING You may not camp along the shoreline, but all the sandbar islands are open to the public. Additionally, you may camp at **Victoria Park** (608-739-2924), along the river in Muscoda.

RENTALS **Eagle Cave** (16320 Cavern Lane, Blue River; 608-537-2988), **River View Hills Canoe Rental** (24678 WI 60, Orion; 608-739-3472), **Wisconsin Canoe Company** (608-432-5058, thebestcanoecompanyever.com), and **Wisconsin Riverside Resort** (S13220 Shifflet Road, Spring Green; 608-588-2826)

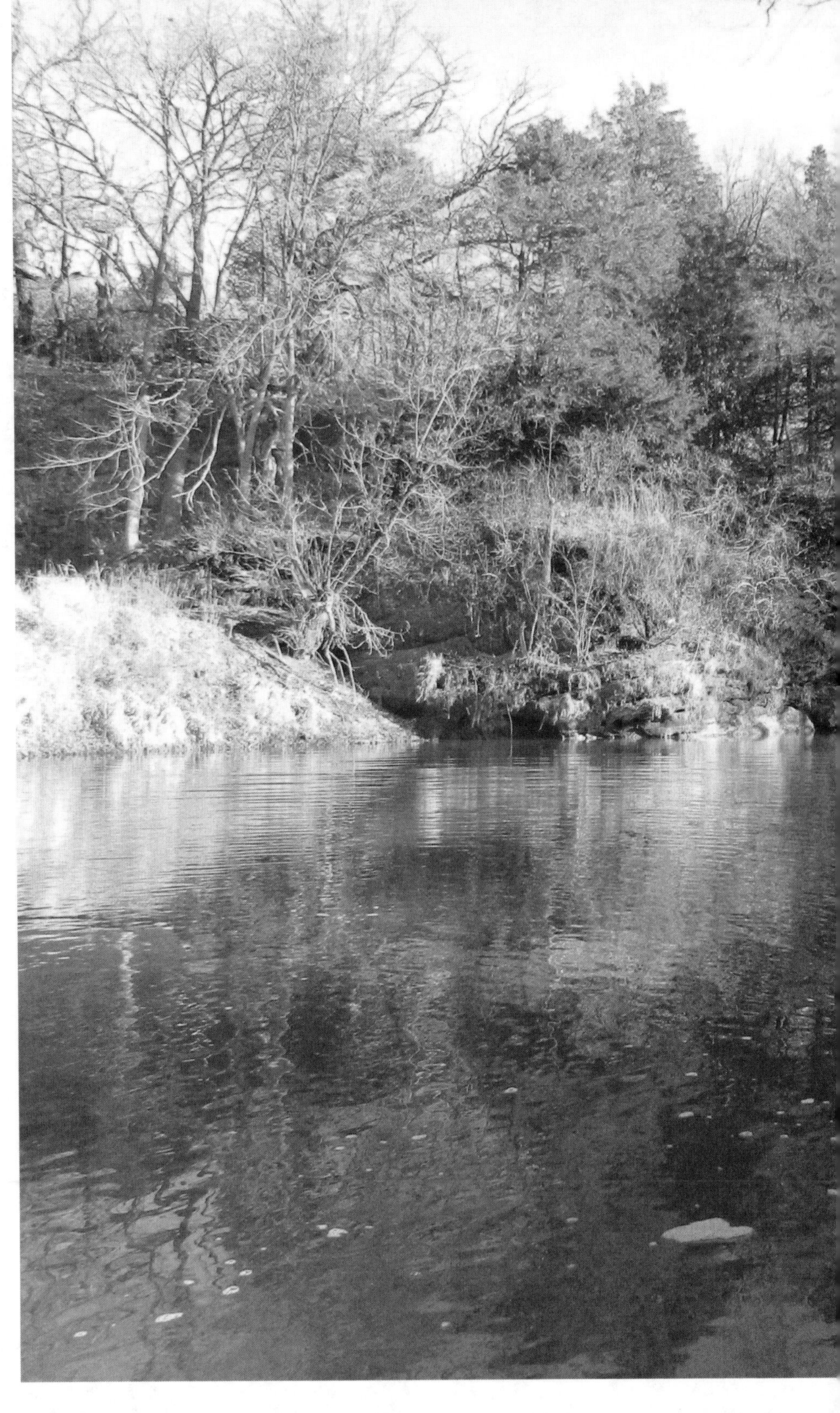

Appendixes

OPPOSITE: Approaching sandstone rock outcrops on the Pecatonica River
(see Trips 36 and 37, pages 190 and 195)

APPENDIX A: Madison Metropolitan Area Trips

Lake Waubesa Wetlands State Natural Area (Fitchburg)

Accessible via Goodland County Park, off Waubesa Avenue and Goodland Park Road in the southwest corner of Lake Waubesa

WAUBESA WETLANDS is one of the highest quality and most diverse wetlands remaining in southern Wisconsin. Nine major springs and numerous smaller ones located within and around the area provide the wetland with an abundance of high-quality water.

Nine Springs Creek (Madison)

Accessible via Syene Road and Moorland Road or Lottes Lane

A NATURAL SPRING bubbling up in between Madison and Verona, the creek features attractive clear water and a very gentle current, and is surrounded by a vast network of public land and trails in a landscape featuring small rolling hills and oak savannas. There are several accesses along the creek, but I recommend launching from Syene Road, which will allow you to see springs but spare you some portaging. The creek is entirely straight, narrow, and channelized, and the long tunnel bridge at US 12 has a very low clearance and is not for the claustrophobic. Take out at the Nine Springs E-Way trailhead on Moorland Road, or continue into Upper Mud Lake and Lake Waubesa via Lottes Lane just north of the beltline.

Pheasant Branch Conservatory (Middleton)

Accessible via Deming Way just west of US 14 or Century Avenue

THIS CREEK HAS TWO BRANCHES: one from the west that tumbles through a mini-gorge along a beautiful dedicated bike/pedestrian path; the other from a hauntingly cool, gurgling spring to the north that empties into Lake Mendota.

The west branch will be difficult to catch with enough water, as its drainage basin is very small and the gradient is at least 10 fpm. Look for no less than 20 cfs at USGS gage 05427948. Unless the water is exceptionally high, you'll need to portage around series of concrete blocks crossing the creek. There's a sizable dam at Park Street that you also need to portage. (Portaging in this case means crossing the road with your boat and reentering through some scraggly woods down a steep bank. There's another required portage at Century Avenue due to a nasty logjam.)

If the water is high enough and you don't mind getting a little dirty, you can paddle/tromp your way through wetlands to the other branch, paddle as close to the bubbling springs as you can, then paddle downstream in a circuit. Otherwise, simply paddle upstream the east branch and back.

Sixmile Creek (Waunakee/Westport)

Accessible via Ripp Park off WI 19 and Waunakee Village Park off Main Street

THE FIRST OF THESE TRIPS will be more open and less shallow (for the most part) but louder, due to nearby roads. The second requires considerable water to float without constant scraping. If the water is high enough, there are many delightful ripples and less development than upstream. There is no good take-out or even a place to leave a vehicle at Mill Road, however.

Starkweather Creek

Accessible via the Olbrich Park boat launch, on the near east side of Madison

DUE TO THE NEGLIGIBLE CURRENT, it's easy to paddle upstream on this creek. About half a mile up, it splits in two; if you go right, you'll paddle to WI 30 and not a whole lot farther due to the many obstructions. It's better to go left; you'll pass beneath several bridges and past some low-income housing units. Depending on how much water is in the creek, you can go as far as the Milwaukee Area Technical College campus and a golf course to your left. It's best to do this after rain to help filtrate the creek, which otherwise gets pretty stinky in the summer.

Wingra Creek and Lake Wingra

Accessible at Lake Wingra via Knickerbocker Street boat launch or at the boat launch (for canoes and kayaks only) at Olin-Turville Park on the near south side of Madison

WINGRA CREEK is a pleasant little strip more like a canal than a creek. Everything south of Fish Hatchery Road is developed, but there's a cool railroad tunnel with a tiny riffle. North of Fish Hatchery, the creek becomes more natural (though flanked on one side by a neighborhood and a local hospital). There's a dam between the creek and the lake that in May is flush with muskies.

Lake Wingra is the prettiest and most intimate of Madison's lakes. With the exception of Edgewood College and a small handful of grandfathered houses, the lake is entirely undeveloped and surrounded by the University of Wisconsin Arboretum. It's a pretty and easy circumnavigation of the lake, with excellent wildlife opportunities. (How often do you see a pair of sandhill cranes or a lone great blue heron flying past a sunset sky with the capitol dome in the near background?)

Yahara River Voyageur

Cherokee Marsh to Riverside Street Park

WHAT MADISON LACKS IN STREAMS it more than makes up for in lakes. That said, it's one river, the Yahara, that links all these lakes. If you like lake paddling and/or want a marathon-type day trip, follow the Yahara as it constricts and expands from Madison to Stoughton.

Put in at Cherokee Marsh on Madison's north side and take out at Riverside Street Park in Stoughton. The Yahara will narrow momentarily after the marsh but then blow out at huge Lake Mendota. Enjoy the novelty of going through the locks by being lowered from Lake Mendota down to the Yahara River, where the river pleasantly connects to Lake Monona a mile downstream.

At Lake Waubesa, the setting again is huge. After portaging around one more lock at Babcock County Park, the river narrows some through a residence, widens at Lower Mud Lake, then narrows again through a brief, pretty section. (There's an attractive iron truss bridge here.) At Lake Kegonsa, things get huge again. The river constricts next at LaFollette County Park and meanders through a wetland before more fluctuations in width, narrowing through downtown Stoughton. Take out at the dam at Riverside Street Park for a total trip of 28 miles. Naturally, this trip can be shortened by using alternative access points—Governor Nelson State Park or Lake Kegonsa State Park, Viking County Park, and so on.

MADISON'S BEST BOAT LAUNCHES	
• **Cherokee Marsh** at School Road	• **Lake Wingra** at Vilas Park
• **Lake Mendota** at Burrows Park	• **Murphy Creek** off of Lake Waubesa via Goodland County Park
• **Lake Mendota** at Governor's Island	• **Starkweather Creek** at Olbrich Park
• **Lake Mendota** at Spring Harbor Park	• **Wingra Creek** at Olin-Turville Park
• **Lake Monona** at Esther Beach Park	• **Yahara River** at Paunuck Park
• **Lake Waubesa** at Lottes Park via Mud Lake	• **Yahara River** at Tenney Park

APPENDIX B: Honorable Mentions

THE FOLLOWING PLACES represent unique paddling experiences that, due to their limited range or level of difficulty, do not merit individual trip profiles for the purpose of this book but are nonetheless worthy of at least a brief mention.

Grand River Marsh State Wildlife Area

Just west of Kingston in Marquette County (off County Road H) to the dam at the western edge of the marsh

COMPRISING 7,000 ACRES of marsh, cattail wetland, upland prairie, and oak savanna with only the occasional Amish farm off in a blurry vista, this is a gorgeous, fun, but long trip at 10 miles, half of which is on the wide-open marsh itself. Finding the inlet from the Grand River can be confusing due to the cattail labyrinth, and sometimes the access roads to the dam are closed.

Lake Columbia

County Road J/County Road V in Dekorra, Columbia County

THE WATER ON LAKE COLUMBIA, a surreal pool of superheated water drawn from the Wisconsin River to cool off the machinery at the coal-fired power plant, remains around 70°F–80°F, even in the dead of winter. Due to the extreme temperature differential, on a particularly cold winter day, there will be a curtain of fog constantly hovering above the water. On a windy day, the fog forms beautiful crystalline figures of hoarfrost along the shore. It's a lot of fun and something totally different. A dedicated few paddle here each New Year's Day on what's dubbed the "Fog Bowl." Just dress warmly—you'll love it!

Maunesha River

Elder Lane to East Branch Road in Bristol, Dane County

ONLY 1.7 MILES from put-in to take-out, the river here follows an eccentric path down the middle of US 151, where there's a random and serendipitous wildlife oasis plumb in the median of the state highway. The setting is attractive, if loud, but the darling highlight of this jaunt is a heron rookery where as many as 20 nests are located in the treetops. The problems for the paddler are poor accesses, extremely shallow water, and numerous obstructions. And then there's the ethical dilemma of not disturbing the birds. If you do try your luck on this, paddle it only after a good douse of rain and not until May, after the chicks have hatched.

Menomonee River

Main Street to Arthur Avenue in Menomonee Falls, Waukesha County

THE LONG AND MOSTLY URBAN Menomonee River falls 53 fpm in a half-mile stretch. Yes, that's right; this whitewater run is only half a mile long, but it rates as Class III–IV. As such, only advanced whitewater paddlers should consider this. Unfortunately, it is runnable only after the snow melts in spring or after a strong rain. Look for between 200–400 cfs at USGS gage 04087030.

Skillet Creek/Pewits Nest State Natural Area

Gasser Road to CR W in West Baraboo, Sauk County

TUMBLING 50 FPM and comprising four total drops in a 2-mile span—the last of which is 15 feet high through a steep-walled gorge with nowhere to exit in case of an accident—this Class III–IV creek is extremely dangerous and so should be considered by none other than advanced whitewater paddlers. It's only runnable after considerable snowmelt or torrential rain. If nothing else, at least go for a hike here and enjoy the spectacular scenery.

Spring Creek/Okee Bay

Just north of Lodi, Columbia County

EVEN THOUGH IT CAN BE PRETTY, I don't recommend paddling upstream of WI 113—there are far too many logjams and dangerous wires (barbed and electric). Instead, put in on the creek at the last WI 113 bridge and paddle into Okee Bay during spring or fall migration. This simple 2.3-mile trip offers some of the absolute best bird-watching to be experienced, including, but not limited to, flocks of pelicans, great blue herons, sandhill cranes, bald eagles, mergansers, cormorants, geese, and loons, all on Okee Bay. Alternatively, you can put in and take out at the boat landing on CR V, west of the bridge separating the bay from Lake Wisconsin, to avoid shuttling. Stop by Fitz's on the Lake for a bite or a beer and a great view of the water.

Wisconsin River

Prairie du Sac Dam, Sauk County

FOR WHITEWATER ENTHUSIASTS and novices, Class I–II standing waves to practice on or play in can usually be found just below the dam, depending on the releases. A long eddy forms on the right, allowing for continual clockwise runs.

APPENDIX C: Illinois Trips Within 60 Miles of Madison

Kishwaukee River: Belvidere to the Rock River

See canoethekish.com and winnebagoforest.org/activities/canoeing for specific information on the river segments.

Lake Le-Aqua-Na State Park: Lena

Consult the Illinois Department of Natural Resources (dnr.illinois.gov) for further information.

Pecatonica River: Winslow to Pecatonica

See paddlethepec.com for in-depth descriptions of specific river segments and information on boat launches.

Piscasaw Creek: Chemung to Boone Township

A tributary of the Kishwaukee River, this popular trout-fishing stream also offers a pretty paddle through two pristine natural areas. For more information, contact the McHenry County Conservation District, mccdistrict.org, or the Boone County Conservation District, boonecountyconservationdistrict.org. Also check out the following video on YouTube: tinyurl.com/piscasawcreek.

Yellow Creek: Florence to Freeport

For a detailed trip report, go to milespaddled.com and choose "Yellow Creek (IL)" from the list of links on the right.

APPENDIX D: How to Read USGS and NOAA Water Level (Gage) Data Online

IN "HOW TO USE THIS GUIDE" (page 5), we discussed the importance of seeking out current data about water levels online before proceeding on trips involving the many streams that may require a certain level to ensure a fun and safe day (as opposed to trips on water with fairly consistent levels). Recall that I've provided notations in the gradient/water-level category of "The Facts" for each trip profile regarding whether to seek out water-level data online from the USGS or the NOAA.

Recall as well that the term *water level,* as we've used it in this guide, encompasses data about flow (also called *streamflow* or *discharge* by the USGS) and height. Discharge, measured in cubic feet per second (cfs), indicates how fast the river is flowing past the fixed gage of the agency that installed and tracks it. Generally speaking, the faster a river flows, the higher its cfs reading will be. Usually, a higher cfs reading also means the river has more water in it, thus its height at the gage will also be higher.

The USGS provides separate graphs for discharge and height, while the NOAA provides graphs that measure *stage* in feet and, in some cases in the same graph, *flow,* in cubic feet per second (cfs). Getting to the pages that display this data is fairly straightforward, but evaluating the data once there can be a bit confounding at first, so follow the steps below to begin getting the hang of it—first for the USGS, then for the NOAA.

Interpreting Current USGS Water-Level Data as Reported Online

FIRST, GO TO waterdata.usgs.gov/nwis and click "Current Conditions"; click on the state of Wisconsin on the national map, then click on the state map once more to expand it. Now that you're looking at the state map in a larger format, hover over dots to see the names of the gage locations, and click on the one that correlates to the trip you're considering.

You can also skip the maps and zoom in immediately on the gage in question by typing into your Internet search engine "USGS," followed by the gage number I've supplied in "The Facts."

If you're looking at the state map and its colored dots, know that dot color communicates current levels in the context of past data. A red dot generally indicates a low level compared with the historical average, green dots indicate "normal" levels, blue denotes levels higher than normal, and black alerts viewers that levels are dangerously high. But it's not a good idea to merely read dot color to determine whether levels are safe, because the colors are determined in comparison to past conditions and are also affected by current weather conditions.

As an example, a higher-than-normal level in summer, if conditions are dry, will usually still be lower than a normal level in spring, when the water is up after rain and snowmelt. This is important to keep in mind, because if the dot is dark blue or even black on a July day, it's probably because of recent rain—and for a river with some whitewater, this will indicate a unique opportunity to run the rapids. Conversely, if the dot is green in August, that doesn't mean that there's necessarily enough water to paddle the river without scraping or even taking your boat for a walk.

While dot color and historical readings are helpful, it's the cfs (discharge/flow) number that's most helpful in conjunction with this guide. So click on the dot for the gage on the river in question—or, again, simply type in the USGS gage I've provided. Let's return to our example from the introduction, the Beaver Dam River trip. Water levels for this trip are not reliable for every paddle jaunt, so I've given you the USGS gage number (05425912) and said you should aim for levels between 200 and 300 cfs.

Scroll down to the "Discharge" graph; you'll see a squiggly blue line that may stay steady or rise and fall, as well as a horizontal line of yellow triangles. The blue line indicates the rate of flow/discharge past the gage for the past seven days; the yellow triangles denote the historical average for that calendar day going back several decades. Use the numbers at left to determine whether discharge falls within the cfs range I've recommended.

Interpreting Current NOAA Water-Level Data as Reported Online

IN THE CASE OF some of the trips recommended here, the NOAA website has a gaging station where the USGS does not. For trips where a NOAA notation appears in the gradient/water-level category, you can type into your Internet search engine "NOAA," the name of the river, and the town location to open the hydrograph closest to your planned trip.

These hydrographs report current and predicted data in terms of *stage* (NOAA term for height) or *stage* and *flow* (NOAA term for streamflow or discharge). Hydrograph color-coding in terms of the flood stages is also provided. Other tabs at the top of the page will take you to a list of other gage locations for the same river/stream and data about the probability of levels in the near future.

You can also access the data above by starting at weather.gov and clicking on the blue "Rivers, Lakes, Rainfall" link above the national map. A new national map will appear, and you can navigate to the Wisconsin state map, and hover over the gaging stations indicated by diamonds and dots to access the hydrographs for each. The benefit of this longer route to the data is that you can quickly compare several gage locations at once.

When evaluating water levels in the context of NOAA flood-stage levels, you'll have to use some common sense. If the river is at 6 feet and flood stage is at 18 feet, you'll be fine. But it's probably best to keep off it when it's closer to 18 feet.

APPENDIX E: Paddling Resources

Websites

THE FOLLOWING WEBSITES offer a treasure trove of information for curious paddlers, ranging from documented canoe/kayak trips to gear reviews and how-to tutorials.

AMERICAN CANOE ASSOCIATION americancanoe.org
A national organization requiring membership that promotes all things paddling and offers a vast number of helpful tidbits.

AMERICAN WHITEWATER americanwhitewater.org
A national nonprofit organization whose mission is to conserve and restore whitewater resources while promoting safe opportunities to enjoy them. The website provides tips, warnings, photos, and videos, as well as real-time recommendations about whether water levels are recommended for paddling.

MILES PADDLED milespaddled.com
An online journal by two Wisconsin paddlers—one of whom is the author of this guide—reports on paddling trips in southern Wisconsin, complete with maps, photos, and videos (plus fun extras like gear reviews and favorite beers). Paddlers are encouraged to share their trip experiences through the website.

PADDLING.NET paddling.net
A comprehensive resource to turn to for almost any paddling question.

Paddling Clubs

THE FOLLOWING CLUBS offer trip outings and social gatherings:

HOOFER OUTING CLUB hooferouting.org
Affiliated with the University of Wisconsin–Madison, the Hoofers plan paddling trips throughout the state and even around the country.

MAD CITY PADDLERS madcitypaddlers.org
This Madison-area group offers a wide variety of trips nearby and in neighboring states.

PRAIRIE STATE CANOEISTS prairiestatecanoeists.wildapricot.org
An extensive group that plans trips statewide, as well as in neighboring states for all levels of paddlers.

STATELINE PADDLERS statelinepaddlers.net

A local group of paddlers who primarily cover northern Illinois and southern Wisconsin.

Broad-Based Preservation Groups

MOSTLY MEMBER-SUPPORTED, the following organizations work to preserve resources and promote stewardship.

NATIONAL RESOURCES FOUNDATION OF WISCONSIN wisconservation.org

Helps protect imperiled species and public lands while facilitating outings for citizens to connect with the state's natural places.

RIVER ALLIANCE OF WISCONSIN wisconsinrivers.org

Helps protect, enhance, and restore Wisconsin's rivers and watersheds.

SIERRA CLUB–JOHN MUIR CHAPTER sierraclub.org/wisconsin

The Madison-based local chapter of the national organization that promotes the exploration and protection of wild places while practicing responsible uses of those resources.

Local Preservation Groups

THE FOLLOWING ORGANIZATIONS provide additional resources for promoting and protecting specific bodies of water discussed in trips in this book. Not only do they do fine work such as cleaning up trash and clearing out debris—for which they can always use new volunteers—they also provide maps and opportunities to meet folks and get involved.

BLACK EARTH CREEK WATERSHED ASSOCIATION becwa.org

Protects and conserves the creek's environmental, cultural, and historical resources while fostering community stewardship.

CAPITOL WATER TRAILS capitolwatertrails.org

Promotes stewardship of the waters in the Madison–Dane County area by restoring habitat and clearing out obstructions.

FOX WISCONSIN HERITAGE PARKWAY heritageparkway.org

Highlights conservation along the Fox and Wisconsin Rivers corridor, also plans paddling events and group tours.

GLACIAL HERITAGE AREA glacialheritagearea.org

A network of parks, natural areas and historical and cultural sites, connected to one other by trails and waterways shaped by the last ice age that today promotes recreation and preservation.

LOWER SUGAR RIVER WATERSHED ASSOCIATION lsrwa.org

Dedicated to empowering citizens to be responsible stewards of the land and water resources in the Lower Sugar River Watershed.

ROCK RIVER TRAIL rockrivertrail.com

Encourages recreational use of the Rock River as well as preservation and restoration of its natural and historic attributes.

UPPER SUGAR RIVER WATERSHED ASSOCIATION usrwa.org

Promotes stewardship as well as advocacy of the Sugar River and its environment by encouraging volunteer projects, citizen science monitoring, and community coalitions between landowners and businesses.

In addition, several local groups have created "friends of" certain creeks, rivers, lakes, and state parks, and advocate on behalf of those natural resources, organizing volunteer cleanup days and paddling events as well as sponsoring social gatherings. Some have their own websites and/or Facebook pages. The following is a list of those groups connected to waterways found in this book, but note that new groups are created all the time.

- **Friends of Badfish Creek Watershed** rockrivercoalition.org/chapters/badfish
- **Friends of Cherokee Marsh** cherokeemarsh.org
- **Friends of Devil's Lake State Park** devilslakefriends.org, facebook.com/friendsofdevilslake
- **Friends of the Fox River** friendsofthefoxriver.org
- **Friends of Governor Dodge State Park** friendsofgovdodge.org
- **Friends of the Horicon National Wildlife Refuge** horiconnwrfriends.org
- **Friends of the Mukwonago River** mukwonagoriver.org
- **Friends of the Pecatonica River** tinyurl.com/friendsofthepeck
- **Friends of the Pine River** friendsofthepine.org
- **Friends of the Platte River** platteriverfriends.org
- **Friends of Turtle Creek** friendsofturtlecreek.com
- **Friends of Vernon Marsh** friendsofvernonmarsh.org
- **Friends of the Yahara River** yahárariver.org

APPENDIX F: Safety Code of American Whitewater

Eric Nise, *Safety Chairman*
Charlie Walbridge, *Safety Vice Chairman*
Mark Singleton, *Executive Director*

ADOPTED 1959, REVISED 2005

Introduction

This code has been prepared using the best available information and has been reviewed by a broad cross section of whitewater experts. The code, however, is only a collection of guidelines; attempts to minimize risks should be flexible, not constrained by a rigid set of rules. Varying conditions and group goals may combine with unpredictable circumstances to require alternate procedures. This code is not intended to serve as a standard of care for commercial outfitters or guides.

I. Personal Preparedness and Responsibility

1. Be a competent swimmer, with the ability to handle yourself under water.
2. Wear a life jacket. A snugly fitting vest-type life preserver offers back and shoulder protection as well as the flotation needed to swim safely in whitewater.
3. Wear a solid, correctly fitted helmet when upsets are likely. This is essential in kayaks or covered canoes, and recommended for open canoeists using thigh straps and rafters running steep drops.
4. Do not boat out of control. Your skills should be sufficient to stop or reach shore before reaching danger. Do not enter a rapid unless you are reasonably sure that you can run it safely or swim it without injury.
5. Whitewater rivers contain many hazards that are not always easily recognized. The following are the most frequent killers:
   a. **High water.** The river's speed and power increase tremendously as the flow increases, raising the difficulty of most rapids. Rescue becomes progressively harder as the water rises, adding to the danger. Floating debris and strainers make even an easy rapid quite hazardous. It is often misleading to judge the river level at the put-in, since a small rise in a wide, shallow place will be multiplied many times where the river narrows. Use reliable gauge information whenever possible, and be aware that sun on snowpack, hard rain, and upstream dam releases may greatly increase the flow.
   b. **Cold.** Cold drains your strength and robs you of the ability to make sound decisions on matters affecting your survival. Cold-water immersion, because of the initial shock and the rapid heat loss that follows, is especially dangerous. Dress appropriately for bad weather or sudden immersion in the water. When the water

temperature is less than 50°F, a wetsuit or drysuit is essential for protection if you swim. Next best is wool or pile clothing under a waterproof shell. In this case, you should also carry waterproof matches and a change of clothing in a waterproof bag. If, after prolonged exposure, a person experiences uncontrollable shaking, loss of coordination, or difficulty speaking, he or she is hypothermic and needs your assistance.

c. **Strainers.** Brush, fallen trees, bridge pilings, undercut rocks, or anything else that allows river current to sweep through can pin boats and boaters against the obstacle. Water pressure on anything trapped this way can be overwhelming. Rescue is often extremely difficult. Pinning may occur in fast current, with little or no whitewater to warn of the danger.

d. **Dams, weirs, ledges, reversals, holes, and hydraulics.** When water drops over a obstacle, it curls back on itself, forming a strong upstream current that may be capable of holding a boat or swimmer. Some holes make for excellent sport; others are proven killers. Paddlers who cannot recognize the difference should avoid all but the smallest holes. Hydraulics around man-made dams must be treated with utmost respect regardless of their height or the level of the river. Despite their seemingly benign appearance, they can create an almost escape-proof trap. The swimmer's only exit from the "drowning machine" is to dive below the surface when the downstream current is flowing beneath the reversal.

e. **Broaching.** When a boat is pushed sideways against a rock by strong current, it may collapse and wrap. This is especially dangerous to kayak and decked-canoe paddlers; these boats will collapse, and the combination of indestructible hulls and tight outfitting may create a deadly trap. Even without entrapment, releasing pinned boats can be extremely time-consuming and dangerous. To avoid pinning, throw your weight downstream toward the rock. This allows the current to slide harmlessly underneath the hull.

6. Boating alone is discouraged. The minimum party is three people or two craft.
7. Have a frank knowledge of your boating ability, and don't attempt rivers or rapids that lie beyond that ability.
8. Be in good physical and mental condition, consistent with the difficulties that may be expected. Make adjustments for loss of skills due to age, health, fitness. Any health limitations must be explained to your fellow paddlers prior to starting the trip.
9. Be practiced in self-rescue, including escape from an overturned craft. The Eskimo roll is strongly recommended for decked boaters who run rapids Class IV or greater, or who paddle in cold environmental conditions.
10. Be trained in rescue skills, CPR, and first aid, with special emphasis on the recognizing and treating hypothermia. It may save your friend's life.

11. Carry equipment needed for unexpected emergencies, including footwear that will protect your feet when walking out, a throw rope, knife, whistle, and waterproof matches. If you wear eyeglasses, tie them on and carry a spare pair on long trips. Bring cloth repair tape on short runs and a full repair kit on isolated rivers. Do not wear bulky jackets, ponchos, heavy boots, or anything else that could reduce your ability to survive a swim.

12. Despite the mutually supportive group structure described in this code, individual paddlers are ultimately responsible for their own safety and must assume sole responsibility for the following decisions:

    a. **The decision to participate on any trip.** This includes an evaluation of the expected difficulty of the rapids under the conditions existing at the time of the put-in.

    b. **The selection of appropriate equipment,** including a boat design suited to their skills and the appropriate rescue and survival gear.

    c. **The decision to scout any rapid,** and to run or portage according to their best judgment. Other members of the group may offer advice, but paddlers should resist pressure from anyone to paddle beyond their skills. It is also their responsibility to decide whether to pass up any walkout or takeout opportunity.

    d. **All trip participants should consistently evaluate** their own and their group's safety, voicing their concerns when appropriate and following what they believe to be the best course of action. Paddlers are encouraged to speak with anyone whose actions on the water are dangerous, whether they are a part of your group or not.

II. Boat and Equipment Preparedness

1. Test new and different equipment under familiar conditions before relying on it for difficult runs. This is especially true when adopting a new boat design or outfitting system. Low-volume craft may present additional hazards to inexperienced or poorly conditioned paddlers.

2. Be sure your boat and gear are in good repair before starting a trip. The more isolated and difficult the run, the more rigorous this inspection should be.

3. Install flotation bags in noninflatable craft, securely fixed in each end and designed to displace as much water as possible. Inflatable boats should have multiple air chambers and be test-inflated before launching.

4. Have strong, properly sized paddles or oars for controlling your craft. Carry sufficient spares for the length and difficulty of the trip.

5. Outfit your boat safely. The ability to exit your boat quickly is an essential component of safety in rapids. It is your responsibility to see that there is absolutely nothing to cause entrapment when coming free of an upset craft, such as the following:

    a. **Spray covers that won't release reliably** or that release prematurely.

    b. **Boat outfitting too tight to allow a fast exit,** especially in low-volume kayaks or decked canoes. This includes low-hung thwarts in canoes lacking adequate clearance for your feet and kayak footbraces which fail or allow your feet to become wedged under them.

c. **Inadequately supported decks** that collapse on a paddler's legs when a decked boat is pinned by water pressure. Inadequate clearance with the deck because of your size or build.

d. **Loose ropes that cause entanglement.** Beware of any length of loose line attached to a whitewater boat. All items must be tied tightly and excess line eliminated; painters, throw lines, and safety-rope systems must be completely and effectively stored. Do not knot the end of a rope, as it can get caught in cracks between rocks.

6. Provide ropes that permit you to hold on to your craft so that it may be rescued. The following methods are recommended:

   a. **Kayaks and covered canoes** should have grab loops of one-quarter-inch-plus rope or equivalent webbing sized to admit a normal-sized hand. Stern painters are permissible if properly secured.

   b. **Open canoes** should have securely anchored bow and stern painters consisting of eight to ten feet of one-quarter-inch-plus line. These must be secured in such a way that they are readily accessible but cannot come loose accidentally. Grab loops are acceptable but are more difficult to reach after an upset.

   c. **Rafts and dories** may have taut perimeter lines threaded through the loops provided. Footholds should be designed so that a paddler's feet cannot be forced through them, causing entrapment. Flip lines should be carefully and reliably stowed.

7. Know your craft's carrying capacity and how added loads affect boat handling in whitewater. Most rafts have a minimum crew size that can be added to on day trips or in easy rapids. Carrying more than two paddlers in an open canoe when running rapids is not recommended.

8. Car-top racks must be strong and attach positively to the vehicle. Lash your boat to each crossbar, then tie the ends of the boat directly to the bumpers for added security. This arrangement should survive all but the most violent vehicle accident.

III. Group Preparedness and Responsibility

1. **ORGANIZATION.** A river trip should be regarded as a common adventure by all participants, except on instructional or commercially guided trips as defined below. Participants share the responsibility for the conduct of the trip, and each participant is individually responsible for judging his or her own capabilities and for his or her own safety as the trip progresses. Participants are encouraged (but are not obligated) to offer advice and guidance for the independent consideration and judgment of others.

2. **RIVER CONDITIONS.** The group should have a reasonable knowledge of the difficulty of the run. Participants should evaluate this information and adjust their plans accordingly. Maps and guidebooks, if available, should be examined if the run

is exploratory or no one is familiar with the river. The group should secure accurate flow information; the more difficult the run, the more important this will be. Be aware of possible changes in river level and how this will affect the difficulty of the run. If the trip involves tidal stretches, secure appropriate information on tides.

3. **GROUP EQUIPMENT SHOULD BE SUITED TO THE DIFFICULTY OF THE RIVER.** The group should always have a throw line available, and one line per boat is recommended on difficult runs. The list may include: carabiners, prussic loops, first-aid kit, flashlight, folding saw, fire starter, guidebooks, maps, food, extra clothing, and any other rescue or survival items suggested by conditions. Each item is not required on every run, and this list is not meant to be a substitute for good judgment.

4. **KEEP THE GROUP COMPACT, BUT MAINTAIN SUFFICIENT SPACING TO AVOID COLLISIONS.** If the group is large, consider dividing into smaller groups or using the "buddy system" as an additional safeguard. Space yourselves closely enough to permit good communication, but not so close as to interfere with one another in rapids.
   a. **A point paddler sets the pace.** When in front, do not get in over your head. Never run drops when you cannot see a clear route to the bottom or, for advanced paddlers, a sure route to the next eddy. When in doubt, stop and scout.
   b. **Keep track of all group members.** Each boat keeps the one behind it in sight, stopping if necessary. Know how many people are in your group, and take head counts regularly. No one should paddle ahead or walk out without first informing the group. Paddlers requiring additional support should stay at the center of a group and not allow themselves to lag behind in the more difficult rapids. If the group is large and contains a wide range of abilities, a "sweep boat" may be designated to bring up the rear.
   c. **Courtesy.** On heavily used rivers, do not cut in front of a boater running a drop. Always look upstream before leaving eddies to run or play. Never enter a crowded drop or eddy when no room for you exists. Passing other groups in a rapid may be hazardous: it's often safer to wait upstream until the group ahead has passed.

5. **FLOAT PLAN.** If the trip is into a wilderness area or for an extended period, plans should be filed with a responsible person who will contact the authorities if you are overdue. It may be wise to establish checkpoints along the way where civilization could be contacted if necessary. Knowing the location of possible help and preplanning escape routes can speed rescue.

6. **DRUGS.** The use of alcohol or mind-altering drugs before or during river trips is not recommended. These substances dull reflexes, reduce decision-making ability, and may interfere with important survival reflexes.

7. **INSTRUCTIONAL OR COMMERCIALLY GUIDED TRIPS.** In contrast to the common adventure-trip format, these trip formats involve a boating instructor or

commercial guide who assumes some of the responsibilities normally exercised by the group as a whole, as appropriate under the circumstances. These formats recognize that instructional or commercially guided trips may involve participants who lack significant experience in whitewater. However, as a participant acquires experience, he or she takes on increasing responsibility for his or her own safety, in accordance with what he or she knows or should know as a result of that increased experience. Also, as in all trip formats, every participant must realize and assume the risks associated with the serious hazards of whitewater rivers. It is advisable for instructors and commercial guides or their employers to acquire trip or personal liability insurance:

a. An **"instructional trip"** is characterized by a clear teacher–pupil relationship, where the primary purpose of the trip is to teach boating skills, and which is conducted for a fee.

b. A **"commercially guided trip"** is characterized by a licensed, professional guide conducting trips for a fee.

IV. Guidelines for River Rescue

1. Recover from an upset with an Eskimo roll whenever possible. Evacuate your boat immediately if there is imminent danger of being trapped against rocks, brush, or any other kind of strainer.

2. If you swim, hold on to your boat. It has much flotation and is easy for rescuers to spot. Get to the upstream end so that you cannot be crushed between a rock and your boat by the force of the current. Persons with good balance may be able to climb on top of a swamped kayak or flipped raft and paddle to shore.

3. Release your craft if this will improve your chances, especially if the water is cold or dangerous rapids lie ahead. Actively attempt self-rescue whenever possible by swimming for safety. Be prepared to assist others who may come to your aid.

   a. **When swimming in shallow or obstructed rapids, lie on your back with feet held high and pointed downstream.** Do not attempt to stand in fast-moving water; if your foot wedges on the bottom, fast water will push you under and keep you there. Get to slow or very shallow water before attempting to stand or walk. Look ahead! Avoid possible pinning situations, including undercut rocks, strainers, downed trees, holes, and other dangers, by swimming away from them.

   b. **If the rapids are deep and powerful, roll over onto your stomach and swim aggressively for shore.** Watch for eddies and slackwater, and use them to get out of the current. Strong swimmers can effect a powerful upstream ferry and get to shore fast. If the shores are obstructed with strainers or undercut rocks, however, it is safer to "ride the rapid out" until a safer escape can be found.

4. If others spill and swim, go after the boaters first. Rescue boats and equipment only if this can be done safely. While participants are encouraged (but not obligated) to

assist one another to the best of their ability, they should do so only if they can, in their judgment, do so safely. The first duty of a rescuer is not to compound the problem by becoming another victim.

5. The use of rescue lines requires training; uninformed use may cause injury. Never tie yourself into either end of a line without a reliable quick-release system. Have a knife handy to deal with unexpected entanglement. Learn to place set lines effectively, to throw accurately, to belay effectively, and to properly handle a rope thrown to you.
6. When reviving a drowning victim, be aware that cold water may greatly extend survival time under water. Victims of hypothermia may have depressed vital signs, causing them to look and feel dead. Don't give up; continue CPR for as long as possible without compromising safety.

V. Universal River Signals

These signals may be substituted with an alternate set of signals agreed upon by the group.

STOP: Potential hazard ahead. Wait for "all clear" signal before proceeding, or scout ahead. Form a horizontal bar with your outstretched arms. Those seeing the signal should pass it back to others in the party (see right).

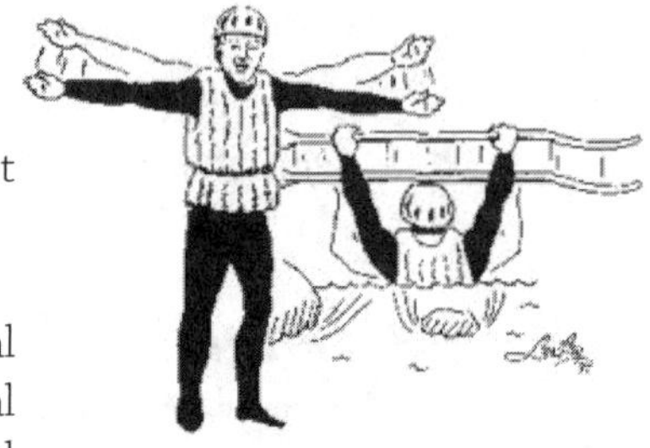

STOP

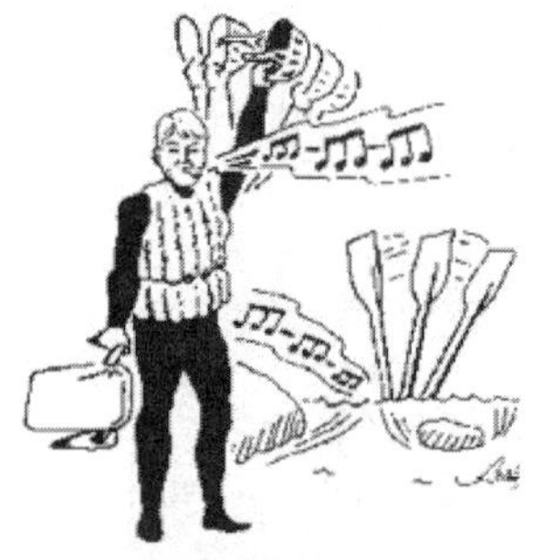

HELP: Emergency.

HELP: Emergency. Assist the signaler as quickly as possible. Give three long blasts on a police whistle while waving a paddle, helmet or life vest over your head. If a whistle is not available, use the visual signal alone. A whistle is best carried on a lanyard attached to your life vest (see left).

ALL CLEAR: Come ahead. In the absence of other directions, proceed down the center. Form a vertical bar with your paddle or one arm held high above your head (see left). Paddle blade should be turned flat for maximum visibility. To signal direction or a preferred course through a rapid around obstruction, lower the previously vertical "all clear" by 45 degrees toward the side of the river with the preferred route. Never point toward the obstacle you wish to avoid (see right).

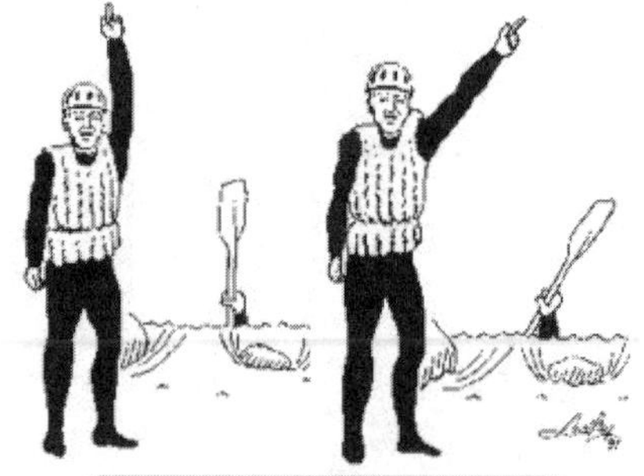

ALL CLEAR

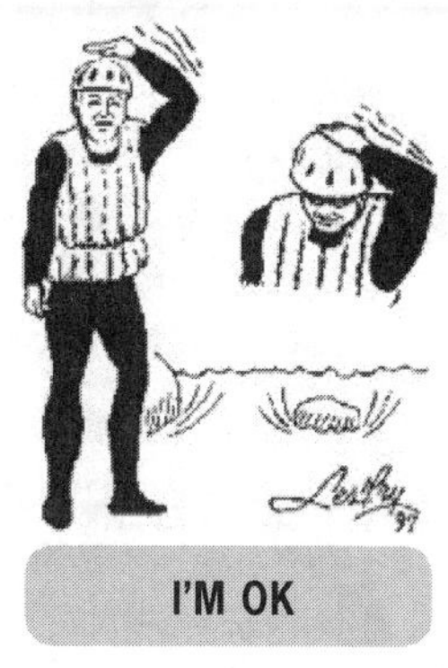
I'M OK

I'M OK: I'm not hurt. While holding an elbow outward toward your side, repeatedly pat the top of your head (see right).

VI. International Scale of River Difficulty

This is the American version of a rating system used to compare river difficulty throughout the world. This system is not exact: Rivers do not always fit easily into one category, and regional or individual interpretations may cause misunderstandings. It is no substitute for a guidebook or accurate first-hand descriptions of a run.

Paddlers attempting difficult runs in unfamiliar areas should act cautiously until they get a feel for the way the scale is interpreted locally. River difficulty may change each year due to fluctuations in water level, downed trees, recent floods, geological disturbances, or bad weather. Stay alert for unexpected problems!

As river difficulty increases, the danger to swimming paddlers becomes more severe. As rapids become longer and more continuous, the challenge increases. There is a difference between running an occasional Class IV rapid and dealing with an entire river of this category. Allow an extra margin of safety between skills and river ratings when the water is cold or if the river itself is remote and inaccessible.

Examples of commonly run rapids that fit each of the classifications are presented in the International Scale of River Difficulty (read it online at tinyurl.com/awriverdifficultyscale). Rapids of a difficulty similar to a rapids on this list are rated the same. Rivers are also rated using this scale. A river rating should take into account many factors, including the difficulty of individual rapids, remoteness, hazards, etc.

The Six Difficulty Classes

CLASS I: EASY. Fast-moving water with riffles and small waves. Few obstructions, all obvious and easily missed with little training. Risk to swimmers is slight; self-rescue is easy.

CLASS II: NOVICE. Straightforward rapids with wide, clear channels that are evident without scouting. Occasional maneuvering may be required, but rocks and medium-sized waves are easily missed by trained paddlers. Swimmers are seldom injured, and group assistance, while helpful, is seldom needed. Rapids that are at the upper end of this difficulty range are designated "Class II+."

CLASS III: INTERMEDIATE. Rapids with moderate, irregular waves that may be difficult to avoid and can swamp an open canoe. Complex maneuvers in fast current and good boat control in tight passages or around ledges are often required; large waves or strainers may be present but are easily avoided. Strong eddies and powerful current effects can be found, particularly on large-volume rivers. Scouting is advisable for inexperienced parties. Injuries while swimming are rare; self-rescue is usually easy, but group assistance may be required to avoid long swims. Rapids that are at the lower or upper end of this difficulty range are designated "Class III–" or "Class III+," respectively.

CLASS IV: ADVANCED. Intense, powerful, but predictable rapids requiring precise boat handling in turbulent water. Depending on the character of the river, it may feature large, unavoidable waves and holes or constricted passages demanding fast maneuvers under pressure. A fast, reliable eddy turn may be needed to initiate maneuvers, scout rapids, or rest. Rapids may require "must" moves above dangerous hazards. Scouting may be necessary the first time down. Risk of injury to swimmers is moderate to high, and water conditions may make self-rescue difficult. Group assistance for rescue is often essential but requires practiced skills. A strong Eskimo roll is highly recommended. Rapids that are at the upper end of this difficulty range are designated "Class IV–" or "Class IV+," respectively.

CLASS V: EXPERT. Extremely long, obstructed, or very violent rapids that expose a paddler to added risk. Drops may contain large, unavoidable waves and holes or steep, congested chutes with complex, demanding routes. Rapids may continue for long distances between pools, demanding a high level of fitness. What eddies exist may be small, turbulent, or difficult to reach. At the high end of the scale, several of these factors may be combined. Scouting is recommended but may be difficult. Swims are dangerous, and rescue is often difficult even for experts. A very reliable Eskimo roll, proper equipment, extensive experience, and practiced rescue skills are essential. Because of the large range of difficulty that exists beyond Class IV, Class 5 is an open-ended, multiple-level scale designated by 5.0, 5.1, 5.2, etc. Each of these levels is an order of magnitude more difficult than the last. Example: increasing difficulty from Class 5.0 to Class 5.1 is a similar order of magnitude as increasing from Class IV to Class 5.0.

CLASS VI: EXTREME AND EXPLORATORY. These runs have almost never been attempted and often exemplify extremes of difficulty, unpredictability, and danger. The consequences of errors are very severe, and rescue may be impossible. For teams of experts only, at favorable water levels, after close personal inspection and taking all precautions. After a Class VI rapids has been run many times, its rating may be changed to an appropriate Class 5.x rating.

APPENDIX G: Glossary of Paddling Terms

BACKROLLER A dangerous recirculation of current at the bottom of a sudden drop (from a ledge or dam), where, instead of flowing forward, the water flows backward toward the drop in a counterclockwise direction. A backroller can also be referred to as a *hydraulic,* and is created by the forceful plunge of water from above hitting water below. Some extremely powerful hydraulics can be deadly. Always portage around if in doubt.

BROACH (OR PIN) The lodging of a boat against an obstacle (like a downed tree) by a strong current. (See the section on running rapids in the Introduction, page 11, for more about what to do in this situation.)

CUBIC FEET PER SECOND (CFS) A measure of the water flow in streams, equal to a volume of water 1 foot high and 1 foot wide flowing a distance of 1 foot in 1 second. One cfs is equal to 7.48 gallons of water flowing each second.

DISCHARGE The volume of water that passes a given location within a given period of time, typically recorded in cubic feet per second (cfs).

DROP A short, downward dip in the streambed that creates a rapid, often caused by the presence of rocks in the water or debris from a removed dam.

EDDY An area of calm water away from an obstruction in the main current (like a boulder garden or a drop), usually located behind or downstream of a boulder or at the bank. To "catch an eddy" while running a set of rapids is to find a spot of water without a current, a skill needed to safely paddle rapids without looking like a runaway train without brakes.

FERRY A maneuver in whitewater conditions whereby the paddler, facing upstream, can safely cross a river sideways without being pushed significantly downstream.

FLATWATER A general term referring to a body of water (usually a lake, estuary, or a river just upstream from a dam) where there is essentially no current.

FLOOD STAGE The point of elevation at which a stream begins to flow over its natural banks.

GAGE (OR GAUGE) The measurement, in cubic feet per second, of height and volume of water at any given time; also, *river gage,* the physical instrument placed in a fixed spot in a river or stream to measure height and flow, usually by the USGS and the NOAA.

GRADIENT The drop in elevation on a stream in between two points, measured in feet, over a distance of a mile (feet per mile, or fpm).

HAYSTACK See *standing wave*, opposite.

HOLE A depression at the base of a drop or ledge into which adjacent water gets sucked and creates a recirculating current called a backroller or hydraulic.

HORIZON LINE A visual effect where, from the perspective of being upstream, one sees a flat horizontal line at the water's edge and either the continuance of the stream below or nothing but the line itself. A horizon line indicates a ledge, steep drop, or dam. If you cannot see the river past this line, get out and scout before running the drop, since you won't know what's below.

HYDRAULIC See *backroller*, above.

LEDGE A partially or wholly submerged rock shelf that a stream flows over, thus forming a drop.

LOW-HEAD DAM A deceptively dangerous (and all too often deadly) type of dam wherein the drop itself may seem insignificant, but the hydraulic below is usually very powerful, with the effect of trapping paddlers in the recirculating current.

PFD Personal flotation device, or life jacket/vest. In Wisconsin, you are not required to wear one at all times, but you must have one per person on your boat.

PIN See *broach*, above.

PORTAGE The act of carrying your boat (and gear) around a difficult rapid, dam, or impassable obstruction.

PUSHY A colloquial term used to describe a current in a stream that is unusually strong and propels the boat forward.

PUT-IN The point at which the boat can be positioned to enter the water.

QUIETWATER Water in which the current is moving at a pleasant, placid pace, usually between 2–4 fpm.

RAPID A splash of water caused by a sudden drop in the streambed (a rise in the gradient), often accompanied by rocks in the water.

READING The act of assessing how water behaves in different environments.

RIFFLE A flicker on the surface of the stream indicating a slight increase in current.

RIPRAP Rock piles used to protect shorelines against scouring and erosion.

SHUTTLE The dry-land transportation route between the put-in and the take-out that all river trips require, lest one paddle from point A to point B and then back upstream to A (which is never recommended).

STANDING WAVE (OR HAYSTACK) Larger rapids one after another that often indicate the main channel. Large standing waves can be dangerous, especially for open canoes.

STRAINER (OR SWEEPER) Typically a tree branch (or branches) in the water, through which water can flow but paddlers cannot.

STREAMFLOW USGS catch-all term that encompasses two types of water data: *discharge* (volume, measured in cfs) and *gage height* (level of water against the bank, measured in feet), as tracked by river gages.

SWEEPER See *strainer,* above.

TAKE-OUT The point at which the boat can be removed from the water.

WATER LEVEL For the purposes of this guide, this term encompasses the height of water against the bank or the volume of water flowing past a river gage at any given time. The USGS refers to this data as *streamflow.*

WAVE TRAIN A series of standing waves (or rapids) that look like the spine of a stream and feel like an amusement park ride. Standing waves often indicate where the water is deepest.

WHITEWATER A general term referring to stream rapids and waves, usually where there is a gradient of 5 or more fpm.

APPENDIX H: Glossary of Geologic/Aquatic Terms

BOG A wetland of spongy ground or peat, often hosting tamaracks and sphagnum moss.

DELL A rock gorge shorn by torrents of water from melting glaciers.

DRIFTLESS AREA The portion of Wisconsin left untouched by glaciers, leaving an ancient landscape deeply cut by streams into narrow, angular valleys and tall ridges.

DRUMLIN An elongated, oval hill sculpted by glacial movement often found in groups known as *swarms*.

ERRATIC A stray boulder deposited in an area of varying bedrock composition.

ESKER A ridge of sand and gravel formed when streams flowed through melting glacial tunnels.

FEN A flat, marshy area where decomposing plants accumulate and form peat.

KAME A conical hill primarily composed of sand and cobbled rock deposited by streams flowing downward through shafts in receding glaciers.

KETTLE A crater-like depression formed by large blocks of melting glacial ice.

KETTLE MORAINE A mostly contiguous tract of state forest roughly 120 miles long but only half a dozen miles wide in southeastern Wisconsin, featuring some of the finest examples of glaciation anywhere in the world.

LOBE A humongous tongue-like extension of a glacier.

MORAINE A ridge ranging from 10 to 300 feet high, formed by glacial deposits.

POTHOLE A smooth cavity gouged into bedrock by the grinding action of stones whirling around in a river eddy.

SEDGE MEADOW A natural wetlands environment dominated by grass-like plants.

SHRUB-CARR A wetlands complex typically dominated by dogwood and willow trees.

SLOUGH A wetland of standing water that usually is cut off from or is a side channel of a more dominant stream.

SWALE A hollow or depression at the foreground of a valley, often composed of wet soils.

Index

About the Author

Water lover and outdoors enthusiast **TIMOTHY BAUER** has been paddling around Wisconsin and the neighboring states with great wanderlust since 2008, always eager to explore uncharted streams but ever grateful for the familiar favorites. Originally from the suburbs of New Jersey (Exit 159), he has gladly made Madison his home since 2003.

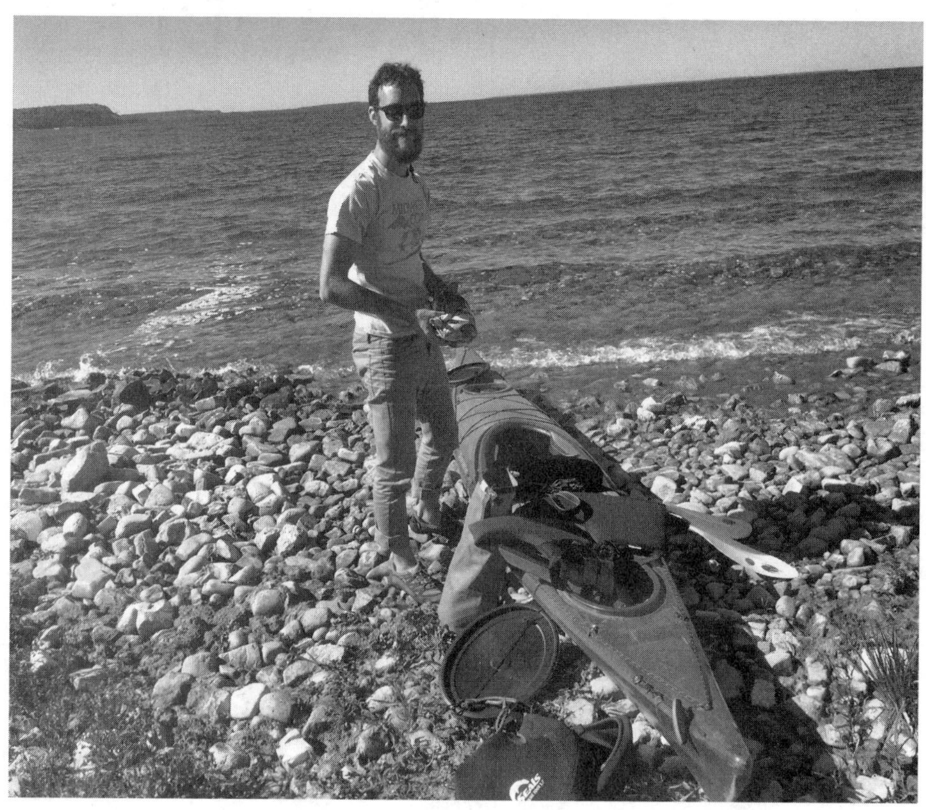